Medical Image Processing for Improved Clinical Diagnosis

A. Swarnambiga
Indian Institute of Technology Madras, India

A volume in the Advances in Medical Technologies and Clinical Practice (AMTCP) Book Series

IGI Global
DISSEMINATOR OF KNOWLEDGE

Published in the United States of America by
IGI Global
Medical Information Science Reference (an imprint of IGI Global)
701 E. Chocolate Avenue
Hershey PA, USA 17033
Tel: 717-533-8845
Fax: 717-533-8661
E-mail: cust@igi-global.com
Web site: http://www.igi-global.com

Library of Congress Cataloging-in-Publication Data

Names: Swarnambiga, A., 1986- editor
Title: Medical image processing for improved clinical diagnosis / A. Swarnambiga, editor.
Description: Hershey PA : Medical Information Science Reference, [2019] | Includes bibliographical references.
Identifiers: LCCN 2017058860| ISBN 9781522558767 (hardcover) | ISBN 9781522558774 (ebook)
Subjects: | MESH: Image Interpretation, Computer-Assisted | Image Processing, Computer-Assisted
Classification: LCC RC78.7.D53 | NLM WN 182 | DDC 616.07/54--dc23 LC record available at https://lccn.loc.gov/2017058860

This book is published in the IGI Global book series Advances in Medical Technologies and Clinical Practice (AMTCP) (ISSN: 2327-9354; eISSN: 2327-9370)

British Cataloguing in Publication Data
A Cataloguing in Publication record for this book is available from the British Library.

Advances in Medical Technologies and Clinical Practice (AMTCP) Book Series

ISSN:2327-9354
EISSN:2327-9370

Editor-in-Chief: Srikanta Patnaik, SOA University, India & Priti Das, S.C.B. Medical College, India

MISSION

Medical technological innovation continues to provide avenues of research for faster and safer diagnosis and treatments for patients. Practitioners must stay up to date with these latest advancements to provide the best care for nursing and clinical practices.

The **Advances in Medical Technologies and Clinical Practice (AMTCP) Book Series** brings together the most recent research on the latest technology used in areas of nursing informatics, clinical technology, biomedicine, diagnostic technologies, and more. Researchers, students, and practitioners in this field will benefit from this fundamental coverage on the use of technology in clinical practices.

COVERAGE

- Clinical Data Mining
- Medical informatics
- Clinical High Performance Computing
- Telemedicine
- Biomedical Applications
- Clinical Studies
- Diagnostic Technologies
- Nursing Informatics
- Neural Engineering
- Biometrics

The Advances in Medical Technologies and Clinical Practice (AMTCP) Book Series (ISSN 2327-9354) is published by IGI Global, 701 E. Chocolate Avenue, Hershey, PA 17033-1240, USA, www.igi-global.com. This series is composed of titles available for purchase individually; each title is edited to be contextually exclusive from any other title within the series. For pricing and ordering information please visit http://www.igi-global.com/book-series/advances-medical-technologies-clinical-practice/73682. Postmaster: Send all address changes to above address.

Titles in this Series

For a list of additional titles in this series, please visit:
https://www.igi-global.com/book-series/advances-medical-technologies-clinical-practice/73682

Microbial Cultures and Enzymes in Dairy Technology
Şebnem Öztürkoğlu Budak (Ankara University, Turkey) and H. Ceren Akal (Ankara University, Turkey)
Medical Information Science Reference • ©2018 • 413pp • H/C (ISBN: 9781522553632) • US $265.00

Multifunctional Nanocarriers for Contemporary Healthcare Applications
Md. Abul Barkat (K.R. Mangalam University, India) Harshita A.B. (K.R. Mangalam University, India) Sarwar Beg (Jubilant Generics, India) and Farhan J. Ahmad (Jamia Hamdard, India)
Medical Information Science Reference • ©2018 • 602pp • H/C (ISBN: 9781522547815) • US $265.00

Biomedical Signal and Image Processing in Patient Care
Maheshkumar H. Kolekar (Indian Institute of Technology Patna, India) and Vinod Kumar (Indian Institute of Technology Roorkee, India)
Medical Information Science Reference • ©2018 • 312pp • H/C (ISBN: 9781522528296) • US $265.00

Next-Generation Mobile and Pervasive Healthcare Solutions
Jose Machado (University of Minho, Portugal) António Abelha (University of Minho, Portugal) Manuel Filipe Santos (University of Minho, Portugal) and Filipe Portela (University of Minho, Portugal)
Medical Information Science Reference • ©2018 • 286pp • H/C (ISBN: 9781522528517) • US $245.00

Innovative Research in Thermal Imaging for Biology and Medicine
Ricardo Vardasca (University of Porto, Portugal) and Joaquim Gabriel Mendes (University of Porto, Portugal)
Medical Information Science Reference • ©2017 • 340pp • H/C (ISBN: 9781522520726) • US $210.00

For an entire list of titles in this series, please visit:
https://www.igi-global.com/book-series/advances-medical-technologies-clinical-practice/73682

Editorial Advisory Board

Table of Contents

Section 5
Study on Fundamentals in Image Processing and Its Advancements

Section 6
Medical Image Registration and Retrieval for Improved Clinical Diagnosis

Detailed Table of Contents

Shoulder arthroplasty is an important operation for the treatment of shoulder joints, with an increasing rate of operations per year around the world. Although this operation is generally achieved successfully, there are a number of complications which increase the risks in the operation. Preoperative planning for a surgery can help reduce the amount of risks resulting from complications and increase the success rate of the operation. Three-dimensional visualization software can be helpful in preoperative planning. This chapter aims to provide such software to help reduce the risks of the operation by visualizing 3D joint anatomy of the specific patient for the surgeon, and letting surgeons observe the geometrical properties of the joint.

Conventional pathology using a light microscope is rapidly shifting towards digital integration. Digital imaging plays an increasing role in clinical diagnosis, biomedical research, and continuing medical education. Currently, pathology platforms are composed of clinical and molecular pathologists and engineers with the sole intention of investigating cellular and molecular basis of human health through applied research in disease aetiology, pathogenesis, diagnosis, and treatment. Molecular diagnosis using technical advances and the application of specific biomarkers in clinical practice are the two main pillars of modern personalized medicine especially in oncology. Thus, it has become evident that accredited clinical and molecular pathology laboratories using digital imaging and advanced technologies can make the most of diagnostic and specific biomarker analyses as well as incorporating other key aspects of translational research and data analysis.

Diagnosis of diseases at the right stage with optimal accuracy is a significant requirement in the medical field. Apart from diagnosis from clinical symptoms, diagnosis based on scanned images of both internal and external organs is playing a vital role in understanding the severity of the disease. Classification is a field of study derived from artificial intelligence, and today it is widely used in medical image classification. These techniques are used to classify the different stages of a disease or different variant diseases possible in an organ from different types of input images such as magnetic resonance imaging (MRI), computed tomography (CT), x-ray, fundus images, iris images, etc. Various preprocessing techniques are used to select the relevant features from the input image to form the feature set. The classifiers are trained using the feature set to generate models. The generated models can be optimized to improve the performance. Various metrics such as accuracy, coverage, precision, recall, and FMeasure are used to measure the accuracy.

This chapter simply encapsulates the basics of image restoration, various noise models, and degradation model including some blur and image restoration filters. The mining of high resolution information from the low-resolution images is a very vital task in several applications of digital image processing. In recent times, a lot of research work has been carried out in this field in order to improve the resolution of real medical images especially when the given images are corrupted with some kind of noise. The displayed images are the result of the various stages that might cause imperfections in the digital images, for instance the so-called imaging and capturing process can itself degrade the original scene. The imperfections present in the image need to be studied and analyzed if the noise present in the images is not modelled properly. There are different types of degradations which are considered such as noise, geometrical degradations, imperfections (due to improper illumination and color), and blur. Blurring in the images is generally caused by the relative motion between the camera and the original object being captured or due to poor focusing of an optical system. In the production of aerial photographs for remote sensing purposes, blurs are introduced by the atmospheric turbulence, aberrations in the optical system, and relative motion between the camera and the ground. Apart from the blurring effect, noise also creates imperfections in the images that corrupt the images under analysis. The noise may be introduced by several factors (e.g., medium, recording or capturing system, or by the quantization process). Due to this noise or blur present in the images, resolution needs to be improved and the image is to be restored from the geometrically warped, blurred, and noisy images.

Ophthalmologists utilize retinal fundus images of humans for the detection, diagnosis, and prediction of many eye diseases. Automatic scrutiny of fundus images are foremost apprehension for ophthalmologists and investigators. The manual recognition of blood vessels is most deceptive because the blood vessels in a fundus image are multifaceted and with low contrast. Unearthing of blood vessels proffers information on pathological transformation and can smooth the progress of rating diseases severity or mechanically diagnosing the diseases. The manual recognition method turns out to be annoying. Consequently, the automatic recognition of blood vessels is also more significant. For extracting the vessel in fundus images unswerving and habitual methods are obligatory. The proposed methodology is designed to effectively diagnose the eye disease by performing feature extraction succeeded by feature selection and to improve the performance factors such as feature extraction ratio, feature selection time, sensitivity, and specificity when compared to the state-of-art methods.

Noise removal in medical images remains a challenge for the researchers because noise removal introduces artifacts and blurring of the image. Developing medical image denoising algorithm is a difficult operation because a tradeoff between noise reduction and the preservation of actual features of image has to be made in a way that enhances and preserves the diagnostically relevant image content. A special member of the emerging family of multiscale geometric transforms is the contourlet transform which effectively captures the image edges and contours. This overcomes the limitations of the existing method of denoising using wavelet and curvelet. But due to down sampling and up sampling, the contourlet transform is shift-variant. However, shift-invariance is desirable in image analysis applications such as edge detection, contour characterization, and image enhancement. In this chapter, nonsubsampled contourlet transform (shift-invariance transform)-based denoising is presented which more effectively represents edges than contourlet transform.

This chapter provides a brief introduction to the various fundamentals and concepts related to the basics of the biomedical image processing. Medical imaging processing comprises various techniques and processes that are used to create images of human body for clinical purposes and medical procedures for the purpose of diagnosis or examination of disease. Digital image processing along with its suitable components and computer-simulated algorithms are implemented using computers to perform the image analysis of digital images. The study of normal anatomy and physiology of human body is made as a part of diagnosis process. Though medical imaging of various organs and tissues can be performed for medical examination purposes, the impact of digital images on modern society is tremendous and image processing has become a critical component of science and technology related to the biomedical image processing.

Preface

WHAT PHYSICIANS, RADIOLOGISTS, AND OTHERS IN THE HEALTH IMAGING PROFESSION CAN EXPECT FOR THE FUTURE: 3D PRINTING – A REVIEW

The development of medical images in medicine are tremendous. It solves the major issues in clinical imaging modalities, with the help of standard image processing operations, focusing on practical issues in assisting clinical diagnosis and prognosis. The book will explain the issue in analyzing the medical image for effectiveness and practical computer based activities.

3D printing is having a great development and impact in the medical field. 3D printing is taking advantage by changing the shape of medical research by duplicating structurally and functionally accurate bio printed human tissue models. Medical institutions across worldwide started the revolutionized printing soft tissue organs for the betterment of human lives. Pandorum technologies, a Bangalore –based biotech start-up has successfully developed artificial 3D printed liver tissue duplicating human liver functions, affordable and eventually loading to full scale, transplantable 3D printed organs. In India, 3D bio printing for patient specific constructs are also progressing. US based Organovo are efficiently dealing with bio printed tissues for volumetric muscle loss injury. They have also succeeded in creating 3D printed kidney tissue. Tissue with blood vessels made a great progress in bio printing blood vessels by researchers at Harvard University, a major and successive breakthrough towards printing tissue with a blood supply. For the development of new anti-cancer drugs, by better understanding how the tumor develops, grows and its spread are analysed by group of researchers in china and US with their printed models of cancerous tumors. Researcher from Cornell University has printed a heart valve and ear cartilage, not only them, but also groups like iLAb/Haiti have taken 3D printing umbilical chord clamps for local hospitals in Haiti. Researcher from Wake forest school of medicine in US came with a developed printer that can print skin straight on to the wounds of burn victims. There are certain questions which will make 3D printing more understandable.

Do I believe this is the solution to repairing damaged tissues? Yes may be. The most important in Bio printing is while printing tissues and organs, keeping those alive. To keep those cells alive, we need a full vascular system like the one that exist in our body, because without oxygen and nutrients cells could not survive. Do I believe that these 3D printing treatments will be safe? Yes. They are used for tissue and organ fabrication, creation of customized prosthetics implants and anatomic models, since tissue engineering is primarily used in reconstructing severely damaged bone and tissue structures. Do I think that this new personalized medical treatment will affect the cost, availability of healthcare? If so, how? Yes, that we can expect to see in the near future. This is going to be a revolution in the healthcare technology. Customisation and personalisation such as custom-made implants, fixtures and surgical tools, increased cost efficiency and enhanced productivity are the top major benefits. But printing of solid organs such as liver, heart and kidney has to go far long for success for benefit of human lives.

OBJECTIVE OF THE BOOK

This book elaborates and endeavours to endow with the recent empirical research findings for diagnosis and prognosis. It is written for professionals who desire to analyze and develop an automated system for assisting clinical diagnosis. This book elaborates the foremost techniques in assisting clinical diagnosis by using image processing techniques. As well as it, includes miscellaneous techniques of various modalities, computer aided diagnosis, hospital management system, etc. It deals, principally with design, analysis and approaches that involve image analysis, retrieval, registration and their algorithm. The most important objectives from this increased research effort in medical imaging are expected in 1) Improved patient care, 2) Cost-efficient healthcare, 3) Socio-economic benefits, 4) Medical imaging highlights, and 5) Diagnosis and prognosis itself has an important role in case of assisting clinical diagnosis and disease entities, in entire processing.

ORGANISATION OF THE BOOK

The book consists of an introductory chapter followed by Twelve chapters that are organised in six sections as shown below. Section 1 focus on medical image analysis for clinical diagnosis, which includes biomedical image processing software development and digital image analysis in clinical and experimental pathology. Section 2 comprises of medical image classification, fundamentals in restoration and way for eye disease diagnosis. Section 3 includes segmentation of colon and removal of opacified fluid for virtual colonoscopy. Section 4 indulge in Medical Data Storage and Compression and in denoising techniques. Section 5 focus on Fundamentals and survey in biomedical image processing for clinical diagnosis. Finally section 6 comprises of Medical image registration and retrieval for improved clinical diagnosis.

Section 1: Medical Image Analysis for Clinical Diagnosis

This section elaborates clinical studies in medicine based on patients and controls using different imaging diagnostic modalities. Clinical trials use medical imaging

Table 1. Organisation of the chapters

<table>
<tr><td colspan="6">Section 1
Medical Image Analysis for Clinical Diagnosis</td></tr>
<tr><td colspan="3">Chapter 1
Biomedical Image Processing Software Development for Shoulder Arthroplasty</td><td colspan="3">Chapter 2
Digital Image Analysis in Clinical and Experimental Pathology: An Ode to Microscopy</td></tr>
<tr><td colspan="6">Section 2
Medical Image Extraction, Classification, and Restoration in Computer-Aided Diagnosis</td></tr>
<tr><td colspan="2">Chapter 3
Medical Image Classification</td><td colspan="2">Chapter 4
The Fundamentals of Medical Image Restoration</td><td colspan="2">Chapter 5
Optimal Feature Selection and Extraction for Eye Disease Diagnosis</td></tr>
<tr><td colspan="6">Section 3
Medical Image Segmentation for Improved Clinical Diagnosis</td></tr>
<tr><td colspan="6">Chapter 6
Certain Investigation Titles on the Segmentation of Colon and Removal of Opacified Fluid for Virtual Colonoscopy</td></tr>
<tr><td colspan="6">Section 4
Study of Compression and Denoising in Clinical Diagnosis</td></tr>
<tr><td colspan="3">Chapter 7
Medical Data Storage and Compression</td><td colspan="3">Chapter 8
Non-Subsampled Contourlet Transform-Based Effective Denoising of Medical Images: Denoising of Medical Images Using Contourlet</td></tr>
<tr><td colspan="6">Section 5
Study on Fundamentals in Image Processing and Its Advancements</td></tr>
<tr><td colspan="3">Chapter 9
The Fundamentals of Biomedical Image Processing</td><td colspan="3">Chapter 10
A Survey on Women Breast Cancer: Computer-Aided Diagnosis Using Digital Breast Tomosynthesis</td></tr>
<tr><td colspan="6">Section 6
Medical Image Registration and Retrieval for Improved Clinical Diagnosis</td></tr>
<tr><td colspan="3">Chapter 11
A Comparative Study of Medical Image Retrieval Using Distance, Transform, Texture, and Shape</td><td colspan="3">Chapter 12
Medical Image Registration in Clinical Diagnosis: An Introduction</td></tr>
</table>

to implement the most suitable diagnostic technique for a particular disease, to validate new diagnostic techniques and to monitor diseases under treatment such as arthroplasty.

Chapter 1

To improve the efficiency and success rate of shoulder arthroplasty which could help the surgeon to identify the challenges and limitations of the surgery on a specific person. This shoulder arthroplasty software creates a 3D virtual environment in which a 3D model of the joint anatomy of the patient. A medical image processing software development procedure is explained, displaying each step of the job needed for enabling a software to read, import, segment, analyze and display anatomical models of the body. By visualizing 3D joint anatomy of the specific patient for the surgeon, and letting surgeons observe the geometrical properties of the joint as a preoperative planning is the major application of this visualization tool.

Chapter 2

This chapter briefly describe the tissue processing and tissue microarrays protocols. Also the main steps for acquiring digital images from tissue samples, and the imaging techniques relevant for this purpose such as whole-slide imaging are discussed. High-throughput vectorial and non-vectorial technologies in molecular pathology, and empathize on their mechanistic details and main applications in diagnostic pathology, oncology and biomedical research are also described.

Section 2: Medical Image Extraction, Classification, and Restoration in Computer-Aided Diagnosis

This section focus on medical imaging that deals with information in image that the medical practitioner and doctors has to evaluate and analyze abnormality in short time for better clinical diagnosis. Analysis of imaging in medical field is very crucial task, because imaging is basic modality to diagnose any diseases at the earliest. Despite, acquisition of image using Imaging techniques like MRI, X-ray, endoscopy, ultrasound, etc. are mostly affected by external or internal phenomenal factors. The techniques to overcome them are discussed in this section.

Chapter 3

Classification plays a vital role in the diagnosis of diseases such as brain tumor and other types of tumors, glaucoma, lung diseases etc. The ensemble classifier techniques such as bagging and boosting has proved to improve the accuracy of medical image classification. A brief survey on classification is well presented in this chapter.

Chapter 4

A brief survey on image restoration is discussed in this chapter. Though, no conclusion is drawn, the fundamentals and various noises were discussed theoretically. This chapter would help academicians and students to understand the basics of one of the major image processing steps.

Chapter 5

To effectively diagnose Diabetic Retinopathy and to improve the performance factors such as extraction feature ratio, feature selection time, sensitivity and specificity are well executed in this chapter. A Deep Learning based Feature Selection (DLFS) procedure is devised. This DLFS method accurately selects pathologies without any human assistance.

Section 3: Medical Image Segmentation for Improved Clinical Diagnosis

Accurate segmentation of medical images is vital in contouring during radiotherapy planning. While selecting a segmentation algorithm one is required to consider partial volume effect, different artifacts: example motion artifacts, ring artifacts, etc and noise due to sensors and related electronic system. This section deals with the measures to avoid those affecting phenomena.

Chapter 6

Segmentation of large intestine using Clustering approach, Automatic segmentation of colon and the removal of Bowels using Neural network approach and Semi automatic segmentation of colon and the removal of opacified fluid using 3D Seeded region growing approach are experimented in this chapter. The first approach focessed on the removal of lungs. The second approach is an automatic approach in which both the removal of lungs and opacified fluid are shown. The third approach reduces the computational time as an semiautomatic approach are achieved.

Section 4: Study of Compression and Denoising in Clinical Diagnosis

Recent developments in the computerized analysis of medical images are expected to aid radiologists and other healthcare professionals in interpretation of medical images. The facors affecting this interpretation are discussed and measures are shown in this section to overcome them. In this section, different noise and denoising algorithm has been explained.

Chapter 7

This chapter focus on survey of compressing medical images. Storing patient information, pathological test results, and medical images in the computer system and digital electronics system assists the medical experts for easy access to medical information. This chapter has discussed various research articles discussing about the novel algorithms or methods related to medical image applications.

Chapter 8

To address the issue of medical image recovery from its noisy counterpart based on the shift invariant contourlet transform is experimented. Experiments are conducted and the performance of Neighshrink with and without bilateral filter is compared. The result shows that proposed Neighshrink with bilateral filter effectively removes noise. The PSNR value is improved and the edges are preserved better in Neighshrink with bilateral method compared to other methods.

Section 5: Study on Fundamentals in Image Processing and Its Advancements

Medical imaging and image processing domains intend to process missing, ambiguous, inconsistent, complementary, contradictory, redundant and distorted data, and information which has a strong structural character. A key distinction exist between (bio)medical imaging and image processing technologies, even though if between these fields of knowledge a strong interrelation may be established.

Chapter 9

This chapter is basically a survey and it discuss the types of medical imaging modalities used for Clinical purposes and its significance in medical procedures i.e. Ultrasound imaging, Mammographic imaging, Radiography, Computed tomography etc. Also focused on various spatial domain and frequency domain methods which could be implied to enhance the medical images.

Chapter 10

This chapter discusses the overview of Breast Cancer, imaging modalities used for Breast Cancer i.e. Ultrasound, Magnetic Resonance Imaging, Digital Mammography and Breast Tomosynthesis. The breast cancer lesions such as micro-calcification, masses, architecture distortion and bilateral symmetry are also well portrayed. Some of the research carried out by other researchers in clinical diagnosis in the mass volume of work are highlighted .

Section 6: Medical Image Registration and Retrieval for Improved Clinical Diagnosis

Medical image registration and fusion processes plays as a valuable assistant for the medical experts. They help the experts in the diagnosis, following up the diseases' evolution, and deciding the necessary therapies regarding the patient's condition. This section also illustrates most well-known toolkits that have been developed to help the working with the registration and retrieval processes. Finally, the section presents the current challenges associated with working with medical image registration and retrieval that were addressed through such an analyzing process.

Chapter 11

This chapter experiments with some basic registration techniques such as Affine, Demons and affine with B-Spline to assist in clinical diagnosis. The simulated results are based on clinical view of the images. To overcome, inter and intra-patient misalignments of the images, orientations and scales in the images, image registration could be helpful. Hence by adopting the registration can solve this problem, which is computationally simple and inexpensive.

Chapter 12

Content-based medical image retrieval (CBMIR) is the application of computer vision techniques to the problem of medical image search in large databases. Three main techniques are applied to check the applicability, such as distance based, transform based and hand crafted feature technique i.e. texture, shape and multi feature techniques are well experimented, executed and justified for clinical diagnosis with the achieved results.

CONCLUSION

This book is expected to assist researchers, academicians, physicians, radiologist and engineering in healthcare informatics, medical imaging, medical image processing and clinical diagnosis. New technology is being developed for all aspects of patient care and the potential benefits in assisting clinical diagnosis. Medical imaging plays vital role in health care system contributing by improved patient outcome and more cost efficient healthcare in all major disease entities. The aim of the book is to develop research based knowledge on how to use medical imaging in healthcare for assisting clinical diagnosis, evidence based reasoning and image guided surgery etc.

A. Swarnambiga
Indian Institute of Technology Madras, India

Acknowledgment

First I would like to thank the lord almighty.

I express my appreciation to My Parents, My Brothers, My husband and My in-laws who always stood behind me for each and every good things happening in my life.

Right from the inception of my career my Parents Mr. Ayyachamy & Mrs. Tharabai, have been my source of strength, my Husband Mr. Raj Goutham, My Siblings Mr. Ganesh Ram, Mr. Ganesh Lakshman and his friend Mr. Anantha Raja have been a second eye on all my works. I was blessed with the opportunity to discuss topics in Medical Science with my Father-in-Law Dr. D. Nagarajan, Prof of Surgery and also a Special Mention to my Mother-In-Law Mrs. Gowri who all have pampered me with their support and affection round the clock. I also thank Prof. Dr. S. Vasuki my Mentor whose guidance and support helped me to learn a lot as a newbie in my research area.

My sincere gratitude goes to the chapters' authors who contributed their time and expertise to this book. Second, I wish to acknowledge the valuable contributions of the reviewers regarding the improvement of quality, coherence, and content presentation of chapters. Most of the authors also served as referees; we highly appreciate their double task.

I would like to express my sincere thanks to Ms. Marianne Caesar, IGI Team, Development and publishing team of IGI Global for their diligence and also to all the people whoever supported in every possible way in publishing this book.

This is my first step as editor. Without IGI Global, USA team, this would not be made possible in a fruitful manner. I owe them in assisting me throughout this entire process in bringing out this book in a very successful way.

Last, but not the least, readers of this book, who gave us their trust and for their belief that this work could inspire and guide them.

Section 1

Medical Image Analysis for Clinical Diagnosis

Chapter 1
Biomedical Image Processing Software Development for Shoulder Arthroplasty

Majid Mohammad Sadeghi
Istanbul Technical University, Turkey

Emin Faruk Kececi
Istanbul Technical University, Turkey

Kerem Bilsel
Bezmialem Vakif University, Turkey

Ayse Aralasmak
Bezmialem Vakif University, Turkey

ABSTRACT

Shoulder arthroplasty is an important operation for the treatment of shoulder joints, with an increasing rate of operations per year around the world. Although this operation is generally achieved successfully, there are a number of complications which increase the risks in the operation. Preoperative planning for a surgery can help reduce the amount of risks resulting from complications and increase the success rate of the operation. Three-dimensional visualization software can be helpful in preoperative planning. This chapter aims to provide such software to help reduce the risks of the operation by visualizing 3D joint anatomy of the specific patient for the surgeon, and letting surgeons observe the geometrical properties of the joint.

DOI: 10.4018/978-1-5225-5876-7.ch001

INTRODUCTION

Shoulder arthroplasty is a shoulder joint replacement surgery, performed when pain prevails or shoulder joint functionality including strength or mobility has deteriorated or has been lost and conservative treatments like analgesics and physiotherapy are not affective (Buck, Jost, & Hodler, 2008).

A great number of shoulder arthroplasty is performed every year around the world. There were 200,000 shoulder arthroplasty surgeries in the USA from 2000 to 2010 (Trofa, Rajaee, & Smith, 2014) and the number of operations performed is increasing (Kim, Wise, Zhang, & Szabo, 2011). In Australia, 37,849 shoulder arthroplasty operations were performed from 2006 to 2016 ("Reported Shoulder Procedures," 2017).

Common issues which can result in shoulder arthroplasty include osteoarthritis, rheumatoid arthritis, complex fractures of the proximal humerus and osteonecrosis of the humeral head. Shoulder arthroplasty is performed also as revisions of failed prosthesis (Buck et al., 2008).

Shoulder arthroplasty operations include humeral hemiarthroplasty, total shoulder arthroplasty, and reverse shoulder arthroplasty (Buck et al., 2008). Humeral hemiarthroplasty is replacing the humeral head with an artificial implant in the joint. Total shoulder arthroplasty is performed by replacing both humeral head and glenoid section of the scapula bone. Major indications for total shoulder arthroplasty are primary and secondary osteoarthritis, as well as early rheumatoid arthritis (Buck et al., 2008). In reverse shoulder arthroplasty, the anatomy of the joint is reversed in a way that the prostheses attached to the glenoid has a ball shape, and the prostheses attached to the humeral bone has a concave shape. Reverse shoulder arthroplasty has been proved as a successful method for treatment in cases with rotator cuff deficiency (Boileau, Watkinson, Hatzidakis, & Hovorka, 2006; Boileau, Watkinson, Hatzidakis, & Balg, 2005).

In Reverse shoulder arthroplasty, medialization and distalisation in the shoulder joint, meaning that the center of rotation is moved downwards and closer to the body, prevents the shoulder from moving upward out of its center and also it increases the force moment that the deltoid muscle can create. As a result, lifting of the arm is improved which is the advantage of this method over previous types of shoulder arthroplasty in many cases (Farshad & Gerber, 2010).

Shoulder arthroplasty is generally achieved successfully, although complications can occur. The number of complications reported varies based on the reporting institution (Hammond, Queale, Kim, & McFarland, 2003; Hasan, Leith, Smith, & Matsen, 2003), however, a meta-analysis has reported a 14.7% rate of complication in a total of 2,810 shoulder arthroplasty operations from 1996 to 2005. The most frequent complication was component loosening (with a higher glenoid loosening rate than humeral loosening), followed by instability, periprosthetic fracture and other less common complications (Bohsali, Wirth, Rockwood, Material, & Surgery, 2010; Matsen et al., 2008). Likewise, in reverse shoulder arthroplasty the most common complication is glenoid component loosening (Deutsch et al., 2007; Walch, Boileau, & Noël, 2010; Zumstein, Pinedo, Old, & Boileau, 2011). Glenohumeral instability, which is the second most common complication, can be caused by a misalignment of the joint prostheses components. Any misplacement of the component in distance or angle can cause instability (Buck et al., 2008). Periprosthetic fracture can be caused during the operation or after the operation resulting from an accident or a fatigue fracture (Buck et al., 2008).

In shoulder arthroplasty, highly experienced surgeons who operate on about 200 patients a year can do their best without preoperative planning, but if the patient's anatomy is much deteriorated or deformed, the risk of complication is higher. For instance, the implant inferior version and tilt angle have shown a 16 and 12 degree variation respectively in traditional surgery methods (Nguyen et al., 2009; Verborgt et al., 2011). Conventional methods in implantation are observed as not being able to restore the retroversion angle when the glenoid is severely damaged (Iannotti, Greeson, Downing, Sabesan, & Bryan, 2012; Karelse et al., 2014).

Preoperative planning of the surgery can greatly help to reduce the risk of complications. In planning, identification of pathology and recognizing challenges are important steps. Identification of limitations in implants and prosthesis, their appropriate sizes and appropriate positioning are likewise very critical.

Correct placement of the glenoid which is one of the main goals of preoperative planning is shown to be crucial for durability of the prosthesis and better functioning results of the arm (Karelse et al., 2014).

Software can be of great help in preoperative planning in different aspects. Viewing a three-dimensional (3D) model of the anatomy of a patient and their specific condition can help a surgeon determine different treatment solutions. Providing the chance for the surgeon to put the implant into the patient's bones in the virtual space can help in deciding the right correction of the glenoid version.

This work aims to create software to help improve the efficiency of shoulder arthroplasty by three-dimensional visualization of the joint anatomy of a specific patient for the surgeon, and letting them observe geometrical properties of the joint. This will also help prevent surprises during the surgery which could happen without a detailed visualization of the patient's anatomy. In the rest of this chapter, software development for the shoulder arthroplasty is explained. The areas which need to be developed and the methods and algorithms used for each are described in the following sections.

SHOULDER ARTHROPLASTY SOFTWARE DEVELOPMENT

To improve the efficiency and success rate of shoulder arthroplasty by helping the surgeon to be able to better identify the challenges and limitations of the surgery on a specific person, this shoulder arthroplasty software creates a 3D virtual environment in which a 3D model of the joint anatomy of the patient is displayed. In this virtual environment, surgeons are given the geometrical properties of the bone and they can manipulate patient's bone model to accurately observe nuance details of the anatomy.

The graphical user interface of the software must include a section in which a three-dimensional model of the patient's bone is displayed. It is in this section that the user of the software should be able to move, rotate and magnify the patient's bone model. This section should also be able to display different geometrical and anatomical features of the bone. Another section needed in the graphical user interface is a control panel for activating and deactivating features to be displayed on the bone model. Numerical geometrical information of the bone can also be displayed in this section, and it can also control the transparency of the model to be displayed. The graphical user interface should also include a section in which cross-sections of a three-dimensional model of the bone is displayed as two-dimensional images. These images should be provided to the surgeon in axial, coronal and sagittal directions, each in a separate subsection. Pan, rotate and zoom operations should also be applicable to these views of the patient's bone.

For the software to support the graphical user interface functionalities, a number of steps must be performed. These steps and the capabilities that each of them provide for the GUI are described in the following sections of this chapter. Figure 1 shows the block diagram of these steps.

Figure 1. Block diagram of the processes performed in the software

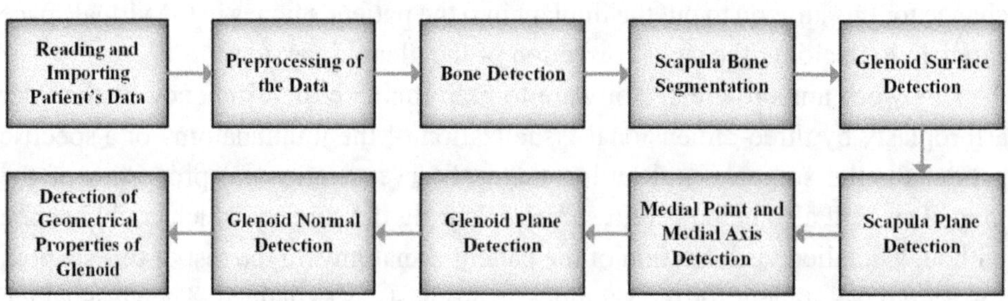

Reading and Importing Patient's Data

The first step in reproducing a three-dimensional joint anatomy of a specific patient is to input the patients data to the software. These data are captured using different medical imaging technologies including Computed Tomography (CT) scan, Magnetic Resonance Imaging (MRI), and Positron Emission Tomography (PET) scan. Different commercial equipment from a variety of manufacturers is used to capture images using each kind of the above technologies. Digital Imaging and Communication in Medicine (DICOM) standard has been created to handle this situation. It is a non-proprietary protocol which helps with safe data exchange in medical fields (Mustra, Delac, & Grgic, 2008). Using DICOM standard enables a shared format between all devices so that regardless of the type of the instrument used for imaging, or the manufacturer of the instrument, images can be accessed. DICOM standard provides data structures which include more types of data besides the image data. Main components of the data structures are Information Object Definitions (IODs), which can include a patient's data, medical device's data, medical institutions data, reports associated with the image and many other optional information (Mildenberger, Eichelberg, & Martin, 2002). These data are stored in a header section, and are of great importance for stable and accurate reading and evaluation of images. DICOM standard images can be accessed and viewed by dedicated DICOM viewers and other third-party viewers which have been available in the recent years. MATLAB has its own specific function for reading DICOM images including the header section information. In this work, the MATLAB's dicomread function has been used to import a patient's image data to the software (Mathworks, 2017).

A patient's image data captured using CT scan or MRI is provided as a set of two-dimensional images. When reading these images into MATLAB it is a good practice to store them in a three-dimensional matrix form, in which each layer of a matrix is a two-dimensional image. The positioning of each image in the three-dimensional matrix is important to be in the original order in which the images are captured from the patient. Naming of the images are not necessarily based on this order and another method is needed to solve this problem. Here DICOM standard helps by providing a series number and an instance number on the header section of each two-dimensional image. This data can be used to insert each image into its specific layer of the three-dimensional image. Figure 2 shows the way that reading and sorting operations are performed.

Figure 2. Simplified algorithm of image reading and sorting method

```
Input: address of the folder containing images
Output: 3D matrix of all images

begin
    Read the first image in the folder
    Find total number of instances in this series from DICOM header file
    Create an empty 3D matrix with sizes of the image and number of instances
        for all images in the folder
            Read current image's instance number
            Insert the image into the proper location of 3D matrix
end
```

Preprocessing of the Data

Image data provided to be used in the software should be preprocessed in order to be usable for more accurate image processing operations. Image intensity contrast is one of the important characteristics of the image, since other image processing methods including bone detection and segmentation will use it. Medical images captured might capture the information of the patient in a narrow range of grayscale values (Battish, 2017). In this case many gray level values will be left empty while a small gray level range will include all the data. Contrast stretching methods (Yang, 2006) are used for enhancement of the image in this case. In this work, medical image contrast is adjusted using MATALB's imadjust function (Mathworks, 2017) which remaps the intensity values of the image by stretching them. Stretching limits are found in a way that one percent of the data is saturated in the lowest intensities and one percent is saturated at the highest intensities and the rest of the data is stretched in between these values.

Medical images captured by different imaging technologies are each affected by different types of noises. The type of noise prevailing in an image depends on the image collection technology and the type of sensor which is used to capture the data. Among different types of noises that can exist in medical images Gaussian noise (Lal, Chandra, & Upadhyay, 2011), Poisson noise (Gravel, Beaudoin, & De Guise, 2004), and Rician noise (Nowak, 1999) are the most prevailing types. MRI images are mostly corrupted by Rician noise (Bhonsle, Chandra, & Sinha, 2012) while noises in Computed Tomography images are found to be of Poisson distribution (Gravel et al., 2004). Noise corrupts medical images in many ways including blurring important details of the image like edges and boundaries of tissue parts, or structural details in an organ. It is important to preserve these features of medical images by reducing the amount of noise presented. In this work, accurate separation of bones from the other tissues presented in the image is of great importance since the software aims at modeling the patient's joint anatomy for the surgeon and the created model geometrical accuracy must be as high as possible. For this reason, noise reduction method used in this work must be able to keep the sharp edges between bone boundaries and other tissues in the image, while trying to remove noises in all parts of the image.

Bilateral noise removal filter is an edge preserving method which is used in medical applications (Tomasi & Manduchi, 1988). Bilateral filter is a non-linear filter and it acts on each pixel of the two-dimensional image by replacing it with an average value of its surrounding pixels. The selection of surrounding pixels to be used in the averaging operation and their corresponding weights in the calculation are of a specific method, which makes the filter an edge preserving filter. In this method, there exist two different criteria for weighting of the surrounding pixels. The first criterion is a spatial kernel with a Gaussian distribution, which assigns higher weights to the pixels closer to the central pixel being proceeded. This part only considers the geometrical distance of pixels. The second criterion is defined in the intensity domain, where pixels with closer intensity values get higher weights. By combining these two criteria, pixels with closer spatial distance and closer intensity values are assigned higher weights, while pixels which are spatially close but have very different intensity values are not greatly considered in the averaging calculation. In this way edges of the image, which by nature have strong difference in intensity on each side, are preserved in the averaging process. Figure 3 describes the filters and their combinational effect on a pixel which is located on an edge in part of the image.

The Bilateral filter also create some side effects. One of the effects is that contrast regions appear in the image and staircase effects can happen. This can create a cartoon-like image (Winnemöller, Olsen, & Gooch, 2006). Gradient reversal artifact near the edges is the other side effect of bilateral filtering (Bae, Paris, & Durand, 2006). Two different improvements over the bilateral filter have been proposed to remove the gradient reversal artifact (Dorsey & Durand, 2002; Buades, Coll, & Morel, 2005). In this specific application where the input image is a grayscale medical image which will be used to extract the bones from the rest of the tissues, the side effects do not create an obstacle in the bone detection process. Figure 4 shows how bilateral noise removal method keeps the edges of bones in the noise removal process on an example CT scan image of a patients shoulder.

Bone Detection

The next step after preprocessing the data is to detect all the bones in the patient's images. There are different methods for segmentation of parts of images in the

Figure 3. The first criteria distributes the weights as shown in the left, it only considers spatial proximity. The second criteria distributes the weights as shown in the center, pixels with high difference in intensity are assigned less weights. The combinational weight assigned is shown on the right.

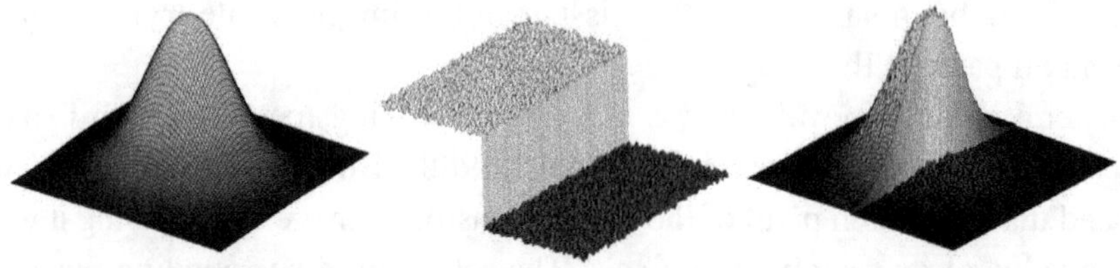

Figure 4. An example of bilateral noise removal method applied to a CT scan image of a shoulder joint

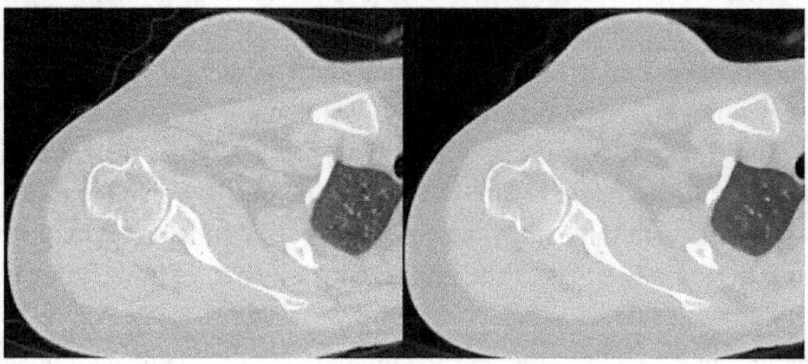

literature. Thresholding, region growing, classification, clustering and using deformable models, are among the mostly used methods (Egmentation, Pham, Xu, & Prince, 2000). Thresholding methods segment the image by using a threshold value in intensity for dividing the pixels in the image into different categories. Using one or more threshold values, pixels with intensity values bigger than the threshold will be categorized as another section from the pixels with intensity values less than the threshold value. Threshold value can be decided manually or can be obtained automatically using different methods (Sezgin & Sankur, 2004). Region growing techniques extract image regions which have pixels connected together by a specific criteria. Similar intensity value, color, or texture are among the criteria for region growing methods (Fan, Yau, Elmagarmid, & Aref, 2001). Region growing segmentation starts by choosing a seed point as the starting point and checks the connectivity of neighboring points by using the given criteria, and either accepts or rejects the neighbors to the current segment.

Classification and clustering are among machine learning methods of image segmentation. In these methods a feature space is derived from the image in which the partitioning is performed. The feature space in its simplest form can be the image intensities themselves (Kamavisdar, Saluja, & Agrawal, 2013). In Classification, previous examples of the desired object to be segmented have been observed by the machine, and their properties in the feature space have been extracted. The segmentation operation compares the extracted features of the new object and the previous examples and decides if the new object can be categorized in the current class. Clustering is different from classification in that no previous example is provided for the evaluation and the definition of classes is extracted as the images are being evaluated. Object classes are determined such a way that in each class objects have high similarity values, and objects of different classes are low in similarity measures (Liu, Zhang, Lu, & Ma, 2007). This method is hence called as an unsupervised segmentation method. Deformable models use curves in two-dimensional applications, or surfaces, in case of a three-dimensional data, located in an image which can move. The motion of model is influenced by two types of forces defined on the model. The first force is the internal force acting within the curve and trying to keep the curve smooth while deforming. The second force is the external force calculated from the image data and tries to push the model towards a specific form or shape (Hegadi, Kop, & Hangarge, 2010).

In this work, the region growing image segmentation method is used to separate the bones form the other tissues of the body in the images. Grayconnected function of the MATLAB image processing toolbox (Mathworks, 2017) which connects image pixels with similar intensity as a region growing method is used. For this region growing operation, the range of image intensities to be considered for the connection of pixels is one of the important parameters to be decided. This parameter is calculated by using the imaging protocol found in the DICOM file header section and the known relationship between the imaging protocol and the grayscale value of the bones in the image. For instance, for a specific computed tomography image, the intensity grayscale value of the bones can be found by considering the image acquisition parameters like tube voltage (kV) (Murakami et al., 2010). Another important parameter of this operation is the seed point position. In order to make a robust algorithm which does not rely on the position of the seed point, the segmentation operation is performed on the sections of the image which do not contain bone. In this way, seed point can be always selected as one corner of the image. After all other sections of the image are selected into a segment, the other parts of the image will include only the bones, which can be easily selected. This operation is performed on all the two-dimensional images of the set and all the areas with no bone material are deleted from the images. Figure 5 shows how the operation is performed.

Figure 5. Simplified algorithm of segmentation of bones from other tissues in the image set

Input: 3D matrix of all images including all tissues
Output: 3D matrix of all images including only bones

```
begin
    for each image in the 3D matrix
        Start from one corner of the image
        Find all connected pixels which their intensity values are out of range of bone's
        intensity value
        Replace their intensity values by zero
end
```

Scapula Segmentation

At this stage all the bones are separated on each two-dimensional image. The next step is to create a three-dimensional model of the bones which will be necessary for the next stages of the work, including scapula segmentation. This three-dimensional model is created through extracting an isosurface from the three-dimensional data of all images. In a scalar volumetric data (Yagel & Cohen, 2000), where each point in three-dimensional space has a scalar value, an isosurface is defined as a surface with all points having a constant value. The constant value is called the isovalue. The three-dimensional data is created from the two-dimensional images inserted on top of each other and given the proper space in the direction of the third dimension. The proper space is found from the DICOM header section of the images, as one of the properties of the image acquisition process. In this work, the isovalue is the value of the intensity of bone pixels, and the isosurface extraction is performed using marching cubes algorithm which is the most popular method for isosurfacing (Newman & Yi, 2006). The basic working principle behind the marching cube algorithm can be described as below. The three-dimensional space of the medical image, which has an intensity value at each point, is divided into different cubes, with each cube having eight neighboring pixels of the image at its corners. All the cubes are evaluated for their corners intensity values. The cubes which have some corners with intensity values in the range of the bone intensity value and some other corners with intensity values outside the bone intensity value, are the cubes which the isosurface will pass through. On these cubes, intersection points are found on the edges which have one corner inside and the other corner outside the object. Next, a surface is drawn in each cube which connects the intersection points. Connecting all the surfaces in all cubes makes the total isosurface.

The isosurface generated can consist of only one object or can include multiple objects. At this step, different bones in the isosurface model must be separated. For this purpose MATLAB's bwconncomp command is used in this work (Mathworks, 2017), which uses a flood-fill algorithm (Law, 2013) to find and label all the connected objects in the isosurface model. Segmentation of the scapula from the other bones is performed based on the fact that scapula bone has the most surface area among all the bones around the shoulder. So after surface area calculation, the bone with the highest surface area is selected as the scapula bone. Figure 6 displays all the bones and the scapula segmented from the rest of the bones.

Glenoid Surface Detection

After segmentation of the scapula bone from the other bones in the patient's image, it is required to understand the position and orientation of the scapula relative to the current three-dimensional image data. For this purpose, a method must be devised to find specific landmarks on the scapula bone. Finding the two most distanced points on the scapula is the first step. The general shape of scapula bone necessitates one of the points to be the inferior point of the scapula and the other point to be located on the outer side of acromion. To find out which of these two points are the inferior point and which one is located on the acromion, the curvature value of the points on the scapula surface are measured and the point with higher curvature is the inferior point of the scapula. This feature is also based on the geometrical properties of the scapula which has a sharper point at the inferior part compared to the outer side of acromion. Having these two points, the process to find the glenoid surface can be started. A line which passes through these two points is drawn in the next step. This line's intersection points on the scapula are found and the intersection point which is closest to the acromion end of the line and is located in the second quarter of the line is on the glenoid surface (Ghafurian, Galdi, Bastian, Tan, & Li, 2016).

Figure 6. Left, All the bones extracted from the other tissues in the image data. Right, Scapula separated from the other bones

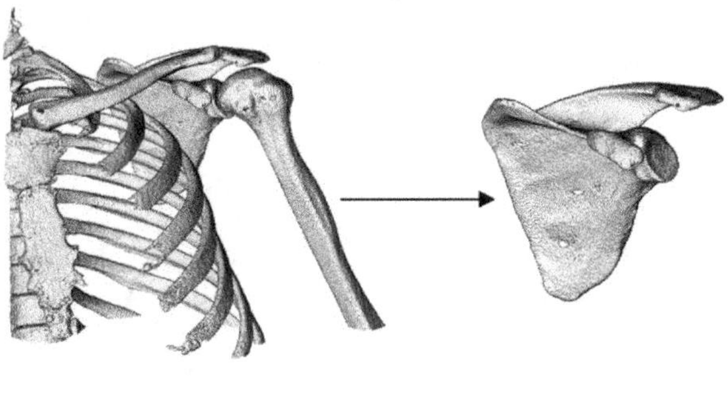

By this method we can detect the first landmark which is located on the glenoid surface. Figure 7 shows the most distanced points detected on the scapula and the line connecting these two points, and the intersection of this line with the glenoid surface which is located by the mentioned method.

Using the point found on the glenoid surface as the starting point, a method is used to find the glenoid surface. In this method, at first the curvature value of all points on the scapula are calculated (figure 9, Left), then an algorithm searches for all the neighbors of the first point found on the glenoid and chooses the neighbor with a minimum curvature value for the next iteration, then it repeats this step until no point with lower curvature value can be found in the neighborhood of the current point. The last point found is considered the point with minimum curvature on the glenoid surface, and is chosen to be the seed point of the next step of the method. Here a curvedness-based region growing algorithm (Moineau, Levigne, Boileau, Young, & Walch, 2012) is used to find all the points on the glenoid surface. This algorithm starts adding neighbors of the seed point to the collection of points which belong to the glenoid surface by checking if their curvature value is below a certain threshold, and on the next iteration it repeats this step for the new points added to the collection. By this method all the points which are connected to each other, and have curvature values in the accepted range will be included in the glenoid surface. This algorithm is shown in figure 8.

Figure 9 on the left shows a section of the scapula containing the glenoid which is color coded for the curvature values of points. In the center it shows the first iteration of the region growing algorithm starting from the minimum curvature point and adding the first set of neighbors and on the right the final set of points comprising the glenoid surface are shown. The threshold curvature value for the points belonging to the glenoid surface, was found experimentally to be 0.4 for this software. After finding the glenoid surface, the center of the glenoid must be found.

Figure 7. The Line connecting the most distanced points on the scapula and the Intersection point of that line and the glenoid surface

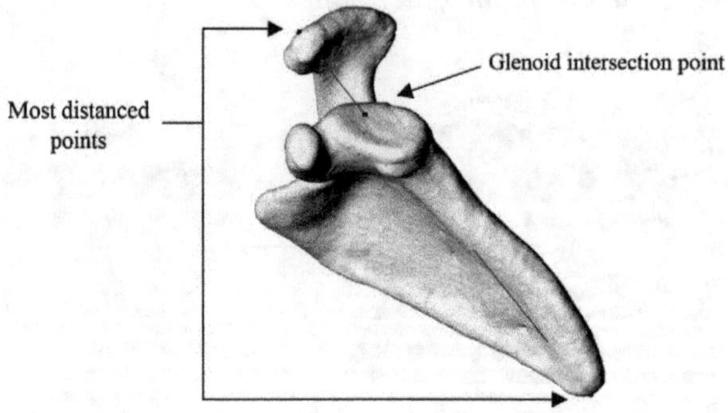

Figure 8. Simplified algorithm of curvedness-based region growing method

Input: 3D matrix including scapula surface points, intersection point found on glenoid surface
Output: set of points comprising the glenoid surface

```
begin
    Find the curvature values of all points
    Start from the intersection point found on the glenoid surface
    while (a point with lower curvature can be found)
        Find neighbors of the current point
        Set the point with lowest curvature value as the current point
    end
    Start from the lowest curvature point found in the last step
    while (new points are added to the glenoid surface point set)
        Find neighbors of the current points
        if (the curvature value of each neighbor is less than the threshold value)
        then add those points to the set of points in the glenoid surface
        end
        Set the newly added points as the current points
    end
end
```

Figure 9. Left, part of the scapula color mapped by curvature value. Center, magnified view of the glenoid, showing the glenoid surface points found in the first iteration of the algorithm. Right, the final set of points comprising the glenoid surface.

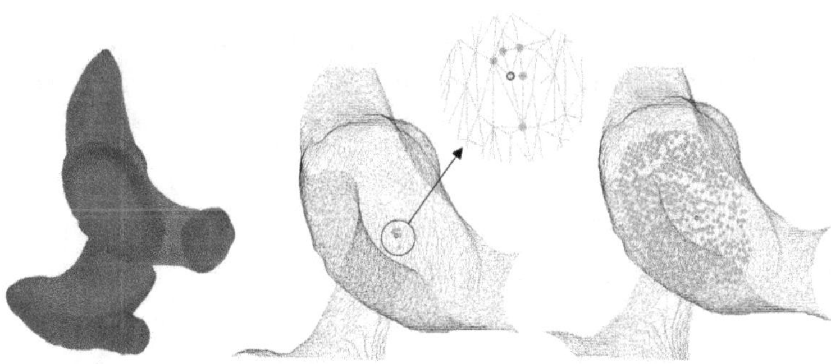

This point is located by finding the average value of all glenoid points and then finding the closest point located on the actual surface of the scapula to this point.

Other GUI Features

After finding the glenoid center as one of the most important features on the scapula, further steps can be performed to find other features which are valuable in demonstrating the patient's bone properties.

- **Scapula Plane:** The scapula plane passes through the center of the glenoid and the inferior point of the scapula, which are already detected in the previous steps of the work. The third point, which is necessary for defining the plane of scapula, is found by the center of weight of all the points on the scapula. The center of weight of all the points is calculated by taking the average of the positions of all the points of the scapula in the three-dimensional space. Using these three points, the plane of the scapula is defined and it is shown in figure 10.
- **Medial Point and Medial Axis of Scapula:** To find the medial point of the scapula, first the intersection of the scapula plane and the scapula surface is found. This intersection is in the form of a contour line which passes through the glenoid center and the inferior point of the scapula. On this contour line, the point which has the furthest distance from the line connecting the glenoid center and the inferior point of the scapula, is the medial point of the scapula (Ghafurian et al., 2016). Finding the furthest distanced point is performed by computing the distance of all the points on the contour line with the line connecting the glenoid center and the inferior point and then choosing the point with the maximum distance. After finding the medial point, the medial axis of the scapula is defined by a line passing through the medial point and the glenoid center. Figure 10 shows the intersection contour on the scapula, the medial point, and the medial axis.
- **Glenoid Plane:** The glenoid plane is the plane which passes through the glenoid center and has the scapula medial axis as its normal. This plane is also perpendicular to the plane of the scapula since it normally lies on the

Figure 10. Scapula bone transparent, Scapula plane, intersection of scapula plane and scapula, medial point, and medial axis

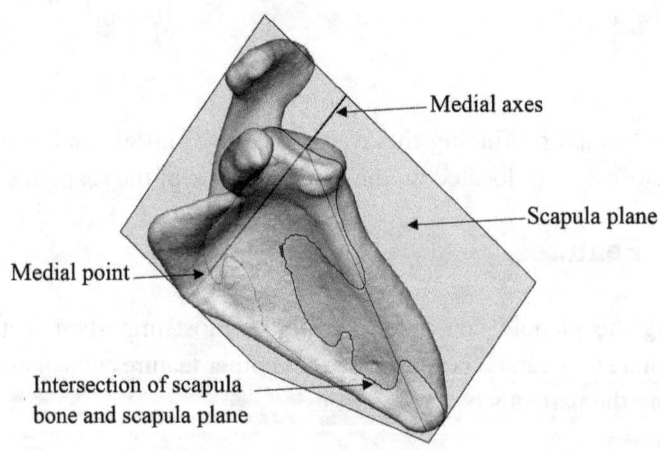

scapula plane. Having found both the scapula plane and the glenoid plane, the transverse scapula plane can also be found since it is perpendicular to both of the previously mentioned planes and passes through the glenoid center. At this step, the coordinate system of the scapula bone model can be defined using the above three planes on the model. Next, the model should be transformed in a way that the orientation of the scapula is properly adjusted for display on the graphical user interface. The transformation consists of three consecutive rotations and a translation. It fits the glenoid plane, the scapula plane, and the transverse scapula plane to xz, yz, and xz planes of the graphical user interface coordinate system respectively, while the glenoid center passes the origin. Using this standard for displaying the model helps with better initial visualization of the scapula. Figure 11 shows three planes of scapula.

- **Glenoid Normal and Geometrical properties:** The glenoid normal is defined as the line connecting the glenoid center to the center point of a best-fit sphere to the glenoid surface (Moineau et al., 2012). The best-fit sphere to the glenoid center is also used to find the average radius of curvature of the glenoid surface. A least squared method (Lewis & Armstrong, 2011) is used to find the best-fit sphere. This method minimizes the sum of squared errors in the distance between the sphere points and the points located on the glenoid surface. The radius of the sphere found is used for estimating the curvature of the total glenoid surface. In figure 12 the best-fit sphere and the glenoid normal are displayed.

Two important geometrical properties of the glenoid surface are its inclination and version angles. The version is the angle between the glenoid normal and the scapula medial axis, when they are projected on transverse scapula plane. The inclination

Figure 11. All three planes of the scapula after the transformation of the model to GUI coordinate system

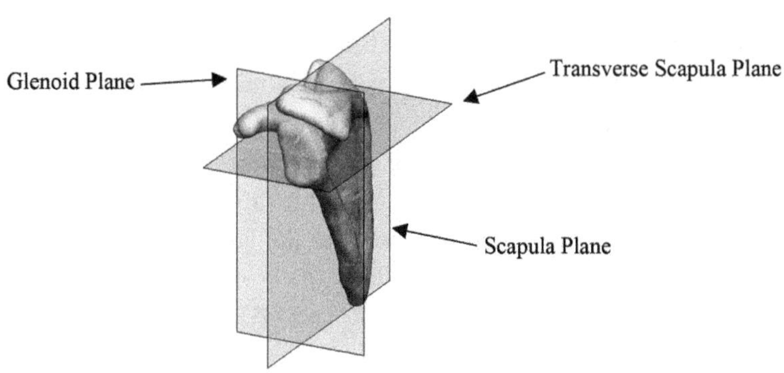

is the angle between the glenoid normal projected on the glenoid plane, and the scapula medial axis. Figure 12 shows the definition of inclination and version angles.

Graphical User Interface

The Graphical User Interface of the software is divided into three main sections as it is shown in Figure 12. In the left section of the graphical user interface, two-dimensional slices of the scapula bone of the patient are displayed in axial, medial and coronal view orientations. These two-dimensional images are sliced from the scapula bone at the scapula plane, glenoid plane and transverse scapula plane, and show the inner structure of the scapula bone. The surgeon can move through the slices in any of the views, using the slide bars on the side of each view window to see other parts of the bone in sections parallel to the initial section. Using the reset button at the bottom of the section, the surgeon can bring the two-dimensional views to the initial position. Zooming and panning operations can be applied to any of the two-dimensional views independently in case closer inspection is needed on a section of the bone.

The central section of the graphical user interface, displays the three-dimensional scapula bone model. In this section different features of the bone model can be observed when activated. When any of the features are activated, the rendering of the model is updated so that the feature is added to the scene, and likewise when the feature is deactivated, the scene is updated again. Like the two-dimensional sections, zooming and panning operations are applicable to the model in this section, so that the surgeon can inspect any section of the bone more accurately. Rotation of the model is also available in this section which is not the case for the two-dimensional views.

The right section of graphical user interface controls different features of the software. On the top of the right section, visualization of the three-dimensional model is controlled. Activation and deactivation of the scapula bone's model's features are performed in this section. These features are as follows: the scapula plane, the glenoid plane, the medial axes of the scapula, the best-fit sphere to the glenoid surface and the glenoid normal. The scapula bone transparency and its amount also can be controlled here, to provide better visualization of other features. In this section, geometrical information of the glenoid, including inclination and version, is also displayed.

There are two other subsections in the right section of graphical user interface, which are provided for future work. One is to enable the software to insert an implant to the anatomy of the joint, which will provide the software with capabilities for displaying different types of implants generally used for shoulder arthroplasty so that the surgeon can better plan the implanting procedure's details. The other is to help with the creation, insertion and saving of the guides to be used with the specific implant. If the software is able to create required guides' models based on the bone and implant geometrical conditions, then many of the factors which are decided during the surgery can be decided preoperatively which is a big help in reducing operation risks.

CONCLUSION

In this work, a medical image processing software development procedure is explained, displaying each step of the job needed for enabling a software to read, import, segment, analyze and display anatomical models of the body. The software helps in preoperative planning of the surgery by creating an environment in which a three-dimensional model of the anatomy of a patient and their specific condition can be observed. Using a software of this kind can help a surgeon determine different treatment solutions, as well as reducing the risk of complications that can happen. As a result, it can improve the efficiency of shoulder arthroplasty operations.

Figure 12. Graphical User Interface of the software with features activated

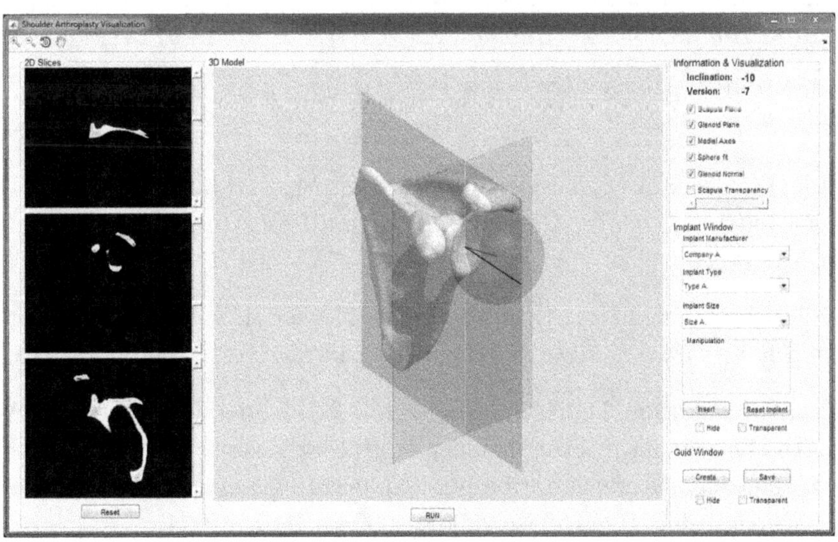

Some other features are planned to be performed for future work. Among those is enabling the software for insertion of an implant of a specific size and type into the three-dimensional model space and allowing the surgeon to adjust the position and orientation of it relative to the bone model. That will greatly help with the surgeons understanding of the operation before starting the surgery. Another feature would be creating a guide system for each patient and each implant type and size so that the implant can be mounted during the surgery with minimum error, and this will greatly improve the preoperative planning support that the software can provide.

ACKNOWLEDGMENT

The first author of this study has been financially supported by TUBITAK 2215 program. This research was supported by the Istanbul Technical University BAP [grant numbers 39686]; and the Bezmialem Vakif University BAP.

The CT scan data used in this study belongs to a patient who received treatment by the authors of this paper previously and the patient has given permission for the medical data to be used in this study.

REFERENCES

Bae, S., Paris, S., & Durand, F. (2006). Two-scale tone management for photographic look. *ACM Transactions on Graphics*, *25*(3), 637. doi:10.1145/1141911.1141935

Battish, N. (2017). *Analysis of Pre-processing Methods using MRI Images*. Academic Press.

Bhonsle, D., Chandra, V., & Sinha, G. R. (2012). Medical Image Denoising Using Bilateral Filter. *I.J. Image, Graphics and Signal Processing, 6*, 36-43. 10.5815/ijigsp.2012.06.06

Bohsali, K. I., Wirth, M. A., Rockwood, C. A., Material, S., & Surgery, J. (2010). *Complications of Total Shoulder Arthroplasty*. Academic Press. 10.2106/JBJS.F.00125

Boileau, P., Watkinson, D., Hatzidakis, A. M., & Hovorka, I. (2006). Neer Award 2005: The Grammont reverse shoulder prosthesis: Results in cuff tear arthritis, fracture sequelae, and revision arthroplasty. *Journal of Shoulder and Elbow Surgery*, *15*(5), 527–540. doi:10.1016/j.jse.2006.01.003 PMID:16979046

Boileau, P., Watkinson, D. J., Hatzidakis, A. M., & Balg, F. (2005). Grammont reverse prosthesis: Design, rationale, and biomechanics. *Journal of Shoulder and Elbow Surgery*, *14*(1S), 147–161. doi:10.1016/j.jse.2004.10.006 PMID:15726075

Buades, A., Coll, B., & Morel, J.-M. J.-M. (2005). A non-local algorithm for image denoising. *Computer Vision and Pattern Recognition, 2005. CVPR 2005. IEEE Computer Society Conference on, 2*, 60–65. 10.1109/CVPR.2005.38

Buck, F. M., Jost, B., & Hodler, J. (2008). Shoulder arthroplasty. *European Radiology*, *18*(12), 2937–2948. doi:10.100700330-008-1093-8 PMID:18618117

Deutsch, A., Abboud, J. A., Kelly, J., Mody, M., Norris, T., Ramsey, M. L., ... Williams, G. R. (2007). Clinical results of revision shoulder arthroplasty for glenoid component loosening. *Journal of Shoulder and Elbow Surgery*, *16*(6), 706–716. doi:10.1016/j.jse.2007.01.007 PMID:17931898

Dorsey, J., & Durand, F. (2002). Fast Bilateral Filtering for the Display of High-Dynamic-Range Images Introduction. *Vine*, 257–266.

Egmentation, S., Pham, D. L., Xu, C., & Prince, J. L. (2000). Current methods in medical image segmentation. *Annual Review of Biomedical Engineering*, *2*(1), 315–337. doi:10.1146/annurev.bioeng.2.1.315 PMID:11701515

Fan, J., & Yau, D. K. Y. (2001). Automatic image segmentation by integrating color-edge extractionand seeded region growing. *IEEE Transactions on Image Processing*, *10*(10), 1454–1466. doi:10.1109/83.951532 PMID:18255490

Farshad, M., & Gerber, C. (2010). Reverse total shoulder arthroplasty-from the most to the least common complication. *International Orthopaedics*, *34*(8), 1075–1082. doi:10.100700264-010-1125-2 PMID:20865260

Ghafurian, S., Galdi, B., Bastian, S., Tan, V., & Li, K. (2016). Computerized 3D morphological analysis of glenoid orientation. *Journal of Orthopaedic Research*, *34*(4), 692–698. doi:10.1002/jor.23053 PMID:26400654

Gravel, P., Beaudoin, G., & De Guise, J. A. (2004). A method for modeling noise in medical images. *IEEE Transactions on Medical Imaging*, *23*(10), 1221–1232. doi:10.1109/TMI.2004.832656 PMID:15493690

Hammond, J. W., Queale, W. S., Kim, T. K., & McFarland, E. G. (2003). Surgeon experience and clinical and economic outcomes for shoulder arthroplasty. *The Journal of Bone and Joint Surgery. American Volume*, *85–A*(12), 2318–2324. doi:10.2106/00004623-200312000-00008 PMID:14668500

Hasan, S. S., Leith, J. M., Smith, K. L., & Matsen, F. A. III. (2003). The distribution of shoulder replacement among surgeons and hospitals is significantly different than that of hip or knee replacement. *Journal of Shoulder and Elbow Surgery*, *12*(2), 164–169. doi:10.1067/mse.2003.23 PMID:12700570

Hegadi, R., Kop, A., & Hangarge, M. (2010). A Survey on Deformable Model and its Applications to Medical Imaging. *International Journal of Computer Applications, RTIPPR*(2), 64–75. Retrieved from http://www.ijcaonline.org/rtippr/number2/SPE101T.pdf%5Cnhttp://files/394/A Survey on Deformable Model and its Applications .pdf%5Cnhttp://files/396/SPE101T.html

Iannotti, J. P., Greeson, C., Downing, D., Sabesan, V., & Bryan, J. A. (2012). Effect of glenoid deformity on glenoid component placement in primary shoulder arthroplasty. *Journal of Shoulder and Elbow Surgery*, *21*(1), 48–55. doi:10.1016/j.jse.2011.02.011 PMID:21600787

Kamavisdar, P., Saluja, S., & Agrawal, S. (2013). A survey on image classification approaches and techniques. *International Journal of Advertising*, *2*(1), 1005–1009. Retrieved from http://ijarcce.com/upload/january/22-A Survey on Image Classification.pdf

Karelse, A., Leuridan, S., Van Tongel, A., Piepers, I. M., Debeer, P., & De Wilde, L. F. (2014). A glenoid reaming study: How accurate are current reaming techniques? *Journal of Shoulder and Elbow Surgery*, *23*(8), 1120–1127. doi:10.1016/j.jse.2013.11.023 PMID:24582954

Kim, S. H., Wise, B. L., Zhang, Y., & Szabo, R. M. (2011). Increasing incidence of shoulder arthroplasty in the United States. *The Journal of Bone and Joint Surgery. American Volume*, *93*(24), 2249–2254. doi:10.2106/JBJS.J.01994 PMID:22258770

Lal, S., Chandra, M., & Upadhyay, G. K. (2011). *Removal of Additive Gaussian Noise by Complex Double Density Dual Tree Discrete Wavelet Transform*. Academic Press.

Law, G. (2013). Quantitative Comparison of Flood Fill and Modified Flood Fill Algorithms. *International Journal of Computer Theory and Engineering*, *5*(3), 503–508. doi:10.7763/IJCTE.2013.V5.738

Lewis, G. S., & Armstrong, A. D. (2011). Glenoid spherical orientation and version. *Journal of Shoulder and Elbow Surgery*, *20*(1), 3–11. doi:10.1016/j.jse.2010.05.012 PMID:20932782

Liu, Y., Zhang, D., Lu, G., & Ma, W. Y. (2007). A survey of content-based image retrieval with high-level semantics. *Pattern Recognition*, *40*(1), 262–282. doi:10.1016/j.patcog.2006.04.045

Mathworks. (2017). *Image Processing Toolbox User's Guide*. Retrieved September 26, 2017, from https://www.mathworks.com/help/images/ref/dicomread.html

Matsen, F. A. III, Clinton, J., Lynch, J., Bertelsen, A., Richardson, M. L., & Matsen Iii, F. A. (2008). Glenoid Component Failure in Total Shoulder Arthroplasty. *The Journal of Bone and Joint Surgery. American Volume*, *90*(4), 885–896. doi:10.2106/JBJS.G.01263 PMID:18381328

Mildenberger, P., Eichelberg, M., & Martin, E. (2002). Introduction to the DICOM standard. *European Radiology*, *12*(4), 920–927. doi:10.1007003300101100 PMID:11960249

Moineau, G., Levigne, C., Boileau, P., Young, A., & Walch, G. (2012). Three-dimensional measurement method of arthritic glenoid cavity morphology: Feasibility and reproducibility. *Orthopaedics & Traumatology: Surgery & Research*, *98*(S6), S139–S145. doi:10.1016/j.otsr.2012.06.007 PMID:22964089

Murakami, Y., Kakeda, S., Kamada, K., Ohnari, N., Nishimura, J., Ogawa, M., ... Korogi, Y. (2010). Effect of tube voltage on image quality in 64-section multidetector 3D CT angiography: Evaluation with a vascular phantom with superimposed bone skull structures. *AJNR. American Journal of Neuroradiology*, *31*(4), 620–625. doi:10.3174/ajnr.A1871 PMID:19942711

Mustra, M., Delac, K., & Grgic, M. (2008). Overview of the DICOM standard. *2008 50th International Symposium ELMAR*, *1*, 39–44.

Newman, T. S., & Yi, H. (2006). A survey of the marching cubes algorithm. *Computers and Graphics (Pergamon)*, *30*(5), 854–879. doi:10.1016/j.cag.2006.07.021

Nguyen, D., Ferreira, L. M., Brownhill, J. R., King, G. J. W., Drosdowech, D. S., Faber, K. J., & Johnson, J. A. (2009). Improved accuracy of computer assisted glenoid implantation in total shoulder arthroplasty: An in-vitro randomized controlled trial. *Journal of Shoulder and Elbow Surgery*, *18*(6), 907–914. doi:10.1016/j.jse.2009.02.022 PMID:19482490

Nowak, R. D. (1999). Wavelet-based Rician noise removal for magnetic resonance imaging. *IEEE Transactions on Image Processing*, *8*(10), 1408–1419. doi:10.1109/83.791966 PMID:18267412

Reported Shoulder Procedures. (2017). Retrieved September 26, 2017, from https://aoanjrr.sahmri.com/shoulders

Sezgin, M., & Sankur, B. (2004). Survey over image thresholding techniques and quantitative performance evaluation. *Journal of Electronic Imaging*, *13*(1), 146–165. doi:10.1117/1.1631315

Tomasi, C., & Manduchi, R. (1988). Bilateral filtering for gray and color images. *Sixth International Conference on Computer Vision* (IEEE Cat. No.98CH36271), 839–846. 10.1109/ICCV.1998.710815

Trofa, D., Rajaee, S. S., & Smith, E. L. (2014). Nationwide trends in total shoulder arthroplasty and hemiarthroplasty for osteoarthritis. *American Journal of Orthopedics (Belle Mead, N.J.)*, *43*(4), 166–172. PMID:24730001

Verborgt, O., De Smedt, T., Vanhees, M., Clockaerts, S., Parizel, P. M., & Van Glabbeek, F. (2011). Accuracy of placement of the glenoid component in reversed shoulder arthroplasty with and without navigation. *Journal of Shoulder and Elbow Surgery*, *20*(1), 21–26. doi:10.1016/j.jse.2010.07.014 PMID:21134663

Walch, G., Boileau, P., & Noël, E. (2010). Shoulder arthroplasty: Evolving techniques and indications. *Joint, Bone, Spine*, *77*(6), 501–505. doi:10.1016/j.jbspin.2010.09.004 PMID:20961793

Winnemöller, H., Olsen, S. C., & Gooch, B. (2006). Real-time video abstraction. *ACM SIGGRAPH 2006 Papers on - SIGGRAPH '06*, 1221. 10.1145/1179352.1142018

Yagel, R., & Cohen, D. (2000). Volume Graphics. In Computer (Vol. 26). London: Springer London. doi:10.1007/978-1-4471-0737-8

Yang, C. C. (2006). Image enhancement by modified contrast-stretching manipulation. *Optics & Laser Technology*, *38*(3), 196–201. doi:10.1016/j.optlastec.2004.11.009

Zumstein, M. A., Pinedo, M., Old, J., & Boileau, P. (2011). Problems, complications, reoperations, and revisions in reverse total shoulder arthroplasty: A systematic review. *Journal of Shoulder and Elbow Surgery*, *20*(1), 146–157. doi:10.1016/j.jse.2010.08.001 PMID:21134666

Chapter 2
Digital Image Analysis in Clinical and Experimental Pathology:
An Ode to Microscopy

Didier Meseure
Curie Institute, France

Kinan Drak Alsibai
Institut de Pathologie de Paris, France

ABSTRACT

Conventional pathology using a light microscope is rapidly shifting towards digital integration. Digital imaging plays an increasing role in clinical diagnosis, biomedical research, and continuing medical education. Currently, pathology platforms are composed of clinical and molecular pathologists and engineers with the sole intention of investigating cellular and molecular basis of human health through applied research in disease aetiology, pathogenesis, diagnosis, and treatment. Molecular diagnosis using technical advances and the application of specific biomarkers in clinical practice are the two main pillars of modern personalized medicine especially in oncology. Thus, it has become evident that accredited clinical and molecular pathology laboratories using digital imaging and advanced technologies can make the most of diagnostic and specific biomarker analyses as well as incorporating other key aspects of translational research and data analysis.

DOI: 10.4018/978-1-5225-5876-7.ch002

INTRODUCTION

Clinical pathologist is a physician who specializes in the diagnosis and management of human diseases using appropriate laboratory methods. Conventional analysis of surgical or core biopsy specimens (histopathology) and body fluids, needle aspiration and exfoliative materials (cytopathology) using a light microscope is rapidly shifting towards digital integration. Digital imaging plays an increasing role in clinical diagnosis, biomedical research, seminar and continuing medical education. Currently, pathology platforms are composed of clinical, molecular, and translational pathologists and engineers with the sole intention of investigating cellular and molecular basis of human health through applied research in disease aetiology, pathogenesis, diagnosis and treatment. Molecular diagnosis using technical advances and the application of specific biomarkers in clinical practice are the two main pillars of modern personalized medicine especially in oncology. There are two levels of biomarker analysis in clinical trials; specific biomarker analysis to determine the patient's stratification and general biomarker analysis to predict patient response to treatment (Salto-Tellez *et al.,* 2014).

Clinical and molecular pathology platforms and translational research laboratories use the same tissue and fluid samples, phenotypic analysis, digital imaging and advanced technologies, under strict standards, in both clinical diagnosis and biomedical research. They play a central role in identifying mechanisms of carcinogenesis, gene expression, signalling aberrations, tumour microenvironment, cancer stem cells, tumour invasion and metastasis, metabolism, extracellular matrix regulation, angiogenesis, autophagy, ribonucleic acid (RNA) and protein expression, deoxyribonucleic acid (DNA) damage, non-coding RNA (ncRNA) deregulation and apoptosis (Meseure *et al.,* 2014; Drak Alsibai & Meseure 2018).

The precision medicine and new scientific research approach of disease generate enormous amounts of information "big data", that require database construction, analysis, storing and managing their storage (i.e. biobanking and bioinformatics). As technique complexity and data increase, so too do the amount and the complexity of data analysis. The complexity of data highlights the importance of integrating an alternative multi-parametric data assays into the clinical practice and scientific research (Gondhalekar *et al.,* 2018).

It has become evident that accredited clinical and molecular pathology laboratories can make the most of specific biomarker analyses as well as incorporating other key aspects of translational research and data analysis. Currently, these laboratories are well equipped by tissue-based techniques {i.e. tissue microarray (TMA), immunohistochemistry (IHC), fluorescence in situ hybridization (FISH), multiplexed hybridisations}, digital image techniques, nucleic acid extractions and polymerase chain reaction (PCR) technologies {i.e. Sanger sequencing, pyrosequencing, quantitative PCR}, and high-throughput technologies {i.e. next-generation sequencing (NGS), high-throughput gene expression arrays, high-throughput methylation, gene copy number variation, high-throughput proteomics and metabolomics, imaging mass spectrometry (IMS) and matrix-assisted laser desorption/ionization-IMS (MALDI-IMS)} (Salto-Tellez *et al.,* 2015).

This chapter will briefly describe the tissue processing and tissue microarrays protocols, and the main steps for acquiring digital images from tissue samples, and the imaging techniques relevant for this purpose such as whole-slide imaging. Then, the chapter will highlight the major high-throughput vectorial and non-vectorial technologies in molecular pathology, and will empathize on their mechanistic details and main applications in diagnostic pathology, oncology and biomedical research (Table 1).

Table 1. Comparative table highlighting the importance and the role of the different imaging modalities (vectorial and non-vectorial technologies) in clinical and experimental pathology and biomedical research.

Vectorial Technologies				Non-Vectorial Technology
IHC	**Multiplexed-IHC**	**RNAscope assay**	**RNA-seq**	**MALD IMS**
• Routine diagnostic in clinical pathology • Experimental pathology • Biomedical research • Detection and quantification of protein expression and tumour biomarkers	• Routine diagnostic in clinical pathology • Experimental pathology • Biomedical research • Detection and quantification of protein expression • Simultaneous detection of multiples biomarkers • Evaluation of single cell coexpression • Monitoring cell signaling pathways • Analyzing of tumour microenvironment	• Experimental pathology • Biomedical research • Simultaneous detection of various target genes to identify co-localization	• Experimental pathology • Biomedical research • Exact sequence and location of transcript • Preserving spatial information • Guiding anti-cancer treatment and drug discovery	• Potential influence in routine pathology's practice • Experimental pathology • Biomedical research • Identification and localization of molecules from the tissue's surface • Imaging pharmacokinetic studies in drug development • Discrimination of normal, neoplasia and tumour tissues. • Classification of tumors based on lipid or protein patterns • Spatial mapping of tumour metabolism • Analyzing of tumour microenvironment • Molecular analysis of tumour margins

CLINICAL PATHOLOGY

Tissue Processing

After reception, tissue specimens should be transferred immediately into fixative (10% neutral buffered formalin) to prevent autolysis. After fixation, specimens are trimmed by pathologist using a scalpel to enable them to fit into an appropriate cassette. Then, the tissue specimens should be passed through multiple changes of dehydrating solvents (increasing concentrations of ethanol) to remove the water and formalin. Next, a clearing solvent such as xylene is used to remove the alcohol and allow infiltration with paraffin wax to obtain a paraffin block, referred to as formalin-fixed, paraffin-embedded (FFPE) tissue. The duration and step details of the tissue processing schedule depend on the nature and size of the tissue specimen. Finally, Paraffin blocks are cut using a microtome, in order to obtain thin tissue sections (4 - 6 μm), mounted on a glass slide and then stained with standard staining {hematoxylin and eosin (H&E)}, special staining and IHC, and/or used for high-throughput technologies. Deparaffinization and hydration processing in xylene and graded ethanol to distilled water are performed prior to any staining protocol or advanced technology (Figure 1A).

Immunohistochemistry

Immunohistochemistry (IHC) is an important application in routine diagnostic pathology that uses monoclonal as well as polyclonal antibodies to determine the tissue distribution of an antigen of interest in tissue samples. To visualize the antibody-antigen interaction the antibody must be conjugated to an enzyme, such as peroxidase, that can catalyse a colour-producing reaction (immunoperoxidase staining) (Figure 1B). Alternatively, the antibody can also be tagged to a fluorophore

Figure 1. Tissue section of breast cancer prepared with conventional tissue processing, mounted on glass slides, and stained with the standard histopathological HE staining (Figure 1A), and with the immunohistochemical antibody HER2 (Figure 1B).

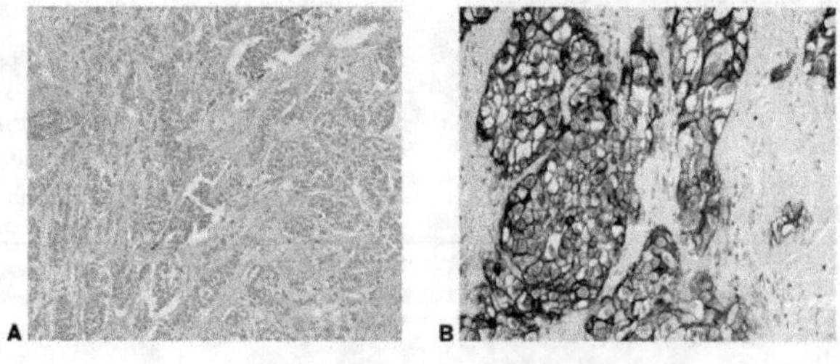

(immunofluorescence), or to radioactive element. IHC is widely used for diagnosis and classification of cancers, as it helps tell the difference between different cancer types and determine the primary origin of metastatic tumours (Duraiyan *et al.*, 2012).

Furthermore, IHC stains of breast cancer biomarkers; oestrogen receptors (ER), progesterone receptors (PR) and human epidermal growth factor 2 receptors (HER2), are able to provide robust, reproducible, and highly predictive information necessary for an appropriate treatment and follow-up (Sheffield *et al.*, 2016).

Tissue Microarray

In the tissue microarray (TMA) technique, a hollow needle is used to remove tissue cores as small as 0.6 mm in diameter and up to 2 mm in diameter from regions of interest in paraffin blocks. These tissue cores are then inserted in a recipient paraffin block in a precisely spaced array pattern contains 40 to 250 cores, which can be subjected to independent tests. Sections from this block are cut using a microtome and mounted on a glass slide to be analysed by any technique. Tests commonly employed in TMA include IHC, FISH and high-throughput technologies (Figure 2). The advantages of using TMA technology are that large amount of data can rapidly be analysed using a single technique protocol, avoid experimental variability, and economize the use of reagents. Thus, TMA is particularly useful in biomedical research analysis, and to study and validate cancer biomarkers in large patient cohorts (Kampf *et al.*, 2012).

Figure 2. Tissue microarray (TMA) technique. This figure shows a TMA glass slide, which contains 88 core sections, all stained with the same immunohistochemical antibody.

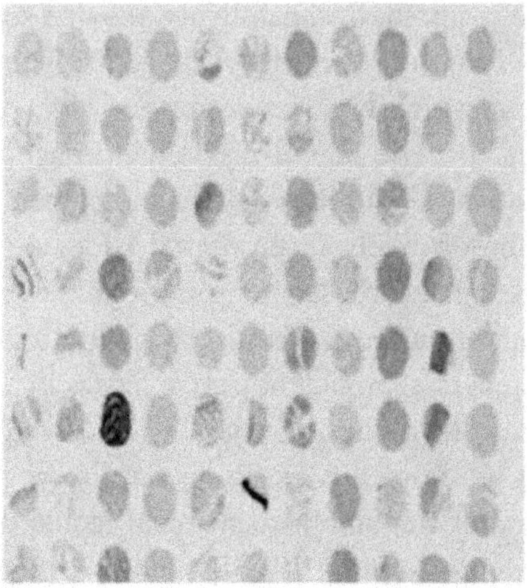

DIGITAL PATHOLOGY

Tissues consist of cells and extra cellular matrix. The small size of these components makes the study of tissues dependent on microscope and other advances techniques. Light microscope is still the gold standard in the interpretation of glass slides in all pathology departments. Currently, most light microscopes are combined with a high-quality digital camera, the so called digital microscope, with an image sensor that records the image on a computer monitor. More recent, the development of the whole slide scanner provides high-throughput and digitization of the entire sample of tissues, thus, light microscope is gradually being replaced by the whole slide imaging (WSI) especially in developed pathology departments, university and research laboratories.

Whole Slide Imaging

Whole slide imaging (WSI) is a new technology that can automate the capturing of the entire conventional glass slides into a digital format, using whole slide scanners to produce digital slides (Pantanowitz *et al.,* 2011). WSI has become an important tool in routine practices of clinical pathology (Farahani *et al.,* 2017). The two main methodologies of whole slide scanners are area scanning and line scanning (Higgins *et al.,* 2015). In area scanners, microscopic tiles are captured using a charge-coupled device (CCD) camera and aligned to make seamless borders between tiles. In a CCD image sensor, pixels are represented by p-doped metal-oxide-semiconductors capacitors, which are biased above the threshold for inversion when image acquisition begins, allowing the conversion of incoming photons into electron charges at the semiconductor-oxide interface. The CCD is then used to read out these charges. CCD image sensors are widely used in medical, and research applications where high-quality images are required. Comparatively, the line scanner uses linear-array detectors combined with motion control components. This technology is ideally suited to applications in which high-resolution, or high-speed image capture is needed. The camera has a single line of pixels that image across a glass slide, to build up a two-dimensional (2D) image, either the camera or the slide is moved perpendicular to the line of pixels. Then digital slides are built up as pyramids of different resolutions created by scanning through several resolution levels at the same spot. The formats allow in-focus navigation and continuous changing magnifications, equivalent to changing objective lenses in a microscope. Recently, three-dimension (3D) reconstruction of whole slide histological data from serial sections (50 – 200) has developed. All sections need to be stained, using standard histological staining and/or immunohistochemical techniques. Next, the stained-glass slides need to be digitized using a WSI scanner, to generate a series of digital images, each corresponding to a different scanned level of the FFPE tissue. These serial digital images are then run through commercially available or custom software, to generate 3D models. WSI system enables automatic sample detection, virtual-Z acquisition and creation of focal maps. Digital slides are layered with multiple resolutions at each location, including the highest resolution needed to allow more detailed review of specific regions of interest. Scans may be acquired at x2, 10, 20, 40, 60 and 100 or a combination of magnifications to highlight important detail. Digital image analysis comprises segmentation, feature extraction, classification and registration (Farahani *et al.,* 2017).

Applications of Digital Imaging

Digitizing of tissue samples has several advantages over viewing the sample through the light and fluorescent microscopes using the conventional glass slides. First advantage is the slide navigation, which enables combining the viewing process with other computer tools for making annotations on interesting parts of a specimen or for measuring lesion or structure sizes. Additionally, digital images provide the ability to apply a highly flexible segmentation and extraction of quantitative features that is easily adapted to the varying appearance of the histopathological images (cell nuclei, cell membranes, cytoplasm and cell clusters) (Kårsnäs *et al.,* 2011; Swamidoss *et al.,* 2013). Second advantage is the comparative analysis between several digital slides from different samples or several techniques from the same sample (i.e., HE, IHC and FISH), which can be opened side-by-side on one monitor. A third important advantage is the transmission of digital imaging. Digital images can be transferred over a computer network, which allows independent viewing by many pathologists at diverse locations, the so called "telepathology". This application has transformed the traditional medical teaching, seminar and exam methods as the reliance on physical space, as well as equipment, is solely dependent upon computers, tablets and internet access (Cucoranu *et al.,* 2014).

Importantly, digital imaging and telepathology have made diagnostic consultation for expert second opinions easier as it is not dependent on local pathologist only (Drak Alsibai *et al.,* 2006). Since many pathology consultation networks have been developed (Cucoranu et al., 2014; Horn *et al.,* 2014; Tabata *et al.,* 2017). Although the acquisition of digital images and the creation of digital files requires a trained pathologist, it has been demonstrated that telepathology using digital slides was sufficient for detection of histopathologic features in dermatitis cases, and for routine diagnosis in cytoplathology (Vyas *et al.,* 2016; Hanna *et al.,* 2015). Finally, the digital files are resistant to being damaged over time and the cost of their creation, replication and storing is minimal (Farahani *et al.,* 2015).

Although digital image analysis involves many applications, the main goal of most applications is to extract quantitative information from these images. Breast cancer biomarkers hormone receptors (ER and PR), and HER2 are the perfect examples of quantitative information relevant to diagnosis of breast cancer. Moreover, the proliferation marker (Ki67) evaluation is considered as a strong surrogate marker for classifying tumours, and is also included in the approved molecular chips dedicated to breast cancer. Although manual evaluation of breast cancer biomarkers using IHC remains the gold standard as it can be used by all pathologists, digital image analysis is currently available in many laboratories using strong electronic algorithm. It is a cost-effective method, as well as time saving. Moreover, digital imaging may help in training pathologists, or when applied on equivoque cases (HER2 score 2) and on low Ki67 proliferative tumours (Figure 3A, 3B and 3C). However, cancers are complex heterogeneous tissues that consists of tumour cells surrounding by a tumour microenvironment, which is composed of extracellular matrix, stromal cells and inflammatory cells. Therefore, the loss of integrity of the interior of nuclear material, the stromal cells, the inflammatory cells, may make the selection of positive nuclei more difficult for image analysis systems (Drak Alsibai *et al.*, 2013a, 2013b).

Figure 3. Whole slide imaging technology using Ventana iScan Coreo and mean of Virtuoso (Ventana Medical Systems, Inc., Roche): (A) digital slides stained by H&E, ER, PR, HER2, and Ki67. (B) Digital image analysis of Ki67 whole slide method, with selection of interesting zones (hot spots). (C) High magnification of the hot spot selected-zone, with quantification of stained nuclei by Ki67
Images from Institut de Pathologie de Paris, Drak Alsibai et al., 2013a and 2013b.

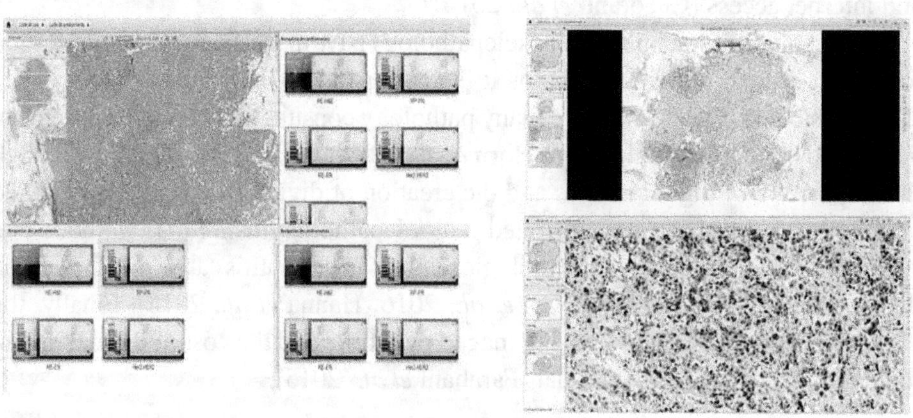

MOLECULAR PATHOLOGY

Human diseases and cancer diagnoses are often performed by using conventional histopathological techniques associated with immunohistochemical staining. However, personalized medicine and patient stratification require the assessment of molecular characterization of cancer (molecular subtypes). Moreover, biomarkers such as DNA, RNA, and proteins are powerful tools in clinical diagnostics and therapeutic development of cancer. Cancer tissue usually contains all genetic and proteomic information and represents the best material sample for molecular technologies, including gene expression analysis by PCR, sequencing, gene mutation and polymorphism detection by NGS, FISH, and fluorescence-activated cell sorting (FACS).

Vectorial Technologies

RNA-FISH and RNAscope® Assay

RNAs have emerged as crucial biomarkers of dynamic genetic expression in cells. Classic techniques that analyze RNA, such as RT-PCR, eliminate cell-to-cell variations in gene expression and single-cell sequencing and transcriptomic analysis require isolation of cells with loss of their spatial relationship. RNA in situ hybridization (RNA ISH) and RNA fluorescent ISH (RNA FISH) allow detection of individual RNA molecules in single cells through a microscope, gaining accurate, absolute single-cell expression data together with information on RNA location down to the subcellular level (Figure 4). A new protocol has been developed for high-content screening microscopy (Querido *et al.*, 2017).

Thus, spatially mapped expression data at the cellular level are pivotal to explore cellular interactions. Although mapping RNA expression to single cells is possible with RNA in situ hybridization (RNA ISH), these techniques present in fact limited performance and technical complexity. The RNAscope® technology (ACB™) provides single-cell expression resolution with spatial and morphological context. It employs a unique signal amplification strategy that allows for the visualization of target RNAs as punctate dots, where each dot represents an individual RNA molecule. The RNAscope® method presents high sensitivity due to its signal amplification strategy, high specificity as a result of the RNAscope® probe design minimizing nonspecific off-target signals, and detection and quantification of RNA with spatial and morphological context. The automated RNAscope® ISH assay can be performed with fresh frozen and FFPE tissues with slide staining systems from BOND RX (Leica Biosystems) and VENTANA DISCOVERY ULTRA and XT (Ventana Medical Systems, Inc., Roche).

Figure 4. RNA florescent in situ hybridization technology. The figure shows an overexpression of the long non-coding RNA MALAT1 (red spots) in breast cancer cells (nuclei in dark blue, DAPI stain).

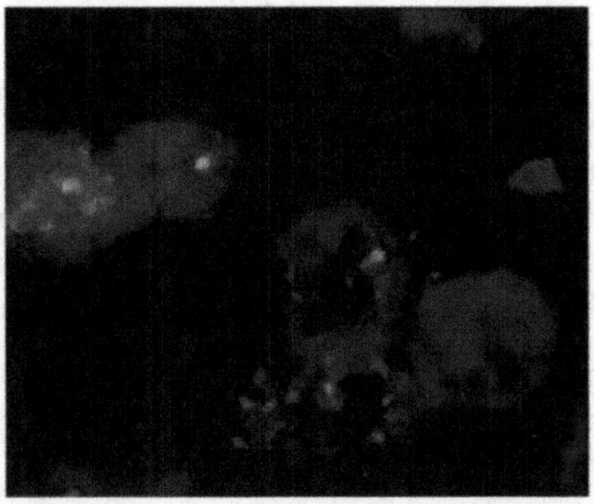

The workflow of the RNAscope® assay includes five main steps (flow diagram 1). The automated RNAscope® ISH assay reveals highly sensitive and specific expression of multiple targets in tissues with a high signal-to-noise ratio, reduces inter-user variability, generates reproducible results, allows simultaneous detection of various target genes to identify co-localization (Anderson *et al.,* 2016). This technology is a new tool for in situ gene expression analysis of cells and tissues with strong potential for utilization in the clinical diagnosis of diseases (Lee JH *et al.,* 2014), thus, it is adaptable to clinical and molecular pathology platforms (Figure 5) (Meseure *et al.,* 2016).

RNA Sequencing

A complete accounting of gene expression in an organism would provide the exact sequence and location of every transcript in every cell. Multiplex sequencing technologies have revolutionized our understanding of biological systems by revealing the complexity of fundamental biological processes such as transcription and translation. RNA sequencing (RNA-seq) has made it possible to measure in cell populations, the gene expression on a genome wide scale (GWS). However, the spatial information associated with gene expression is important for elucidating the context-dependent transcriptional regulation and NGS methods lose all spatial information of detected molecules. Moreover, classic in situ methods, although preserving spatial information, are typically low-throughput and cannot detect numerous genes in a same tissue sample. Recent high-resolution sampling technologies, such as RNA

Figure 5. RNAscope® in situ hybridization technology. The figure shows an overexpression of the long non-coding RNA HOTAIR (brown spots) in breast cancer cells (nuclei in bleu).

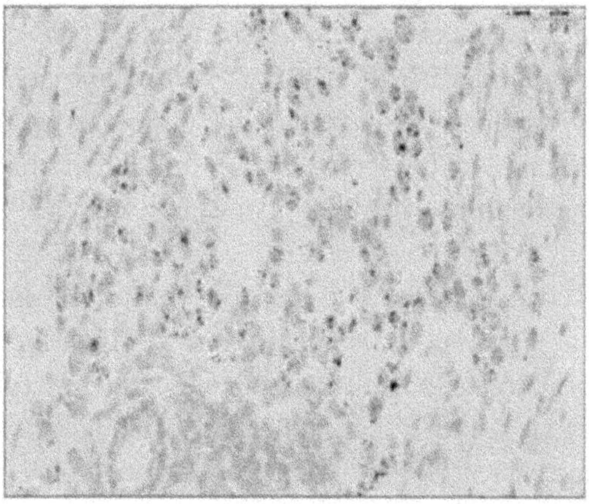

Figure 6. A diagram shows the five main steps of RNAscope® assay

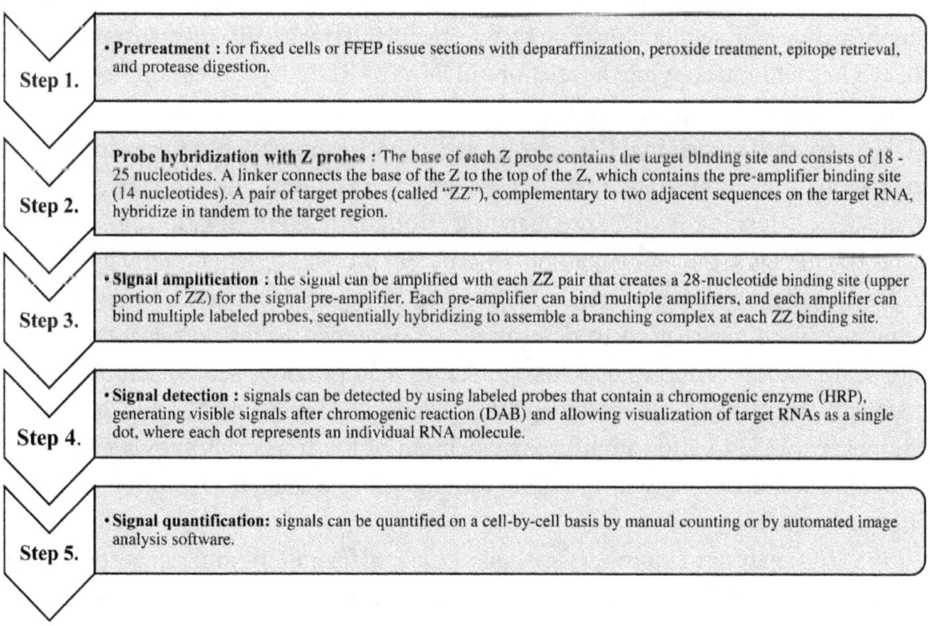

tomography or single-cell RNA-seq combined with FISH, have provided indirect ways to view global gene expression patterns in three dimensions.

The introduction of in situ sequencing methods, such as fluorescent in situ sequencing, allows visualization of the genetic signature directly in microscope images. Firstly, Larsson and colleagues (Larsson *et al.,* 2004) constructed a padlock probe and rolling circle amplification (RCA)-based approach to capture, amplify, and image the DNA with single nucleotide resolution in fixed tissues. Then, they incorporated padlock probes for targeted NGS and targeted RNA detection using in situ sequencing to identify a small number of transcripts and mutations in tissue sections.

Later, Lee and colleagues have combined both NGS and FISH methods to sequence RNA in single cells in situ. Their approach, called fluorescence in situ RNA sequencing (FISSEQ), treats the cell as a sequencing chip while preserving spatial information about RNA location (Lee *et al.,* 2014). Thus, FISSEQ is considered as a next-generation in situ technology that can sequence DNA or RNA within fixed cells without destroying their spatial context, and can be used to directly correlate spatial patterns to genetic and molecular events in fresh frozen and FFPE tissue sections (Mignardi *et al.,* 2015).

FISSEQ comprises 3 principal steps, including in situ RNA library edification, amplification, and sequencing. The authors begin by fixing cells, reverse transcribing the RNA in situ and copying the resulting cDNAs by RCA to generate single-stranded DNA ‘nanoballs’. Each nanoball, about 200–400 nm in diameter, consists of many cDNA copies of an original RNA sequence. The large number of repeats means that the nanoballs can withstand repeated sequencing reactions, allowing the authors to analyze them inside cells using sequencing by oligonucleotide ligation and detection (SOLiD). In this sequencing method, fluorescent probes are sequentially hybridized to the nanoballs, with a color corresponding to a pair of adjacent bases, and the sequence of colors is used to determine the sequence of the transcript. FISSEQ allows for digital counting of RNA molecules, and provides sequence information necessary to identify alleles or splice variants via image processing platforms. Moreover, FISSEQ allows multiplex detection of the transcriptome, genome, and proteome simultaneously in the same sample with molecular resolution of 10 nm (Lee *et al.,* 2015).

FISSEQ analysis of a tumuor tissue may be useful for guiding anti-cancer treatment, in which multiple drugs might be chosen for different components of the tumour. However, FISSEQ in its current form does not provide a complete accounting of the RNA within single cells and may miss lower-abundance transcripts because it produces a spatially localized subsampling of the transcriptome. Nevertheless, FISSEQ represents an enormous step forward in the ability to measure gene expression in its spatial context, single nucleotide polymorphism (SNP), structural variation discovery, mRNA and ncRNA profiling, and protein-nucleic acid interaction assays, which may potentially transform several areas of cancer and biomedical research, and drug discovery (Yadav *et al.,* 2014).

Multiplexed Immunochemistry

Although immunoblotting technique is considered as the gold standard for investigating protein expression, IHC is still widely used for detection of protein expression and localization in both research and routine clinical pathology. However, compartment-specific expression is difficult without other complementary techniques such as laser capture microdissection. Furthermore, evaluation of IHC staining is often semi-quantitative and subjectivity in analysis still remains, although immunohistochemical scores incorporating staining intensity and frequency, and subcellular location, are currently performed. Using fluorescent antibodies on glass slides offers a reasonable compromise, but background autofluorescence due to NADPH, lipofuscins, collagen, and elastin can create interpretation errors. Automated computational pathology platforms are a promising direction for more objective quantitation of pathology staining.

Multiplexed immunohistochemistry (multiplexed-IHC) facilitates high-throughput study of protein expression in large tissue samples, protein co-localization, heterogeneity, and subcellular localization. Multiplexed workflow enables imaging and analysis of up to six immunofluorescence markers within the same tissue section. Quantitative assessment of cellular phenotype is performed in a way that is similar to flow cytometry, while simultaneously providing information on tissue and cell-to-cell interactions. When combined with TMAs, multiplexed-IHC allow for faster and more objective quantitation of protein expression than allowed by manual analysis by a pathologist. A significant advantage of measuring protein expression via automated platforms using multispectral imaging for is reproducibility of results with data from computerized pathology platforms correlating highly with manual analysis. Furthermore, studies have shown high overall concordance in results between different multispectral platforms and staining results are highly reproducible. Multiplexed-IHC is of pivotal importance, particularly in limited samples, in phenotyping cells while retaining tissue context, evaluating single cell coexpression, monitoring cell signaling pathways and analyzing the tumour microenvironment (Stack *et al.,* 2014).

The Phenoptics™ workflow allows simultaneous detection of multiple biomarkers in tissue by incorporating three essential steps:

- Multiplex fluorescent immunohistochemistry (multiplex-fIHC) (Opal™ method) is performed for 4 or 7-color IHC on FFPE tissue. Opal method uses unlabeled primary antibodies, followed by addition of anti-species-HRP conjugate and detection substrate. Opal fluorescent detection substrates bind covalently near the epitope. After labeling is complete, antibodies are removed, allowing the next target to be detected without fear of antibody cross reactivity. The approach involves detection with Opal reactive fluorophores that covalently label the epitope, followed by heat-induced stripping for removal of primary and secondary antibodies. The Opal signal is largely unaffected by stripping and antibody removal. After stripping step, another round of staining can be performed for additional target detection without risk of antibody cross reactivity (Zheng *et al.,* 2017).
- Multispectral imaging (Vectra® and Mantra™ multiplexed biomarker imaging systems, PerkinElmer) allows edification of a spectral library from control slides stained with only one chromogen, measurement of each fluorescence signal and separates all the signals for quantitative analysis. These imaging systems eliminate spectrally overlapping fluorophores and tissue autofluorescence (Esbona *et al.,* 2016).
- Image analysis software (InForm™ Tissue Finder™) determines per-cell and per-subcellular compartment intensity values. This information is used in combination with user-trainable machine learning algorithms to tissue and cell segmentation, cellular immunophenotyping and cell counting. Data may be exported from inForm™ for additional analysis such as distance mapping between selected cellular phenotypes. In addition to fluorescent composite images, inForm™ provides simulated brightfield monoplex IHC from the same data for visual interpretation and data validation. This method can be useful in analyzing, quantification and phenotypig of immune and other cells *in situ* in tumour microenvironment (Mlecnik *et al.,* 2016).

The ability to interrogate multiple immunohistochemical markers within a single tissue section is often a complicated assay, which can be performed using either chromogenic or fluorescent detection methods (Figure 7A, 7B and 7C). The Opal multiplex-IHC method also offers a significant improvement in pathology workflow, in part by reducing the need for multiple tissue sections to support several individual stains. With multiplex-IHC and multispectral analysis integrated into the pathologist workflow, this methodology can offer unparalleled pathology support, enabling deeper insight into tissue and cellular processes (Remark *et al.,* 2016).

Figure 7. Fluorescent multiplex immunohistochemistry. Section from invasion margin of breast cancer tissue shows tertiary lymphoid structure stained with standard HE staining (Figure A), and with fluorescent IHC panel (Figure B); CD20 (B cells, in green), CD3 ($CD3^+$ T lymphocytes, in purple), DC-Lamp (dendritic cells 'DCs', in bleu), CD21 (follicular DCs) and PNAd (High endothelial venules, in yellow). The images are interpreted using digital microscope and can be opened side-by-side on one monitor (Figure C).

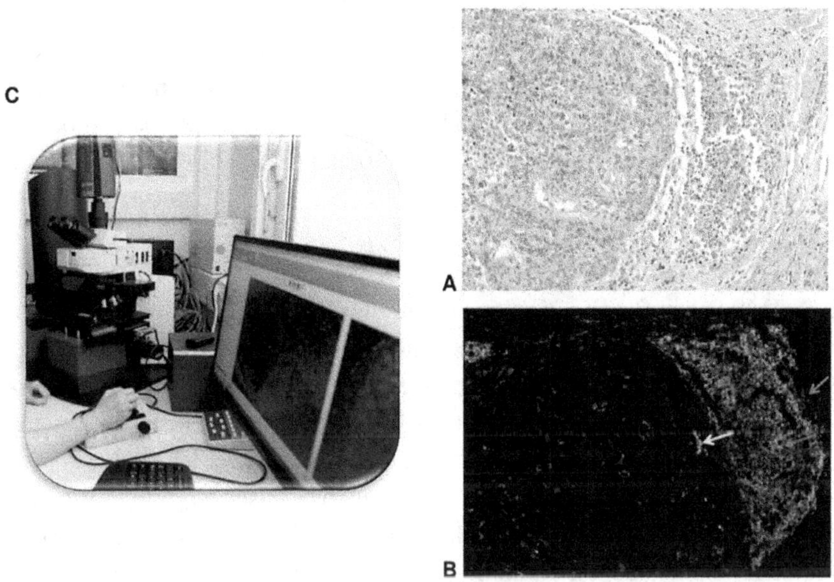

Non-Vectorial Technology

Matrix-Assisted Laser Desorption/Ionization-Imaging Mass Spectrometry

Cancer tissues represent the best material for morphological and molecular technologies. In the setting of personalized medicine and patient stratification, cancer characterization requires molecular techniques, including gene expression analysis by PCR, gene mutation or polymorphism detection by NGS, FACS and DNA/RNA-FISH. These major technological improvements have essentially concerned genes expression, although proteins are known to be the executing molecules. Therefore, characterization of cancer proteome is warranted to improve tumour typing and classification, prognosis and prediction to therapy. Mass spectrometry (MS)-based proteomic technologies identify and quantify proteins, peptides, lipids or phospholipids, carbohydrates or glycoconjugates and exogenous or endogenous small molecules involved in drug metabolism in tissue compartments (Reyzer *et al.*, 2003; Chaurand *et al.*, 2003; Schwartz *et al.*, 2003). However, conventional proteomic approaches do not provide topological information. Imaging mass spectrometry (IMS) combined with conventional proteomic techniques has overcome this problem and represents an ideal method correlating biochemical data with morphological histopathology. Matrix-assisted laser desorption/ionization-IMS (MALDI IMS) is a high-throughput analytical tool that does not require homogenization prior to sample preparation and links biochemical identification, quantitative evaluation and spatial distribution of numerous molecules in tissues. When compared to other in situ molecular techniques, MALDI-IMS does not require target-specific reagents such as antibodies or DNA/RNA probes and allows evaluation of hundreds of molecules on the same slide (Kriegsmann *et al.*, 2015; McDonnell *et al.*, 2014; Maier *et al.*, 2013).

Methodology of MALDI IMS

MALDI-IMS is a soft ionization technique that identifies and localizes molecules of interest from the surfaces of tissue samples by measuring the mass to charge ratios (m/z) of their ionized forms, through conversion of molecules into ions by the ionizing laser, separation of ions according to their m/z ratios in a mass analyzer and detection of separated ions via an ion detector. Molecules are co-crystallized with the matrix to form sample–matrix crystals. UV laser targeting of the crystals results in vaporization of the matrix that carries molecules with it. The matrix acts as a proton donor or acceptor, ionizing molecules. Proton transfer between the matrix and the molecules renders neutral molecules protonated or deprotonated that are thus detectable as positive or negative ions, respectively. MALDI IMS, is coupled with time-of-flight (TOF) mass analysis and detection by ion-to electron conversion. In TOF, ions accelerated by an electrostatic field are allowed to drift in a neutral field. Smaller particles move faster through the flight tube and reach the detector in shorter periods of time than heavy particles. The time required to reach the detector determines the ion's m/z ratio. A mass spectrum is generated at each position irradiated the laser. The tissue distribution and relative intensity of individual ions can be visualized using a color scale corresponding to the relative intensity of each ion at every pixel. Positions of individual or clusters of molecules visualized on the image can be co-localized with histolopathology. Since its introduction in the 90´s, MSI technique has greatly evolved in terms of sample preparation, instrumentation, and data processing (Eriksson *et al.*, 2013). MSI can be performed on fresh/frozen (fr/fr), as well as on FFPE tissue, TMA (Casadonte, 2017), and combined with laser microdissection-based microproteomics. An improvement of the method has consisted of automation for the acquisition of spectra through areas of interest and combination with mathematical calculations that give semi quantitative information on tissue sections. Direct identification of proteins in situ via MALDI MS/MS is possible but difficult, thus liquid chromatography Tandem mass spectrometry (LC-MS/MS) can be required to complement MSI in identification analysis. Typical workflow for MALDI IMS experiments comprises (i) cutting, mounting on a target and matrix application for fresh frozen samples and paraffin removal, antigen retrieval and enzymatic digestion for FFPE samples, (ii) generation of mass spectra in an ordered array at each x, y coordinate, (iii) visualization of individual spectral pattern within the tissue to generate protein images and correlation with stained sections, (iv) protein/peptide identification through MS/MS analysis, (v) statistical analysis to visualize classification results on tissue sections and validation by IHC, multiplex-fIHC or western blot (Lai YH *et al.,* 2017; Casadonte *et al.,* 2017; Longuespée *et al.,* 2016; Nirmalan *et al.,* 2009).

Applications of MALDI IMS in Oncology

MALDI IMS is considered as a powerful technique that has the potential to influence decision processes in pathology's practice by evaluating tumour margins and heterogeneity, and by providing morphomolecular information on tumour typing, grading, prognosis and prediction of treatment response (Table 2). Therefore, mass spectrometry based proteomic technologies are highly warranted to improve tumour classification, and help assessment of prognosis and prediction to therapy, as they can be used to identify and quantify proteins in body fluids and tissue samples Therefore, IMS techniques have been applied to a variety of tumours (Longuespée, 2018).

MALDI IMS is a powerful technology that fills the gap between high-throughput technologies and classical histopathology and integrates biochemical approach with the already established molecular and morphologic features and allows pathologists and researchers to visualize, localize and quantify molecules in situ in tissue sections. The possibility to measure hundreds of molecules at the cellular level with direct correlation to histological features could overcome a multitude of the limitations of other approaches in identification and evaluation of new biomarkers and molecular profiles. Although Introduction of MALDI IMS to clinical practice for diagnostic and prognostic purposes is inevitable in the field of cancer and great progress concerning sample preparation and instrumentation has been made within the last decade, large scale studies proving the technology to be reliable in a clinical setting and establishing robust sample preparation and measurement strategies that show high agreement between different laboratories are still lacking. Moreover, identification and absolute quantification directly from tissue sections is required and MALDI-IMS data must be validated for biomarker discovery and clinical use by using multiplex-f or chromatography-based MS. Recently, a rapid evaporative ionization mass spectrometry (REIMS) was developed by the direct combination of

Table 2. Applications of vectorial and non-vectorial technologies in oncology and cancer research.

Tumour Type	Clinical and Vectorial Technologies (IHC, WSI, Multiplexed-IHC, RNAscope® ISH, and RNA-seq)	References	Non-Vectorial Technologies (MALDI IMS)	References
Brain	Multiplexed exome sequencing supports evaluation and classification of adult low-grade gliomas with a single clinical test	Cryan *et al.*, 2014	• Visualization of brain and tumour distribution of PI3K-inhibitors in glioblastoma • Monitoring therapeutic monoclonal antibodies (bevacizumab) in brain tumor. • Grading of meningioma • Classification of brain tumours based on lipid signatures • Demonstration of drug transit of small molecules through the blood-brain barrier	Salphati *et al.*, 2014 Ait-Belkacem *et al.*, 2014 Agar *et al.*, 2010 Eberlin *et al.*, 2013 Liu X *et al.*, 2013
Thyroid	RNAscope® ISH: monoclonal PAX8 antibody showed high specificity to thyroid tumours and is superior to the polyclonal antibody).	Toriyama *et al.*, 2014	• S100A10, thioredoxin, and S100-A6 as biomarkers in metastatic papillary carcinomas • Distinction between different thyroid lesions; follicular lesions and papillary carcinoma, and characterization of proteomic profile of medullary carcinoma	Nipp *et al.*, 2012 Pagni *et al.*, 2015
Head and neck	• Multiplexed-IHC and computational image processing workflows: identify differential immune profiles based on lymphoid and myeloid cell densities, correlating with human papilloma virus status and prognosis in head and neck squamous cell carcinomas (SCC) • RNAscope®: presence of transcriptionally active HPV rarely occurs in oral SCC suggesting that p16 is not an appropriate surrogate marker for HPV in this case	Tsujikaxa *et al.*, 2017 Gafeer *et al.*,	Identification of SCARA5 as a potential biomarker for oral SCC	Liu Y et al., 2018
Lung	• IHC and RNAscope®: Determinants of variability of five PDL-1 immunohistochemistry assays in non-small cell lung cancer samples • RNAscope: provides sensitive and specific detection of PD-L1 in lung adenocarcinoma (ADC)	Soo *et al.*, 2018	• Classification of protein peaks in non-small cell lung cancer (NSCLC) according to histological type, and discrimination of primary cancer from metastases and patients with good and poor prognosis • Distinction of NSCLC subtypes; adenocarcinoma from SCC • Classification of NSCLC according to lipid profile • Imaging pharmacokinetic studies in drug development: o I - Study of heterogeneous distribution of erlotinib in xenograft and patients with NSCLC o II - Study of erlotinib in combination with bevacizumab in xenograft mice bearing B901L, EGFR-mutated NSCLC cells	Yanagisawa, 2003 Groseclose et al., 2008 Lee GK *et al.*, 2012 Tsubata *et al.*, 2017 Nishidate *et al.*, 2017
Oesophagus	RNAscope®: High protein and mRNA expression levels of TUBB3 (class III ß-tubulin) are associated with aggressive tumor features in esophageal ADC	Loeser *et al.*, 2017	Identification of COX7A2, TAGLN2 and S100-A10 as prognostic markers in Barrett's adenocarcinoma	Elsner *et al.*, 2012

continued on following page

Table 2. Continued

Tumour Type	Clinical and Vectorial Technologies (IHC, WSI, Multiplexed-IHC, RNAscope® ISH, and RNA-seq)	References	Non-Vectorial Technologies (MALDI IMS)	References
Stomach	IHC and RNAscope®: PD-L1 expression is higher in intestinal type than in diffuse type of gastric ADC (by RNAdcope) RNAscope and DISH are suitable methods to evaluate FGFR2 status in gastric cancer.	Yuan J *et al.*, 2016 Kuboki *et al.*, 2017	• Distinguished gastric cancer from normal mucosa with overexpression of defensins and calgranulins in tumours • Classification of signals which could discern between normal gastric tissue and adenocarcinoma; signal specific to poor differentiation corresponds to histone H4 (by IMS on TMA) • Identification of prognostic seven protein signatures in intestinal-type gastric adenocarcinoma • Identification of S100A8 and S100A9 as negative regulators for lymph node metastasis of adenocarcinoma	Kim *et al.*, 2010 Morita *et al.*, 2010 Balluff *et al.*, 2011 Choi *et al.*, 2012
Colon/rectum	Multiplexed fluorescence microscopy method enables multiplexed, in situ microscopic analysis of biological molecules in individual cells (study performed in 747 colorectal cancer FFPE tissues)	Gerdes *et al.*, 2013	Mutational analysis for KRAS and NRAS in colorectal carcinoma	Kriegsmann *et al.*, 2015
Pancreas	IHC and WSI: Quantitative assessment of pancreatic cancer precursor lesions	Aeffner F, 2016	• Imaging of glucose-regulated protein in pancreatic adenocarcinoma • Modeling therapy response and spatial tissue distribution of erlotinib in pancreatic cancer	Djidja *et al.*, 2009 Grüner *et al.*, 2016
Liver	IHC and RNAscope®: preliminary study suggests that Podoplanin contributes to the malignant potential of hepatocellular carcinoma (HCC)	Cioca *et al.*, 2017	• Protein profiles of HCC and liver cirrhosis • Ubi (1-74) and kallikrein 6 as biomarkers of cancer risk	Le Faouder *et al.*, 2011 Laouirem *et al.*, 2014
Kidney	RNA-seq enables utilization of FFPE biopsies with clear cell renal cell carcinoma (RCC) for exploration of disease biology and biomarker development	Eikrem *et al.*, 2016	• Molecular analysis of tumour margins in RCC • Detection of race disparities in Wilms' tumours • Discrimination of papillary and clear cell RCC using MALDI on TMA samples. • Study of dysregulated Sulfoglycosphingolipids in RCC tissues.	Oppenheimer *et al.*, 2010 Axt *et al.*, 2011 Steurer *et al.*, 2014 Jirasko 2017
Bladder	• IHC and RNAscope®: concordance of PD-L1 expression in primary and metastatic bladder carcinomas between commonly used antibodies and RNA expression. • RNAscope® assay: Comparison of fibroblast growth-factor receptor gene alterations at the DNA versus messenger RNA level in advanced urothelial cancer.	Tretiakova *et al.*, 2017 Necchi *et al.*, 2017	Signals associated with tumour aggressiveness, histological phenotype and proliferation of bladder carcinoma	Steurer *et al.*, 2014

continued on following page

Table 2. Continued

Tumour Type	Clinical and Vectorial Technologies (IHC, WSI, Multiplexed-IHC, RNAscope® ISH, and RNA-seq)	References	Non-Vectorial Technologies (MALDI IMS)	References
Breast	• Using microfluidic multiplexed immunohistochemistry in breast cancer diagnostics. • Using multiplexed ion beam imaging (MIBI) to analyse FFPE tissue of human breast tumour stained with ten labels simultaneously. • A multiplex IHCμA with 180 spots targeting 8 cancer proteins was performed on a breast cancer FFPE tissue section. • Multiplexed fluorescent immunohistochemistry: perform quantitative and simultaneous analyses of tumor-infiltrating lymphocytes (TILs) and their spatial distribution in medullary carcinoma of breast (Igari F 2017). • IHC and RNAscope® ISH: PD1 protein expression in tumor infiltrated lymphocytes rather than PDL1 in tumor cells predicts survival in triple-negative breast cancer. • RNA ISH: detection of specific the LncRNA *MALAT1* in breast carcinoma cells.	Kim *et al.*, 2013 Angelo et al., 2014 Li H *et al.*, 2017 Igari *et al.*, 2017 Ren *et al.*, 2018 Meseure *et al.*, 2016	• Proteomic differences between normal tissue, ductal carcinoma in situ, invasive cancer and tumour microenvironment • Lymph node status of breast carcinoma and prediction of response to chemotherapy • Localization of choline metabolites in viable and necrotic tumour compartments in metastatic breast tumor xenograft models • Classification of Her2 status of breast carcinomas by protein identification using MALDI IMS • Acylcarnitines and sphingomyelin differentially expressed in tumour and necrotic compartments in breast tumour models) • Identification of protein signals in intratumoral and extratumoral microenvironment stroma • Study of Poly(ADP-ribose) polymerase inhibitors (PARPi) tumour penetration in triple negative breast cancer	Cornett *et al.*, 2006 Seeley and Caprioli 2011 Amstalden van Hove et al., 2010 Rauser et al., 2010 Chughtai *et al.*, 2013 Dekker *et al.*, 2014 Bartelink *et al.*, 2017
Ovary	RNAscope®: decreased gene and protein expression levels of ARID1A are related to the occurrence and development of endometriosis-associated ovarian cancer, especially clear cell carcinoma.	Wang Q *et al.*, 2017	• MALDI: Reg alpha fragment of 11S proteasome activator complex as a biomarker for ovarian carcinoma • Discrimination of interface between serous carcinoma and normal tissue • Integrated transcriptomic and lipidomic analysis of sulfatides • Platinum anticancer imaging in ovarian carcinomas	Lemaire *et al.*, 2007 Kang *et al.*, 2010 Liu Y *et al.*, 2010 Bianga *et al.*, 2014
Cervix	RNAscope®: detection of E6/E7 mRNA of seven high risk HPV subtypes (HPV 16, 18, 31, 33, 35, 52, and 58) in FFPE tissue samples.	Pandey *et al.*, 2018	Automated classification of intraepithelial neoplasia lesions on cervical Pap smears cytology.	Schwamborn *et al.*, 2011
Prostate	IHC and WSI: simultaneous analysis of androgen receptor (AR) and alpha-methylacyl-CoA (AMACR) expression at cell-level resolution in prostate cancer with analysis of T cell subpopulations in tumour microenvironment.	Blom et al., 2017	• Discrimination of cancer from normal tissue based on protein profile • Distinction between cancer and uninvolved prostate tissue on the basis of specific fragment of mitogen-activated protein kinase/extracellular signal regulated kinase • Detection of signals associated with favourable tumour phenotype	Schwamborn *et al.*, 2007 Cazares *et al.*, 2009 Steurer *et al.*, 2013
Testis	Quantitative multiplexed-IHC: exploration of the immune infiltrate and outcome prediction in testicular cancer (myeloid-inflamed tumour-immune complexity associated with poor prognosis.	Siska *et al.*, 2017	Identification of human testicular embryonal carcinoma proteins	Li F *et al.*, 2009
Skin	RNA-seq: EZH2 is a promising therapeutic avenue for a substantial fraction of melanoma patients.	Tiffen *et al.*, 2016	• Detection of protein signatures for survival and recurrence in malignant melanoma • Differential diagnosis of Spitz nevi from Spitzoid malignant melanoma • Identification of vemurafenib in malignant melanoma • Visualize the spatial distribution of various proteins in melanoma and healthy skin tissue.	Hardesty *et al.*, 2011 Lazova *et al.*, 2012 Sugihara *et al.*, 2014 Guran *et al.*, 2017

continued on following page

Table 2. Continued

Tumour Type	Clinical and Vectorial Technologies (IHC, WSI, Multiplexed-IHC, RNAscope® ISH, and RNA-seq)	References	Non-Vectorial Technologies (MALDI IMS)	References
Soft tissue	RNAscope®: preserves tissue morphology and reduces "false positives" related to detection of endogenous FGF23 mRNA expression by osteocytes, in phosphaturic mesenchymal tumors of the mixed connective tissue type.	Carter *et al.*, 2015	• Proteins and lipids signatures in myxoid sarcomas specific to tumour type and grade • Subtyping 4 different high-grade sarcomas	Willems *et al.*, 2010 Lou S *et al.*, 2017
Neuroblastoma	IHC with WSI using a grid quantification for detection of phenotypic alterations.	Shirinifard *et al.*, 2016	Pharmacokinetic studies in drug development and the mechanism of action of drugs by clarifying their distribution: Heterogeneous distribution of alectinib in neuroblastoma xenografts.	Shoraku Ryu *et al.*, 2018
Lymphoma	A multiplexed immunofluorescence: simultaneous scoring of markers and quantitative imaging of a multiplexed panel of cellular markers in FFPE sections of a cellularly heterogenous lymphoma.	Ng SB *et al.*, 2017	Discrimination of Hodgkin's lymphoma and lymphadenitis	Schwamborn *et al.*, 2010

electrosurgical devices and MS to enable the spatial mapping of tumour metabolism. REIMS can also offer an alternative to frozen section for intraoperative tissue identification and surgical margin assessment (Takats *et al.,* 2017).

CONCLUSION

For over 150 years, pathology has relied upon a description of cellular and tissue morphology for tumour classification and grading. The rapid introduction of digital imaging, next-generation sequencing and other high-complexity molecular technologies has modified our understanding of cancer biology and our capability for detecting, stratifying and selecting treatment in the setting of personalized medicine. We are over the digital revolution in the field of experimental and diagnostic pathology. During the last decade, new in situ technologies, including digital pathology, vectorial (multiplexed-IHC, RNAscope®, RNA-seq in situ) and non-vectorial ionizing techniques (MALDI IMS) have found their way from research laboratories into clinical pathology laboratories, bringing together researchers from a wide spectrum of disciplines, such as physics, biochemistry, medicine, and mathematics. A key feature of these new technologies is the ability to combine molecular signatures with tissue morphology. However, combining these new technologies with state of the art tissue morphology evaluation and maintaining close collaboration between pathologists, molecular biologists, and technology developers is mandatory. As such, introduction of these technologies into pathology laboratories will extend their capabilities and revolutionize management and treatment of cancer.

DISCLOSURE: CONFLICT OF INTEREST

The authors declare that they have no competing interests.

ACKNOWLEDGMENT

André Nicolas, Laëtitia Lesage, Renaud Leclère, and Gabriel Champenois from the platform of experimental pathology, of Curie institute contributed to this work, concerning the development of methodology, technical approach, and material support.

REFERENCES

Aeffner, F., Martin, N. T., Peljto, M., Black, J. C., Major, J. K., Jangani, M., ... Young, G. D. (2016). Quantitative assessment of pancreatic cancer precursor lesions in IHC-stained tissue with a tissue image analysis platform. *Laboratory Investigation*, *96*(12), 1327–1336. doi:10.1038/labinvest.2016.111 PMID:27775692

Agar, N., Malcolm, J. G., Mohan, V., Yang, H. W., Johnson, M., Tannenbaum, A., ... Black, P. M. (2010). Imaging of meningioma progression by matrix-assisted laser desorption ionization time-of-flight mass spectrometry. *Analytical Chemistry*, *82*(7), 2621–2625. doi:10.1021/ac100113w PMID:20196536

Ait-Belkacem, R., Berenguer, C., Villard, C., Ouafik, L., Figarella-Branger, D., Beck, A., ... Lafitte, D. (2014). Monitoring therapeutic monoclonal antibodies in brain tumor. *mAbs*, *6*(6), 1385–1393. doi:10.4161/mabs.34405 PMID:25484065

Amstalden van Hove, E. R., Blackwell, T. R., Klinkert, I., Eijkel, G. B., Heeren, R. M., & Glunde, K. (2010). Multimodal mass spectrometric imaging of small molecules reveals distinct spatio-molecular signatures in differentially metastatic breast tumor models. *Cancer Research*, *70*(22), 9012–9021. doi:10.1158/0008-5472.CAN-10-0360 PMID:21045154

Anderson, C. M., Zhang, B., Miller, M., Butko, E., Wu, X., Laver, T., ... Ma, X.-J. (2016). Fully Automated RNAscope In Situ Hybridization Assays for Formalin-Fixed Paraffin-Embedded Cells and Tissues. *Journal of Cellular Biochemistry*, *117*(10), 2201–2208. doi:10.1002/jcb.25606 PMID:27191821

Angelo, M., Bendall, S. C., Finck, R., Hale, M. B., Hitzman, C., Borowsky, A. D., ... Nolan, G. P. (2014). Multiplexed ion beam imaging (MIBI) of human breast tumors. *Nature Medicine*, *20*(4), 436–442. doi:10.1038/nm.3488 PMID:24584119

Axt, J., Murphy, A. J., Seeley, E. H., Martin, C. A., Taylor, C., & Lovvorn, H. N. III. (2011). Race disparities in Wilms tumor incidence and biology. *The Journal of Surgical Research*, *170*(1), 112–119. doi:10.1016/j.jss.2011.03.011 PMID:21529835

Balluff, B., Rauser, S., Meding, S., Elsner, M., Schone, C., Feuchtinger, A., ... Walch, A. (2011). MALDI imaging identifies prognostic seven-protein signature of novel tissue markers in intestinal-type gastric cancer. *American Journal of Pathology*, *179*(6), 2720–2729. doi:10.1016/j.ajpath.2011.08.032 PMID:22015459

Bianga, J., Bouslimani, A., Bec, N., Quenet, F., Mounicou, S., Szpunar, J., ... Larroque, C. (2014). Complementarity of MALDI and LA ICP mass spectrometry for platinum anticancer imaging in human tumor. *Metallomics*, *6*(8), 1382–1386. doi:10.1039/C4MT00131A PMID:24984817

Calligaris, D., Caragacianu, D., Liu, X., Norton, I., Thompson, C. J., Richardson, A. L., ... Agar, N. Y. R. (2014). Application of desorption electrospray ionization mass spectrometry imaging in breast cancer margin analysis. *Proceedings of the National Academy of Sciences of the United States of America*, *111*(42), 15184–15189. doi:10.1073/pnas.1408129111 PMID:25246570

Carter, J. M., Caron, B. L., Dogan, A., & Folpe, A. L. (2015). A novel chromogenic in situ hybridization assay for FGF23 mRNA in phosphaturic mesenchymal tumors. *The American Journal of Surgical Pathology*, *39*(1), 75–83. doi:10.1097/PAS.0000000000000290 PMID:25025444

Casadonte, R., & Caprioli, R. M. (2011). Proteomic analysis of formalin- fixed paraffin-embedded tissue by MALDI imaging mass spectrometry. *Nature Protocols*, *6*(11), 1695–1709. doi:10.1038/nprot.2011.388 PMID:22011652

Casadonte, R., Longuespée, R., Kriegsmann, J., & Kriegsmann, M. (2017). MALDI IMS and Cancer Tissue Microarrays. *Advances in Cancer Research*, *134*, 173–200. doi:10.1016/bs.acr.2016.11.007 PMID:28110650

Cazares, L. H., Troyer, D., Mendrinos, S., Lance, R. A., & Nyalwidhe, J. O. (2009). Imaging mass spectrometry of a specific fragment of mitogen-activated protein kinase/extracellular signal-regulated kinase 2 discriminates cancer from uninvolved prostate tissue. *Clinical Cancer Research*, *15*, 5541–5551. doi:10.1158/1078-0432.CCR-08-2892 PMID:19690195

Chaurand, P., Fouchécourt, S., DaGue, B. B., Xu, B. J., Reyzer, M. L., Orgebin-Crist, M. C., & Caprioli, R. M. (2003). Profiling and imaging proteins in the mouse epididymis by imaging mass spectrometry. *Proteomics*, *3*(11), 2221–2239. doi:10.1002/pmic.200300474 PMID:14595821

Choi, J. H., Shin, N. R., Moon, H. J., Kwon, C. H., & Kim, G. H. (2012). Identification of S100A8 and S100A9 as negative regulators for lymph node metastasis of gastric adenocarcinoma. *Histology and Histopathology*, *27*, 1439–1448. PMID:23018243

Chughtai, K., Jiang, L., Greenwood, T. R., Glunde, K., & Heeren, R. M. (2013). Mass spectrometry images acylcarnitines, phosphatidylcholines, and sphingomyelin in MDA-MB-231 breast tumor models. *Journal of Lipid Research*, *54*(2), 333–344. doi:10.1194/jlr.M027961 PMID:22930811

Cornett, D. S., Mobley, J. A., Dias, E. C., Andersson, M., Arteaga, C. L., Sanders, M. E., & Caprioli, R. M. (2006). A novel histology- directed strategy for MALDI-MS tissue profiling that improves throughput and cellular specificity in human breast cancer. *Molecular & Cellular Proteomics*, *5*(10), 1975–1983. doi:10.1074/mcp.M600119-MCP200 PMID:16849436

Cryan, J. B., Haidar, S., Ramkissoon, L. A., Bi, W. L., Knoff, D. S., Schultz, N., ... Ramkissoon, S. H. (2014). Clinical multiplexed exome sequencing distinguishes adult oligodendroglial neoplasms from astrocytic and mixed lineage gliomas. *Oncotarget*, *5*(18), 8083–8092. doi:10.18632/oncotarget.2342 PMID:25257301

Cucoranu, I. C., Parwani, A. V., Vepa, S., Weinstein, R. S., & Pantanowitz, L. (2014). Digital pathology: A systematic evaluation of the patent landscape. *Journal of Pathology Informatics*, *5*(1), 16. doi:10.4103/2153-3539.133112 PMID:25057430

Dekker, T. J., Balluff, B. D., Jones, E. A., Schöne, C. D., Schmitt, M., Aubele, M., ... McDonnell, L. A. (2014). Multicenter matrix-assisted laser desorption/ionization mass spectrometry imaging (MALDI MSI) identifies proteomic differences in breast-cancer-associated stroma. *Journal of Proteome Research*, *13*(11), 4730–4738. doi:10.1021/pr500253j PMID:24762205

Djidja, M. C., Claude, E., Snel, M. F., Francese, S., Scriven, P., Carolan, V., & Clench, M. R. (2010). Novel molecular tumour classification using MALDI-mass spectrometry imaging of tissue micro-array. *Analytical and Bioanalytical Chemistry*, *397*(2), 587–601. doi:10.100700216-010-3554-6 PMID:20204332

Djidja, M. C., Claude, E., Snel, M. F., Scriven, P., Francese, S., Carolan, V., & Clench, M. R. (2009). MALDI-ion mobility separation-mass spectrometry imaging of glucose-regulated protein 78 kDa (Grp78) in human formalin-fixed, paraffin-embedded pancreatic adenocarcinoma tissue sections. *Journal of Proteome Research*, *8*(10), 4876–4884. doi:10.1021/pr900522m PMID:19673544

Drak Alsibai, K., Azoulay, S., Languille-Mimoune, O., Poulet, B., Barres, A., & Adem, C. (2013a). Digital Imaging in Breast Cancer: An Ode to Microscopy. USCAP Poster Session V (Abstract 2048). *Modern Pathol*ogy, *26*(S2), 489-504. doi:10.1038/modpathol.2013.26

Drak Alsibai, K., Azoulay, S., Languille-Mimoune, O., Poulet, B., Barres, A., & Adem, C. (2013b). Ki67 Evaluation in Breast Cancer: Molecular Pathology Using Digital Imaging. USCAP, Poster Session V (Abstract 2047). *Modern Pathology*, *26*(S2), 489-504. doi:10.1038/modpathol.2013.26

Drak Alsibai, K., Denis, B., Bottlaender, J., Kleinclaus, I., Straub, P., & Fabre, M. (2006). Impact of cytopathologist expert on diagnosis and treatment of pancreatic lesions in current clinical practice. A series of 106 endoscopic ultrasound-guided fine needle aspirations. *Cytopathology*, *17*(1), 18–26. doi:10.1111/j.1365-2303.2006.00312.x PMID:16417561

Drak Alsibai, K., & Meseure, D. (2018). Tumor microenvironment and noncoding RNAs as co-drivers of epithelial-mesenchymal transition and cancer metastasis. *Developmental Dynamics*, *247*(3), 405–431. doi:10.1002/dvdy.24548 PMID:28691356

Duraiyan, J., Govindarajan, R., Kaliyappan, K., & Palanisamy, M. (2012). Applications of immunohistochemistry. *Journal of Pharmacy & Bioallied Sciences*, *4*(6Suppl 2), S307–S309. doi:10.4103/0975-7406.100281 PMID:23066277

Eberlin, L. S., Norton, I., Orringer, D., Dunn, I. F., Liu, X., Ide, J. L., ... Cooks, R. G. (2013). Ambient mass spectrometry for the intraoperative molecular diagnosis of human brain tumors. *Proceedings of the National Academy of Sciences of the United States of America*, *110*(5), 1611–1616. doi:10.1073/pnas.1215687110 PMID:23300285

Eikrem, O., Beisland, C., Hjelle, K., Flatberg, A., Scherer, A., Landolt, L., ... Marti, H.-P. (2016). Transcriptome Sequencing (RNAseq) Enables Utilization of Formalin-Fixed, Paraffin-Embedded Biopsies with Clear Cell Renal Cell Carcinoma for Exploration of Disease Biology and Biomarker Development. *PLoS One*, *11*(2), e0149743. doi:10.1371/journal.pone.0149743 PMID:26901863

Elsner, M., Rauser, S., Maier, S., Schone, C., Balluff, B., Meding, S., ... Walch, A. (2012). MALDI imaging mass spectrometry reveals COX7A2, TAGLN2 and S100-A10 as novel prognostic markers in Barrett's adenocarcinoma. *Journal of Proteomics*, *75*(15), 4693–4704. doi:10.1016/j.jprot.2012.02.012 PMID:22365974

Eriksson, C., Masaki, N., Yao, I., Hayasaka, T., & Setou, M. (2013). MALDI Imaging Mass Spectrometry—A Mini Review of Methods and Recent Developments. *Mass Spectrometry (Tokyo, Japan)*, *2*(Spec Iss), S0022. doi:10.5702/massspectrometry.S0022 PMID:24349941

Esbona, K., Inman, D., Saha, S., Jeffery, J., Schedin, P., Wilke, L., & Keely, P. (2016). COX-2 modulates mammary tumor progression in response to collagen density. *Breast Cancer Research : BCR*, *18*(1), 35. doi:10.118613058-016-0695-3 PMID:27000374

Farahani, N., Braun, A., Jutt, D., Huffman, T., Reder, N., Liu, Z., ... Pantanowitz, L. (2017). Three-dimensional Imaging and Scanning: Current and Future Applications for Pathology. *Journal of Pathology Informatics*, *8*(1), 36. doi:10.4103/jpi.jpi_32_17 PMID:28966836

Farahani, N., Parwani, A. V., & Pantanowitz, L. (2015). Whole slide imaging in pathology: Advantages, limitations, and emerging perspectives. *Pathology and Laboratory Medicine International: PLMI*, *7*, 23–33.

Gerdes, M. J., Sevinsky, C. J., Sood, A., Adak, S., Bello, M. O., Bordwell, A., ... Ginty, F. (2013). Highly multiplexed single-cell analysis of formalin-fixed, paraffin-embedded cancer tissue. *Proceedings of the National Academy of Sciences of the United States of America*, *110*(29), 11982–11987. doi:10.1073/pnas.1300136110 PMID:23818604

Gondhalekar, C., Rajwa, B., Patsekin, V., Ragheb, K., Sturgis, J., & Robinson, J.P. (2018). Alternatives to current flow cytometry data analysis for clinical and research studies. *Methods*, *1*(134-135), 113-129. doi: 10.1016/j.ymeth.2017.12.009

Groseclose, M. R., Massion, P. P., Chaurand, P., & Caprioli, R. M. (2008). High-throughput proteomic analysis of formalin-fixed paraffin- embedded tissue microarrays using MALDI imaging mass spectrometry. *Proteomics*, *8*(18), 3715–3724. doi:10.1002/pmic.200800495 PMID:18712763

Grüner, B. M., Winkelmann, I., Feuchtinger, A., Sun, N., Balluff, B., Teichmann, N., ... Siveke, J. T. (2016, May). Modeling Therapy Response and Spatial Tissue Distribution of Erlotinib in Pancreatic Cancer. *Molecular Cancer Therapeutics*, *15*(5), 1145–1152. doi:10.1158/1535-7163.MCT-15-0165 PMID:26823494

Hanna, M.G., Pantanowitz, L., & Evans, A.J. (2015). Overview of contemporary guidelines in digital pathology: what is available in 2015 and what still needs to be addressed? *Journal of Clinical Pathology, 68*(7), 499-505. doi: 10.1136/jclinpath-2015-202914

Hardesty, W. M., Kelley, M. C., Mi, D., Low, R. L., & Caprioli, R. M. (2011). Protein signatures for survival and recurrence in metastatic melanoma. *Journal of Proteomics*, *74*(7), 1002–1014. doi:10.1016/j.jprot.2011.04.013 PMID:21549228

Higgins, C. (2015, July). Applications and challenges of digital pathology and whole slide imaging. *Biotechnic & Histochemistry*, *90*(5), 341–347. doi:10.3109/10520295.2015.1044566 PMID:25978139

Horn, C. L., DeKoning, L., Klonowski, P., & Naugler, C. (2014). Current usage and future trends in gross digital photography in Canada. *BMC Medical Education*, *14*(1), 11. doi:10.1186/1472-6920-14-11 PMID:24422898

Kampf, C., Olsson, I., Ryberg, U., Sjöstedt, E., & Pontén, F. (2012). Production of Tissue Microarrays, Immunohistochemistry Staining and Digitalization Within the Human Protein Atlas. *Journal of Visualized Experiments*, *3620*(63). doi:10.3791/3620 PMID:22688270

Kang, S., Shim, H. S., Lee, J. S., Kim, D. S., Kim, H. Y., Hong, S. H., ... Cho, N. H. (2010). Molecular proteomics imaging of tumor interfaces by mass spectrometry. *Journal of Proteome Research*, *9*(2), 1157–1164. doi:10.1021/pr900666q PMID:19821573

Kårsnäs, A., Dahl, A. L., & Larsen, R. (2011). Learning histopathological patterns. *Journal of Pathology Informatics*, *2*(2), S12. doi:10.4103/2153-3539.92033 PMID:22811956

Kim, H. K., Reyzer, M. L., Choi, I. J., Kim, C. G., Kim, H. S., Oshima, A., ... Green, J. E. (2010). Gastric cancer-specific protein profile identified using endoscopic biopsy samples via MALDI mass spectrometry. *Journal of Proteome Research*, *9*(8), 4123–4130. doi:10.1021/pr100302b PMID:20557134

Kim, M. S., Kwon, S., & Park, J. K. (2013). Breast cancer diagnostics using microfluidic multiplexed immunohistochemistry. *Methods in Molecular Biology (Clifton, N.J.)*, *949*, 349–364. doi:10.1007/978-1-62703-134-9_22 PMID:23329453

Kriegsmann, J., Kriegsmann, M., & Casadonte, R. (2015, March). MALDI TOF imaging mass spectrometry in clinical pathology: A valuable tool for cancer diagnostics. *International Journal of Oncology*, *46*(3), 893–906. doi:10.3892/ijo.2014.2788 PMID:25482502

Kriegsmann, M., Arens, N., Endris, V., Weichert, W., & Kriegsmann, J. (2015). Detection of KRAS, NRAS and BRAF by mass spectrometry - a sensitive, reliable, fast and cost-effective technique. *Diagnostic Pathology*, *10*(1), 132. doi:10.118613000-015-0364-3 PMID:26220423

Kuboki, Y., Schatz, C. A., Koechert, K., Schubert, S., Feng, J., Wittemer-Rump, S., ... Ochiai, A. (2017, August 29). In situ analysis of FGFR2 mRNA and comparison with FGFR2 gene copy number by dual-color in situ hybridization in a large cohort of gastric cancer patients. *Gastric Cancer*. doi:10.100710120-017-0758-x PMID:28852882

Lai, Y-H., & Wang, Y-S. (2017). Matrix-Assisted Laser Desorption/Ionization Mass Spectrometry: Mechanistic Studies and Methods for Improving the Structural Identification of Carbohydrates. *Mass Spectrometry*, *6*(2), S0072. doi:.10.5702/massspectrometry.S0072

Laouirem, S., Le Faouder, J., Alexandrov, T., Mestivier, D., Léger, T., Baudin, X., ... Bedossa, P. (2014). Progression from cirrhosis to cancer is associated with early ubiquitin post-translational modifications: Identification of new biomarkers of cirrhosis at risk of malignancy. *The Journal of Pathology*, *234*(4), 452–463. doi:10.1002/path.4398 PMID:24979321

Larsson, C., Koch, J., Nygren, A., Janssen, G., Raap, A. K., Landegren, U., & Nilsson, M. (2004). In situ genotyping individual DNA molecules by target-primed rolling-circle amplification of padlock probes. *Nature Methods*, *1*(3), 227–232. doi:10.1038/nmeth723 PMID:15782198

Lazova, R., Seeley, E. H., Keenan, M., Gueorguieva, R., & Caprioli, R. M. (2012). Imaging mass spectrometry - a new and promising method to differentiate Spitz nevi from Spitzoid malignant melanomas. *The American Journal of Dermatopathology*, *34*(1), 82–90. doi:10.1097/DAD.0b013e31823df1e2 PMID:22197864

Le Faouder, J., Laouirem, S., Chapelle, M., Albuquerque, M., Belghiti, J., Degos, F., ... Bedossa, P. (2011). Imaging mass spectrometry provides fingerprints for distinguishing hepatocellular carcinoma from cirrhosis. *Journal of Proteome Research*, *10*(8), 3755–3765. doi:10.1021/pr200372p PMID:21675781

Lee, G. K., Lee, H. S., Park, Y. S., Lee, J. H., Lee, S. C., Lee, J. H., ... Kim, H. K. (2012). Lipid MALDI profile classifies non-small cell lung cancers according to the histologic type. *Lung Cancer (Amsterdam, Netherlands)*, *76*(2), 197–203. doi:10.1016/j.lungcan.2011.10.016 PMID:22099218

Lee, J. H. (2017). Quantitative approaches for investigating the spatial context of gene expression. *Wiley Interdisciplinary Reviews. Systems Biology and Medicine*, *9*(2), e1369. doi:10.1002/wsbm.1369 PMID:28001340

Lee, J. H., Daugharthy, E. R., Scheiman, J., Kalhor, R., Ferrante, T. C., Terry, R., ... Church, G. M. (2015). Fluorescent in situ sequencing (FISSEQ) of RNA for gene expression profiling in intact cells and tissues. *Nature Protocols*, *10*(3), 442–458. doi:10.1038/nprot.2014.191 PMID:25675209

Lee, J. H., Daugharthy, E. R., Scheiman, J., Kalhor, R., Yang, J. L., Ferrante, T. C., ... Church, G. M. (2014). Highly multiplexed subcellular RNA sequencing *in situ*. *Science*, *343*(6177), 1360–1363. doi:10.1126cience.1250212 PMID:24578530

Lemaire, R., Menguellet, S. A., Stauber, J., Marchauadon, V., & Lucot, J. P. (2007). Specific MALDI imaging and profiling for biomarker hunting and validation: Fragment of the 11S proteasome activator complex, Reg alpha fragment, is a new potential ovary cancer biomarker. *Journal of Proteome Research*, *6*(11), 4127–4134. doi:10.1021/pr0702722 PMID:17939699

Li, F., Zou, Y. G., Zhou, Q. Z., Li, T. Q., Guo, W. B., Jing, X. W., ... Zheng, S. B. (2009). Identification of human testicular embryonal carcinoma proteins by two-dimensional gel electrophoresis and mass spectrometry. *Nan Fang Yi Ke da Xue Xue Bao*, *29*(8), 1585–1587. PMID:19726299

Liu, X., Ide, J.L., Norton, I., Marchionni, M.A., Ebling, M.C., ... Agar, N.Y.R. (2013) Molecular imaging of drug transit through the blood-brain barrier with MALDI mass spectrometry imaging. *Sci Rep.*, *4*(3), 2859. doi: 10.1038rep02859

Liu, Y., Chen, Y., Momin, A., Shaner, R., Wang, E., Bowen, N. J., ... Merrill, A. H. (2010). Elevation of sulfatides in ovarian cancer: An integrated transcriptomic and lipidomic analysis including tissue-imaging mass spectrometry. *Molecular Cancer*, *9*(1), 186. doi:10.1186/1476-4598-9-186 PMID:20624317

Liu, Y., Tan, Y. R., Sun, W. W., Ju, W. T., Fu, Y., Wang, L. Z., ... Zhong, L. P. (2018, February 20). Identification of SCARA5 as a potential biomarker for oral squamous cell carcinoma using MALDI TOF MS analysis. *Proteomics. Clinical Applications*. doi:10.1002/prca.201700180 PMID:29461673

Loeser, H., Schallenberg, S., von Winterfeld, M., Tharun, L., Alakus, H., Hölscher, A., ... Quaas, A. (2017). High protein and mRNA expression levels of TUBB3 (class III ß-tubulin) are associated with aggressive tumor features in esophageal adenocarcinomas. *Oncotarget*, *8*(70), 115179–115189. doi:10.18632/oncotarget.23112 PMID:29383151

Longuespée, R., Casadonte, R., Kriegsmann, M., Pottier, C., Picard de Muller, G., Delvenne, P., ... De Pauw, E. (2016). MALDI mass spectrometry imaging: A cutting-edge tool for fundamental and clinical histopathology. *Proteomics. Clinical Applications*, *10*(7), 701–719. doi:10.1002/prca.201500140 PMID:27188927

Longuespée, R., Casadonte, R., Schwamborn, K., Reuss, D., Kazdal, D., Kriegsmann, K., ... Kriegsmann, M. (2018). Proteomics in Pathology. *Proteomics*, *18*(2), 1700361. doi:10.1002/pmic.201700361 PMID:29236356

Lou, S., Balluff, B., Cleven, A. H. G., Bovée, J. V. M. G., & McDonnell, L. A. (2017). Prognostic Metabolite Biomarkers for Soft Tissue Sarcomas Discovered by Mass Spectrometry Imaging. *Journal of the American Society for Mass Spectrometry*, *28*(2), 376–383. doi:10.100713361-016-1544-4 PMID:27873216

Maier, S. K., Hahne, H., Gholami, A. M., Balluff, B., Meding, S., Schoene, C., ... Kuster, B. (2013). Comprehensive identification of proteins from MALDI imaging. *Molecular & Cellular Proteomics*, *12*(10), 2901–2910. doi:10.1074/mcp.M113.027599 PMID:23782541

McDonnell, L. A., Walch, A., Stoeckli, M., & Corthals, G. L. (2014). MSiMass list: A public database of identifications for protein MALDI MS imaging. *Journal of Proteome Research*, *13*(2), 1138–1142. doi:10.1021/pr400620y PMID:24313301

Meding, S., Martin, K., Gustafsson, O. J., Eddes, J. S., Hack, S., Oehler, M. K., & Hoffmann, P. (2013). Tryptic peptide reference data sets for MALDI imaging mass spectrometry on formalin-fixed ovarian cancer tissues. *Journal of Proteome Research*, *12*(1), 308–315. doi:10.1021/pr300996x PMID:23214983

Meseure, D., Drak Alsibai, K., & Nicolas, A. (2014). Pivotal Role of Pervasive Neoplastic and Stromal Cells Reprogramming in Circulating Tumor Cells Dissemination and Metastatic Colonization. *Cancer Microenvironment*, *7*(3), 95–115. doi:10.100712307-014-0158-2 PMID:25523234

Meseure, D., Vacher, S., Lallemand, F., Drak Alsibai, K., Hatem, R., Chemlali, W., ... Bieche, I. (2016). Prognostic value of a newly identified MALAT1 alternatively spliced transcript in breast cancer. *British Journal of Cancer*, *114*(12), 1395–1404. doi:10.1038/bjc.2016.123 PMID:27172249

Mignardi, M., Mezger, A., Qian, X., La Fleur, L., Botling, J., Larsson, C., & Nilsson, M. (2015). Oligonucleotide gap-fill ligation for mutation detection and sequencing *in situ*. *Nucleic Acids Research*, *43*(22), e151. doi:10.1093/nar/gkv772 PMID:26240388

Mlecnik, B., Bindea, G., Kirilovsky, A., Angell, H. K., Obenauf, A. C., Tosolini, M., ... Galon, J. (2016). The tumor microenvironment and Immunoscore are critical determinants of dissemination to distant metastasis. *Science Translational Medicine*, *8*(327), 327ra26. doi:10.1126citranslmed.aad6352 PMID:26912905

Morita, Y., Ikegami, K., Goto-Inoue, N., Hayasaka, T., Zaima, N., Tanaka, H., ... Konno, H. (2010). Imaging mass spectrometry of gastric carcinoma in formalin-fixed paraffin-embedded tissue microarray. *Cancer Science*, *101*(1), 267–273. doi:10.1111/j.1349-7006.2009.01384.x PMID:19961487

Nipp, M., Elsner, M., Balluff, B., Meding, S., Sarioglu, H., Ueffing, M., ... Zitzelsberger, H. (2012). S100-A10, thioredoxin, and S100-A6 as biomarkers of papillary thyroid carcinoma with lymph node metastasis identified by MALDI imaging. *Journal of Molecular Medicine*, *90*(2), 163–174. doi:10.100700109-011-0815-6 PMID:21938494

Nirmalan, N.J., Harnden, P., Selby, P.J., & Banks, R.E. (2009). Development and validation of a novel protein extraction methodology for quantitation of protein expression in formalin-fixed paraffin-embedded tissues using western blotting. *J Pathol*, *217*, 497-506.

Oppenheimer, S. R., Mi, D., Sanders, M. E., & Caprioli, R. M. (2010). Molecular analysis of tumor margins by MALDI mass spectrometry in renal carcinoma. *Journal of Proteome Research*, *9*(5), 2182–2190. doi:10.1021/pr900936z PMID:20141219

Pagni, F., Mainini, V., Garancini, M., Bono, F., Vanzati, A., Giardini, V., ... Magni, F. (2015). Proteomics for the diagnosis of thyroid lesions: Preliminary report. *Cytopathology*, *26*(5), 318–324. doi:10.1111/cyt.12166 PMID:25040579

Pantanowitz, L., Valenstein, P. N., Evans, A. J., Kaplan, K. J., & Pfeifer, J. D. (2011). Review of the current state of whole slide imaging in pathology. *Journal of Pathology Informatics*, *2*(1), 36. doi:10.4103/2153-3539.83746 PMID:21886892

Querido, F., Dekakra-Bellili, L., & Chartrand, P. (2017). RNA fluorescence in situ hybridization for high-content screening. *Methods (San Diego, Calif.)*, *15*(126), 149–155. doi:10.1016/j.ymeth.2017.07.005 PMID:28694064

Remark, R., Merghoub, T., Grabe, N., Litjens, G., Damotte, D., Wolchok, J.D., … Gnjatic, S. (2016). In-depth tissue profiling using multiplexed immunohistochemical consecutive staining on single slide. *Science Immunology, 14*(1). doi: 10.1126ciimmunol.aaf6925

Reyzer, M. L., Hsieh, Y., Ng, K., Korfmacher, W. A., & Caprioli, R. M. (2003). Direct analysis of drug candidates in tissue by matrix-assisted laser desorption/ionization mass spectrometry. *Journal of Mass Spectrometry*, *38*(10), 1081–1092. doi:10.1002/jms.525 PMID:14595858

Salphati, L., Shahidi-Latham, S., Quiason, C., Barck, K., Nishimura, M., Alicke, B., ... Phillips, H. S. (2014). ... Distribution of the phosphatidylinositol 3-kinase inhibitors Pictilisib (GDC- 0941) and GNE-317 in U87 and GS2 intracranial glioblastoma models-assessment by matrix-assisted laser desorption ionization imaging. *Drug Metabolism and Disposition: the Biological Fate of Chemicals*, *42*(7), 1110–1116. doi:10.1124/dmd.114.057513 PMID:24754926

Salto-Tellez, M., James, J. A., & Hamilton, P. W. (2014). Molecular pathology – The value of an integrative approach. *Molecular Oncology*, *8*(7), 1163–1168. doi:10.1016/j.molonc.2014.07.021 PMID:25160635

Salto-Tellez, M., & Kennedy, R. D. (2015, December). Integrated molecular pathology: The Belfast model. *Drug Discovery Today*, *20*(12), 1451–1454. doi:10.1016/j.drudis.2015.10.011 PMID:26499202

Schwamborn, K., Krieg, R. C., Jirak, P., Ott, G., Knuchel, R., Rosenwald, A., & Wellmann, A. (2010). Application of MALDI imaging for the diagnosis of classical Hodgkin lymphoma. *Journal of Cancer Research and Clinical Oncology*, *136*(11), 1651–1655. doi:10.100700432-010-0823-x PMID:20865362

Schwamborn, K., Krieg, R. C., Reska, M., Jakse, G., Knuechel, R., & Wellmann, A. (2007). Identifying prostate carcinoma by MALDI-Imaging. *International Journal of Molecular Medicine*, *20*, 155–159. PMID:17611632

Schwamborn, K., Krieg, R. C., Uhlig, S., Ikenberg, H., & Wellmann, A. (2011). MALDI imaging as a specific diagnostic tool for routine cervical cytology specimens. *International Journal of Molecular Medicine*, *27*(3), 417–421. doi:10.3892/ijmm.2010.587 PMID:21174066

Schwartz, S. A., Reyzer, M. L., & Caprioli, R. M. (2003). Direct tissue analysis using matrix-assisted laser desorption/ionization mass spectrometry: Practical aspects of sample preparation. *Journal of Mass Spectrometry*, *38*(7), 699–708. doi:10.1002/jms.505 PMID:12898649

Seeley, E. H., & Caprioli, R. M. (2011). MALDI imaging mass spectrometry of human tissue: Method challenges and clinical perspectives. *Trends in Biotechnology*, *29*(3), 136–143. doi:10.1016/j.tibtech.2010.12.002 PMID:21292337

Sheffield, B. S. (2016). Immunohistochemistry as a Practical Tool in Molecular Pathology. *Archives of Pathology & Laboratory Medicine*, *140*(8), 766–769. doi:10.5858/arpa.2015-0453-RA PMID:27472235

Shirinifard, A., Thiagarajan, S., Vogel, P., & Sablauer, A. (2016). Detection of Phenotypic Alterations Using High-Content Analysis of Whole-Slide Images. *The Journal of Histochemistry and Cytochemistry*, *64*(5), 301–310. doi:10.1369/0022155416639884 PMID:27026297

Stack, E. C., Wang, C., Roman, K. A., & Hoyt, C. C. (2014). Multiplexed immunohistochemistry, imaging, and quantitation: A review, with an assessment of Tyramide signal amplification, multispectral imaging and multiplex analysis. *Methods (San Diego, Calif.)*, *70*(1), 46–58. doi:10.1016/j.ymeth.2014.08.016 PMID:25242720

Stack, E. C., Wang, C., Roman, K. A., & Hoyt, C. C. (2014). Multiplexed immunohistochemistry, imaging, and quantitation: A review, with an assessment of Tyramide signal amplification, multispectral imaging and multiplex analysis. *Methods (San Diego, Calif.)*, *70*(1), 46–58. doi:10.1016/j.ymeth.2014.08.016 PMID:25242720

Steurer, S., Borkowski, C., Odinga, S., Buchholz, M., Koop, C., Huland, H., ... Schlüter, H. (2013). MALDI mass spectrometric imaging based identification of clinically relevant signals in prostate cancer using large-scale tissue microarrays. *International Journal of Cancer*, *133*(4), 920–928. doi:10.1002/ijc.28080 PMID:23381989

Steurer, S., Seddiqi, A. S., Singer, J. M., Bahar, A. S., & Eichelberg, C. (2014). MALDI imaging on tissue microarrays identifies molecular features associated with renal cell cancer phenotype. *Anticancer Research*, *34*, 2255–2261. PMID:24778028

Steurer, S., Singer, J. M., Rink, M., Chun, F., & Dahlem, R. (2014). MALDI imaging-based identification of prognostically relevant signals in bladder cancer using large-scale tissue microarrays. *Urologic Oncology*, *32*(8), 1225–1233. doi:10.1016/j.urolonc.2014.06.007 PMID:25131659

Sugihara, Y. (2014). A new look at drugs targeting malignant melanoma - an application for mass spectrometry imaging. *Proteomics*, *14*, 1963–1970. doi:10.1002/pmic.201300476 PMID:25044963

Swamidoss, I. N., Kårsnäs, A., Uhlmann, V., Ponnusamy, P., & Kampf, C. (2013). Automated classification of immunostaining patterns in breast tissue from the human protein atlas. *Journal of Pathology Informatics*, *4*(2Suppl), S14. doi:10.4103/2153-3539.109881 PMID:23766936

Tabata, K., Mori, I., Sasaki, T., Itoh, T., Shiraishi, T., Yoshimi, N., ... Fukuoka, J. (2017, November). Whole-slide imaging at primary pathological diagnosis: Validation of whole-slide imaging-based primary pathological diagnosis at twelve Japanese academic institutes. *Pathology International*, *67*(11), 547–554. doi:10.1111/pin.12590 PMID:28980740

Takats, Z., Strittmatter, N., & McKenzie, J. S. (2017). Ambient Mass Spectrometry in Cancer Research. *Advances in Cancer Research, 134*, 231–256. doi:10.1016/bs.acr.2016.11.011 PMID:28110652

Thomas, A., Patterson, N. H., Marcinkiewicz, M. M., Lazaris, A., Metrakos, P., & Chaurand, P. (2013). Histology-driven data mining of lipid signatures from multiple imaging mass spectrometry analyses: Application to human colorectal cancer liver metastasis biopsies. *Analytical Chemistry, 85*(5), 2860–2866. doi:10.1021/ac3034294 PMID:23347294

Tiffen, J., Wilson, S., Gallagher, S. J., Hersey, P., & Filipp, F. V. (2016). Somatic Copy Number Amplification and Hyperactivating Somatic Mutations of EZH2 Correlate With DNA Methylation and Drive Epigenetic Silencing of Genes Involved in Tumor Suppression and Immune Responses in Melanoma. *Neoplasia (New York, N.Y.), 18*(2), 121–132. doi:10.1016/j.neo.2016.01.003 PMID:26936398

Toriyama, A., Mori, T., Sekine, S., Yoshida, A., Hino, O., & Tsuta, K. (2014). Utility of PAX8 mouse monoclonal antibody in the diagnosis of thyroid, thymic, pleural and lung tumours: A comparison with polyclonal PAX8 antibody. *Histopathology, 65*(4), 465–472. doi:10.1111/his.12405 PMID:24592933

Vyas, N. S., Markow, M., Prieto-Granada, C., Gaudi, S., Turner, L., Rodriguez-Waitkus, P., ... Jukic, D. M. (2016). Comparing whole slide digital images versus traditional glass slides in the detection of common microscopic features seen in dermatitis. *Journal of Pathology Informatics, 7*(1), 30. doi:10.4103/2153-3539.186909 PMID:27563489

Willems, S. M., van Remoortere, A., van Zeijl, R., Deelder, A. M., McDonnell, L. A., & Hogendoorn, P. C. (2010). Imaging mass spectrometry of myxoid sarcomas identifies proteins and lipids specific to tumour type and grade, and reveals biochemical intratumour heterogeneity. *The Journal of Pathology, 222*(4), 400–409. doi:10.1002/path.2771 PMID:20839361

Yadav, N.K., Shukla, P., Omer, A., Pareek, S., & Singh, R.K. (2014). Next Generation Sequencing: Potential and Application in Drug Discovery. *The Scientific World Journal*. doi:10.1155/2014/802437

Yanagisawa, K., Shyr, Y., Xu, B. J., Massion, P. P., Larsen, P. H., White, B. C., ... Carbone, D. P. (2003). Proteomic patterns of tumour subsets in non-small-cell lung cancer. *Lancet, 362*(9382), 433–439. doi:10.1016/S0140-6736(03)14068-8 PMID:12927430

Yuan, J., Zhang, J., Zhu, Y., Li, N., Tian, T., Li, Y., ... Shen, L. (2016). Programmed death-ligand-1 expression in advanced gastric cancer detected with RNA in situ hybridization and its clinical significance. *Oncotarget, 7*(26), 39671–39679. doi:10.18632/oncotarget.9381 PMID:27191996

Zheng, Y., Coltharp, C., Dilworth, R., Liu, L., Unfricht, D., Hoyt, C., … Miller, P. (2017). Optimization strategy for fluorescent multiplex immunohistochemistry tissue staining. Abstract 3832. *Cancer Research, 77*(13S), 3832.

Zheng, Y., Coltharp, C., Dilworth, R., Liu, L., Unfricht, D., Hoyt, C., ... Peter Miller, P. Optimization strategy for fluorescent multiplex immunohistochemistry tissue staining. In *Proceedings of the American Association for Cancer Research Annual Meeting 2017*. Philadelphia: AACR. doi:10.1158/1538-7445.AM2017-3832

Section 2

Medical Image Extraction, Classification, and Restoration in Computer-Aided Diagnosis

Chapter 3
Medical Image Classification

Jesu Vedha Nayahi J.
Anna University Tirunelveli, India

Gokulakrishnan K.
Anna University Tirunelveli, India

ABSTRACT

Diagnosis of diseases at the right stage with optimal accuracy is a significant requirement in the medical field. Apart from diagnosis from clinical symptoms, diagnosis based on scanned images of both internal and external organs is playing a vital role in understanding the severity of the disease. Classification is a field of study derived from artificial intelligence, and today it is widely used in medical image classification. These techniques are used to classify the different stages of a disease or different variant diseases possible in an organ from different types of input images such as magnetic resonance imaging (MRI), computed tomography (CT), x-ray, fundus images, iris images, etc. Various preprocessing techniques are used to select the relevant features from the input image to form the feature set. The classifiers are trained using the feature set to generate models. The generated models can be optimized to improve the performance. Various metrics such as accuracy, coverage, precision, recall, and FMeasure are used to measure the accuracy.

INTRODUCTION

In medical field there is a lot of challenge with regard to diagnosis of different diseases. Magnetic Resonance Imaging (MRI) (Geethu & Monica, 2005), Computed Tomography (CT) (Yang et al., in press), X-Ray, fundus images (Andres et al., 2017), iris images and other type of images are acting as an important aid for the physician

DOI: 10.4018/978-1-5225-5876-7.ch003

to diagnose a particular disease. Human processing of these images may be erroneous and varies from one person to other. Traditionally the medical images are analyzed with the help of pixel based or region based segmentation. Today medical images are processed using a branch of study in artificial intelligence namely classification in order to improve the accuracy of prediction.

Classification is playing a vital role in the diagnosis of diseases such as brain tumor and other types of tumors, glaucoma, lung diseases etc. Decision Tree classifier, Naive Bayes classifier, Neural Network classifier, Support Vector Machine, k-Nearest Neighbour (k-NN) classifier etc. are some of the classification techniques used for data classification. Recently different modified versions of neural network, support vector machine, k-NN are widely used in image classification. There are also ensemble classifier techniques such as bagging and boosting which has proved to improve the accuracy of medical image classification.

The first phase of medical image classification is feature extraction. Many of the filters and other transforms are used for feature extraction. Feature extraction will identify all the possible features and as the next step feature selection can be used to identify the most relevant features. Feature selection will play a significant role in improving the accuracy of classification by selecting the most relevant features for further classification.

The best features selected are fed to classifiers and most of the classifiers work by assigning weightage to the different features. One of the most promising techniques used for image classification is neural network classifier. Neural network classifier assigns initial weights and biases to each of the features and the edges connecting the different layers respectively. The weight and bias are adjusted based on the error in the output layer. The best weight and bias which would have very negligible error rate is fixed for future classification.

Support vector machine (SVM) classifier is also another significant technique used for image classification. This classifier is suitable for all types of linear or non linear data and hence widely used in image classification. The support vectors are identified by choosing the maximal margin hyperplane used to separate the different classes. These support vectors are then used as reference to classify the future values.

Optimization is also playing a key role nowadays in medical image classification. Different optimization techniques such as genetic algorithm, particle swarm optimization etc are integrated with the classifier to optimize the weights of the features used for classification. Neural network or SVM can be combined with optimization techniques to improve the accuracy, specificity, sensitivity of the classification.

The use of ensemble classifiers or classifiers combined with optimization techniques would improve the result of classification. Since the success of medical image classification lies in the accuracy of classification different preprocessing techniques and post processing techniques can be applied to improve accuracy.

Clustering techniques can be employed before classification and this would definitely improve the accuracy of classification. The use of optimization techniques to improve the generated classifier model can also improve accuracy.

The objective of this chapter would be to explain the key steps in the process of image classification by concentrating more on the various classification techniques available in machine learning that can be incorporated for image classification. It discussed the other ways in which the accuracy of the classification process can be improved.

BACKGROUND

Medical image classification is used in place of segmentation techniques owing to the high level of accuracy possible with the of classification techniques. The main limitation is the requirement of large number of input images to form the training set (Geethu & Monica, 2005). Normally classification techniques are applied to diagnose any particular type of disease in an internal organ. Classification techniques are also applied to predict the different stages of some fatal diseases. Geethu and Monica, (2005) have made extensive survey on the various classification techniques used to predict the stages of brain tumor.

Artificial Neural Network (ANN) classifier is widely used in medical image classification. Today several variations of neural networks such as convolutional neural networks are used to improve the accuracy and efficiency of neural networks. Geert et al. (2017) has compared the deep learning algorithms used for brain images, retinal images, chest x-ray, chest CT, pathology images, breast images, cardiac images, abdominal images, musculoskeletal images, and other applications. Jefferson et al. (in press) has examined colonoscopy images and used several machine learning techniques such as decision tree, Naive Bayes, SVM, back propagation. They have predicted whether the colonoscopy images of patients are normal or abnormal.

Sharif et al. (2015) has extracted various statistical features from corneal images and used ANN, Artificial Neuro Fuzzy Inference System (ANFIS) and Committee Machine (CM) to predict the abnormality in the different layers of cornea. The accuracy of CM was better than the other two individual classifiers. Yang et al. (2015) proposed locally constrained subcluster ensemble model for predicting lung image classification. Spectral clustering is used to generate similar subcluster in the lung image and then an ensemble of classifiers is used to improve the accuracy of prediction.

Ahmed et al. (in press) compared the used of decision tree and ANN classifiers for leukemia diseases using color, shape, geometric and size features. ANN is proved to be performing better than decision tree classifier for predicting leukemia from microscopic images. Zhang et al. (2017) proposed multi-scale non negative sparse coding to represent the image using multi-scale decomposition. SVM classifier is used to predict the medical image class label. Tanvi et al. (2017) used MRI images to predict cerebral tumors. Discrete Wavelet Transform (DWT) is used for feature extraction and Principal Component Analysis (PCA) is used for feature selection. Among the different classifiers used for predicting the neuro diagnosis, SVM is proven to be performing better than Classification and Regression Trees (CART), k-Nearest Neighbour (k-NN) and Random Forest classifier.

There are a lot of other research works that are also aimed at optimizing the accuracy of prediction of diseases. The accuracy can be improved by using better methods for feature extraction, feature selection, optimized classifiers etc. The other sections in this chapter would discuss about the various steps involved in medical image classification and the ways in which the accuracy can be estimated and optimized.

STEPS IN MEDICAL IMAGE CLASSIFICATION

Figure 1 shows the block diagram of the steps in the process of medical image classification. Any image processing technique involves preprocessing techniques. There are number of filters in literature that are used as preprocessing tools. Feature extraction and feature selection are the preprocessing techniques used and this is followed by classifier. The classifier produces the model and the results can be optimized using optimization techniques.

The input image quality depends on the preciseness of the instrument used to capture those images. Depending on that an optional image enhancement technique can be used to improve the quality of the images. Feature extraction is one of the preprocessing technique and most of the image classification starts with feature

Figure 1. Steps in medical image classification

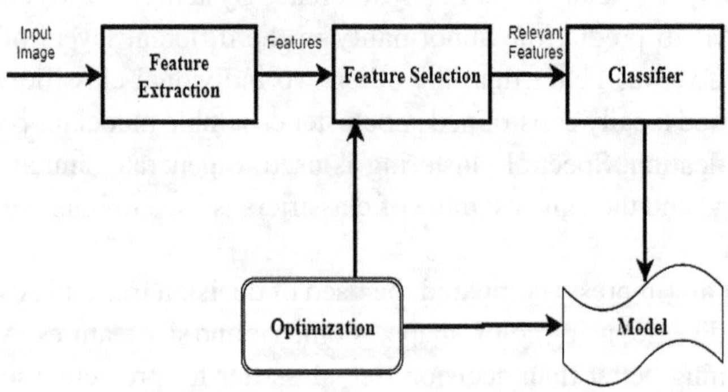

extraction (Mark & Alberto, 2008). There are methods that are used to extract the color features, texture features and shape features.

Some of the feature extraction techniques are

1. Color histogram
2. Local binary patterns
3. Principal Component analysis
4. Canny edge detection
5. Gabor filter
6. Edge and corner detection
7. Hough transform
8. Active Contours

One or more of these techniques can be used to extract the features from the given input image I. Feature extraction helps to represent an image in a non pictorial representation using other internal characteristics of the image. The feature extracted image is represented in the form of a feature vector consisting of features. Let (x_1, x_2, …. x_n) denote a feature vector with *n* features representing an image.

The training set is formed by the feature vectors of the given set of images. Let the number of input image samples be *m*. The size of the training data set would be m X n.

Table 1 shows a sample training feature set created from *m* images each with *n* features. x_{ij} represents the jth feature value of ith image and C represents any particular class.

The features extracted may be redundant or irrelevant to the target. The irrelevant features in the input would affect the accuracy of prediction. In some cases the features extracted may be redundant i.e. few features may convey the same information. The redundant features can be eliminated and would reduce the time taken for processing and storage cost. Hence feature extraction has to be followed by either feature selection or dimensionality reduction or both. Feature selection is a preprocessing technique

Table 1. Training feature set

$Feature_1$	$Feature_2$	$Feature_3$	…….	$Feature_n$	Class/Target
x_{11}	x_{12}	x_{13}	…….	x_{1n}	C
x_{21}	x_{22}	x_{23}	…….	x_{2n}	C
x_{31}	x_{32}	x_{33}	…….	x_{3n}	C
…….	…….	…….	…….	……..	……..
x_{m1}	x_{m2}	x_{m3}	…….	x_{mn}	C

used to select the best or most relevant features that are highly correlated with the class label. Feature selection is broadly classified into three categories

1. **Filter Based Methods:** These are the most basic techniques that are used to retrieve the most relevant features. The relevance of each feature to the target is estimated using information measures. The features are ranked based on the value of these information measures and the best features are selected. Entropy measure, Pearson correlation coefficient, chi-squared analysis and mutual information are some of the filter based techniques used to retrieve the relevant data from the given feature set.
2. **Wrapper Based Methods:** These set of methods apply learning/classification algorithms on the whole set of features and determine a subset of features that gives the maximum accuracy (Rattanawadee & Anongnart, 2015). This subset of features forms the reduced data set. Forward selection, backward elimination and hybrid techniques are some of the techniques used to determine the best subset of features that improves the accuracy.
3. **Hybrid Methods:** Hybrid methods are used to exploit the advantage of both filter based and wrapper based techniques (Ivan et al., 2016). Filter based techniques are simple and less time consuming whereas wrapper based methods consume more time. Wrapper based methods achieve high accuracy because actual classification is performed before choosing relevant features. The filter based techniques can be used to get a reduced set of features over which wrapper can be used to refine further to reduce the features and also improve accuracy.

Dimensionality reduction techniques are used to reduce the size of the training set. Dimensionality reduction is suitable for high dimensional data. This reduction technique can be applied when the number of features extracted and the number of input images are too large. The entire data can be represented in a smaller dimension. Principal component analysis, wavelet transform are some of the dimensionality reduction techniques. The reduced set of most relevant features is given as input to the learning algorithm.

Learning is an important aspect in the field of Artificial Intelligence. The learning algorithms are used to train the machines. Normally learning is classified into two types, supervised learning and unsupervised learning. Supervised learning is analogous to the process of human learning with the help of a supervisor or a teacher. The supervisor or teacher is substituted by the history of data and it is called as training set. Unsupervised learning is analogous to the process of human learning called as self learning or learning without a supervisor. Classification is a supervised learning technique used to predict the target label.

Classification can optionally be followed by optimization techniques that are used to optimize the results of classification. Genetic algorithm, particle swarm optimization, ant colony optimization are some of the optimization techniques that can be used to optimize the prediction accuracy. Optimization techniques are also used to choose the best features or to optimize the weight of the chosen features.

Optimization for Feature Selection

Optimization consists of a group of techniques that are normally used to optimize the results. In classification problems optimization is either used to choose the best input features (preprocessing) or optimization can be combined with the classification algorithms to improve the predicted result (post processing). Genetic algorithm, particle swarm optimization, ant colony optimization etc are used to select the best features. This section would describe the different techniques in literature that are used to optimize the feature selection process which in turn would enhance the classified results.

Djaafar and Fouad, (2018) have proposed a swarm intelligence algorithm for selecting the best feature subset based on quantum computing. It is a combination of Firefly algorithm and Particle Swarm Optimization. The best set of features is selected based on the fitness function. Majdi and Seyedali, (2018) proposed Whale optimization algorithm for wrapper based feature selection. The best features are selected using the fitness function with two objectives. One objective is to improve the classification accuracy based on K-Nearest Neighbour (KNN) classifier and the other objective is to reduce the number of features selected. The optimization is done by mapping the feature set to the position of the whale. Exploitation and exploration are the two phases of the algorithm which are mapped to the whales nature of trapping the prey and searching the prey respectively.

Bolun et al. (2013) employed ant-colony optimization mechanism for selecting the best feature subset for images. The best set of features that increases the accuracy is determined by mapping feature selection to the ant's best solution path. Each feature is represented as a node in the graph and the shortest solution path from one node to the other is determined. Forest optimization algorithm is normally used for continuous search space problem but in this problem the authors have used the algorithm for discrete search space problem (feature selection). Initially trees are randomly generated with n features and age of the tree as variables. In the next phase local seeding is done by identifying some neighbors for each tree. Based on the fitness function value the trees are removed from the forest. The tree with the highest fitness value is selected as the best tree (Manizheh & Mohammad-Reza, 2016).

FUNDAMENTALS OF CLASSIFICATION

Any classifier requires an input training data set. In the case of images the features that are extracted from several images are considered as the training data set which here after will be denoted as feature set.

Example

Fundus images are used for ophthalmic disease prediction. Glaucoma is a common syndrome and it can cause blindness if not diagnosed earlier. Classification techniques are widely used to identity glaucoma based on segmentation of the optic disc and cup. Some of the common features extracted from fundus photographs are intensity, centre, radius, contrast, other spatial features, intra retinal features.

First step of any classifier is to generate a model using the feature set. The generated model is used to predict the test data. The accuracy of the prediction is the ratio between the number of correctly classified instances and the total number of instances. If the accuracy is acceptable then the model is used to predict new data (new image).

The input feature set is normally divided into two, namely the training feature set and the test feature set. The training feature set is formed by different approaches such as random sampling, percentage split, k-fold cross validation etc. Cross validation is proven to be best way to form the training set and test set. The most popular form of cross validation is 10-fold cross validation. The given input feature set is divided into 10 independent partitions. The experiment is repeated for ten times and in each iteration, one partition is considered as the test feature set and the remaining nine are considered as training feature set. The accuracy achieved using 10-fold cross validation is proved to be the best.

DECISION TREE CLASSIFICATION

Decision tree classification is one of the very basic techniques in classification. The famous decision tree classifiers are ID3, C4.5. The feature extracted training set of images are used as input to the decision tree classifier. The first step in decision tree learning is feature evaluation. The features are evaluated using different techniques such as information gain, gain ratio and Gini index. A decision tree consists of nodes and edges. The nodes are either internal nodes or leaf nodes. The internal nodes are nothing but the features of given training set of images. The leaf nodes are the class label that is the target value to be predicted. In our case it is the diagnosis label (name of the disease).

Feature Selection

Each feature is evaluated using any of the above mentioned feature selection measures. These metrics are used to estimate the purity of the feature set formed after partitioning the data using the given feature. When the image samples in each partition belong to the same class it is said to be pure. The purity of partitioning using a given feature is measured using these measures. The features are ranked based on their calculated values of information gain. The best feature is one with the maximum information gain and this feature is chosen as the root of the decision tree.

Information of the given feature set is calculated using the Equation 1, p denotes the number of classes and S_i denotes the probability of a class.

$$Inf = -\sum_{i=1}^{p} S_i \log_2 S_i \, . \tag{1}$$

The information of the given feature, Inf_A is given by Equation 2. r represents the total number of possible values of the given feature A. $|I|$ denotes the cardinality of the given feature set and $|I_j|$ represents the cardinality of the jth possible value of feature A. $Inf(I_j)$ is the information value of a particular partition.

$$Inf_A = \sum_{j=1}^{r} \frac{|I_j|}{|I|} X Inf(I_j) \tag{2}$$

Information gain, $Gain(A)$ .s the difference between the information value of the whole feature set and the information value obtained by partitioning using feature A.

$$Gain(A) = Inf - Inf_A \tag{3}$$

Growing a Decision Tree

The first step in the construction of the tree is to identify the root node from among the available features. Each node has branches equal to the number of possible values of that feature. Originally decision tree classifier is not used for numerical features because it is impossible to form as many branches as the number of possible values of a numerical feature. It is applicable only for categorical data. Binary feature can be partitioned into two branches, one for yes and the other for no. Numerical data can be discretized using various preprocessing techniques used for concept hierarchy generation. With the help of discretization techniques decision tree classifier can also be used with numerical attributes. Without discretizing the numerical feature can be partitioned by choosing a split point value. All those samples whose values are less than or equal to the split point value belongs to one branch and those values that are larger than the split point value belongs to the other branch. The spilt point is chosen in such a way to make the samples in each partition pure to the extent possible.

The root node is the best node that can partition the image samples such that each branch has only samples belonging to one class i.e. pure samples. The image samples satisfying a particular feature value will be grouped in each branch. If all the samples belong to one class then the branch is returned with a leaf node labeled with a class. Otherwise another feature is chosen to partition the samples into pure. This process is repeated until there are no more samples or until there are no more features or each branch is returned with a leaf node.

Figure 2 shows a decision tree whose root node is Feature1 and there are two branches one for value V1 and V2. The samples with V1 for Feature 1 are not pure and hence Feature2 is used to partition again. In this branch, samples with values V1 are pure and hence returned with class label C1. Similarly the other branches that are pure are returned with class label and impure branches are partitioned again with new features.

Figure 2. Decision tree example

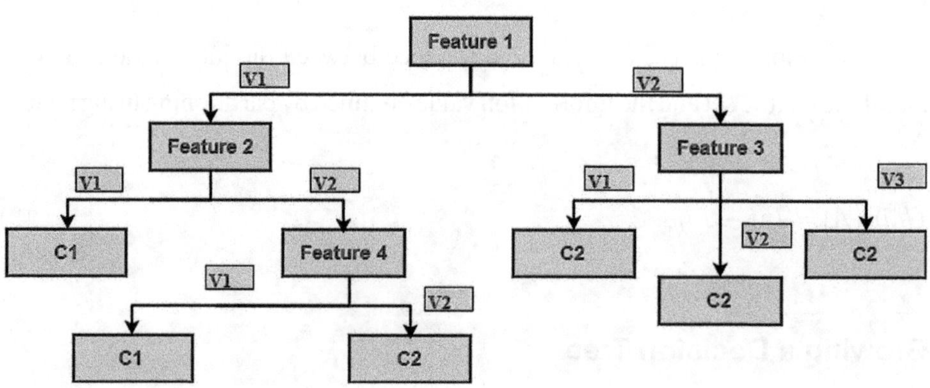

Rule Generation

The rules used for classification are generated from the fully grown decision tree. Each path of the tree is converted into a rule. The antecedent of the decision rule is the conjunction of each node value and the consequent of the decision rule is the class label in the leaf node of that path. The total rules formed from the tree are equal to the total number of paths in the decision tree. The rule that matches the test data value is triggered and the class label is returned as the predicted class value of the test data. The strong rules are one with maximum coverage and accuracy. Eq 4 is a decision rule extracted from the tree in Figure tracing first path.

$$Feature1\left(V_1\right) and Feature2\left(V_2\right) => C1 \tag{4}$$

NAIVE BAYES CLASSIFIER

Naive Bayes classifier is a probability based classification technique and it involves only simple mathematical calculation for estimating the class. This technique is based on Bayes theorem. Naive Bayes works under the assumption that a feature is independent of other features. The probability of each sample (X) belonging to every class (C) is determined using prior and posterior probabilities. Two prior probabilities estimated are probability of a class P(C) and probability of a sample P(X). Posterior probability is the conditional probability of occurrence of a variable with respect to another. Here two conditional probabilities are considered namely P(C|X) and P(X|C). P(C|X) is the probability of a class conditioned on the particular combination of X (sample). P(X|C) is the probability of a sample conditioned on the occurrence of a class.

$$P\left(C|X\right) = \frac{P\left(C\right) * P(X \mid C)}{P\left(X\right)} \tag{5}$$

The denominator P(X) is a constant and it does not change with respect to the given number of classes. Hence P(C|X) is determined only with $P\left(C\right) * P(X \mid C)$. P(C|X) is determined for all the possible classes in the given training set. The test set is assigned to the class whose P(C|X) value is maximum.

P(C) is the probability of the class which is the ratio between the number of occurrence of C and the total number of samples. Assume X is a combination of n features and then X is represented by x_1, x_2, x_3....x_n. Then P(X|C) is given by the product of the probability of each features i.e. $P(x_1) * P(x_2) * ...... * P(x_n)$. This is suitable for discrete valued features. The computation of P(X|C) is possible under the assumption that each feature is independent of each other. But in real world scenario that may not be true. There will be inter dependence among the various features and the class. In the case of continuous valued features the probability is determined using probability distribution function. Bayesian belief network classifier incorporates the inter dependence among the features with respect to the class.

NEURAL NETWORK CLASSIFIER

Neural Network classifier is based on the study of biological neurons in human brain. Each neuron gets input and depending on the activation function is produces output. Human brain consists of numerous neurons each connected with one another to form a network. Analogous to this the neural network classifier consists of three layers of neurons. The first layer is a single input layer, the second layer is one or more hidden layer and the third layer is a single output layer. The input layer consists of neurons called as input neurons and the number of input neurons is mapped to the number of input features in the given training set. The hidden layer consists of hidden neurons each connected to the input neurons. The number of hidden layers is chosen based on trial and error method. The number of hidden neurons is usually less than are equal to the number of input neurons. The output layer consists of output nodes and the number of output nodes depends on the number of classes. Two classes can be represented by a single output node. More number of output nodes is included for predicting more number of classes. Figure 3 shows a neural network with three input neurons and three hidden neurons in a single hidden layer and a output layer with two neurons. Neural network classifier can handle noisy data. Normalization is a preprocessing technique use to scale the input data into new narrower range such as +1 to -1. The input feature values can be normalized and then it can be fed to the network to improve the results.

Weight and Bias

The input neurons are connected to the hidden neurons and the hidden neurons are connected to the output neurons. Each edge is assigned a weight and each hidden neuron is allocated a bias. The weight and bias are initialized to very small values such as +0.5 to -0.5, +1 to -1 etc.

Figure 3. Neural network

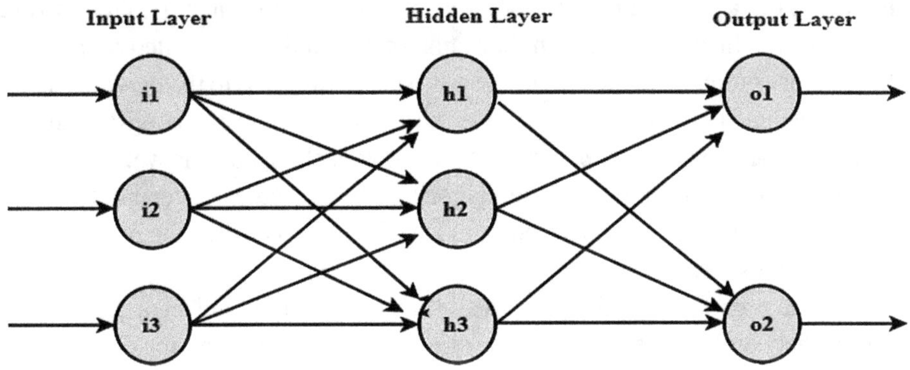

Activation Function

The input at the hidden layer or output layer is determined by the output from the previous layer. The input at the hidden node and the output nodes are calculated using Equation 5. O represents the output from a node, W is the weight, I is the input and B is the bias.

$$I = W * O + B \tag{5}$$

$$O = \frac{1}{1 + e^{-I}} \tag{6}$$

Activation function is used to determine the output at each node which will be eventually the input of the next node. It combines the input with weight and bias and determines the output for the next node. It is similar to our human brain responding in different ways for the same input because the brain chooses different activation function depending on the situation. Example is a person is hit by his teacher and by his younger one the response would not be same. Equation 6 shows the sigmoid function used to convert the input I to output O.

Back Propagation

The neural network is of different types and the most basic is the feed forward network. The input from each layer is fed to the next layers by applying suitable activation function. The output is fed forward and the final output is available at the output node. If the class value is discrete then the error is 1 when the predicted value is not the actual value and 0 otherwise. In the case of numerical class value the error is the difference between the actual output and the predicted output.

The error computed at the output layer is back propagated to the previous layers. The error value is estimated at each layer based on the error at the next layer. The weight and bias are adjusted based on the error at each layer. This weight and bias correction helps the back propagation algorithm to converge to actual output. This process is repeated for a predefined number of iterations or till the error value is lesser than threshold.

The same process is continued with all the input samples and an optimum value is set for the weight and bias. This network is used for predicting the class label of test data and future instances. Neural network classifier implicitly makes feature evaluation and ranks the features. The features that influence the target are assigned higher weights when compared to the features that have less influence on the target.

CONVOLUTIONAL NEURAL NETWORKS

Image processing using ANN without feature extraction is very tedious because of the huge number of pixels possible even in the case of smaller images. Convolutional Neural Networks (CNN) are used tin image and video processing that involves a very large number of pixels. In ANN every input unit is connected to every other unit and this would increase the number of weights and bias. Convolutional neural networks are also similar to ANN except for few differences. CNN has an input layer and output layer similar to ANN. But in place of hidden layer there are additional convolutional layer and pooling layer. To minimize the number of weights in the network the weights are shared among a group of pixels. The input image is convoluted with a smaller size of weight matrix. This would produce a convoluted image of size smaller than the input image. The convoluted image is given as input to the pooling layer and aggregation operations such as maximum, average etc. are used to determine the maximum or the average value among a group of pixels. The convolutional and pooling layers are repeated and the finally the activation function is used to produce a single class value at the output layer.

SUPPORT VECTOR MACHINE

Support Vector Machine (SVM) is a popular technique and it is widely used in image processing. SVM is used for classifying any type of data. They support both linear and non linear models for classification. Each sample is considered as a point in n dimensional space. SVM finds maximum margin hyperplane that separates the points belonging to different classes. There may many hyperplanes that can separate set of points but the objective is to choose the hyperplane that has maximum between the support vectors. Support vectors are points belonging to each class located on the marginal hyperplane.

$$y = w_0 + w_1 x_1 + w_2 x_2 + \ldots . + w_n x_n \tag{7}$$

Eq.7 represents the hyperplane used to separate data points. y stands for response variable i.e. the variable whose value is to be predicted. x1, x2.... Xn stands for the input vector of n dimensions. w0, w1, w2, ... wn is the weight vectors.

Figure 4 shows a set of points belonging to two different classes. The two classes are shown with different symbols. The two classes can be separated by a line with maximum margin. The boundary separating the two classes is called as maximal margin hyperplane.

K-NEAREST NEIGHBOUR CLASSIFIER

Basically the learners can be classified into two types lazy learner and eager learner. All the previous classifiers are eager learners because they generate model based on the training set and they are ready to predict the test data based on the generated model. Lazy learners are methods which do nothing until the test data is released. Once the test set is available it analyses the training set to determine the best class. K-Nearest Neighbour (KNN) classifier is a lazy learner. The classifier works by determining k best neighbours of the given test data. The neighbours are determined by any distance metrics such as Euclidean distance and the training data that are at the least distance is chosen as neighbours. k is an input parameter and the results of classification is dependent on the k value.

Figure 4. Lineraly separable points

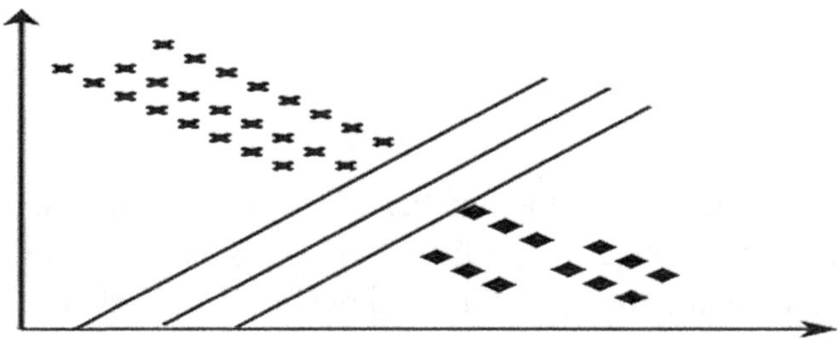

Data points in some real world problems cannot be separated using a linear separator. In this scenario the given data in one space is converted into another space. This would convert the data into linearly separable.

CLASSIFIER EFFICIENCY

Accuracy of the given classifier is estimated using the Equation 8. It is the ratio between the number of instances correctly classified by the classifier and the total number of instances in the data set.

$$Accuracy = \frac{Correctly\ classified\ instances}{Total\ instances} \tag{8}$$

Coverage is another parameter used to determine the quality of a rule and it is determined by the ration between the total number of instances triggered by the rule and the total number of instances.

$$Coverage = \frac{Total\ number\ of\ instances\ covered}{Total\ instances} \tag{9}$$

Precision and Recall are two other measures used to measure the accuracy of the classifier in a detailed manner and are given in Equation 10 and Equation 11. Recall is the ratio between number of true positives and the sum of true positive and false negative. Precision is the ration between the number of true positives and the sum of true positives and false positives.

$$Precision = \frac{TP}{TP + FP} \tag{10}$$

$$Recall = \frac{TP}{TP + FN} \tag{11}$$

TP, FP, TN, FN represents the number of true positives, false positives, true negatives and false negatives respectively. True positives (TP) are samples that are actually positive and the algorithm also predicted as positive. True negatives

(TN) are samples that are actually negative and also predicted as negative. False positives (FP) are samples that are actually negative but predicted as positive and False negatives (FN) are samples that are actually positive but predicted as negative.

FMeasure is a accuracy measure computed using recall and precision and is given in Equation 12.

$$FMeasure = \frac{2\, X\, recall\, X\, precision}{recall + precision} \tag{12}$$

Consider any type of scan image taken as input that will be used to predict a presence of a disease. MRI and CT images are typically of size 512 X 512. The first preprocessing required in any image classification technique is feature extraction.

Comparison of Classification Algorithms

This section compares the performance of the five classification algorithms namely decision tree classifier, Naive Bayes classifier, neural network classifier, support vector machine and K-Nearest Neighbour classifier. Table 2 shows the classification results of experiments conducted in Weka 3.8.1. Three feature extracted medical image data sets that are available at the UCI machine learning repository (Lichman, 2013) are used to compare the results. The performance is compared using five metrics such as Accuracy, Root Mean Square Error (RMSE), FMeasure, Precision and Recall. KNN shows the best performance on all the three data sets. Decision tree classifier also shows a comparatively better performance on all the three data sets.

SOLUTIONS AND RECOMMENDATIONS

The accuracy of the medical image classification should be near 100% because they are going to predict diseases. The accuracy of classifiers can be improved by incorporating optimization techniques to select the best features that can improve the accuracy of the results. Particle Swarm Optimization (PSO) can be combined with different classifiers to generate the best features. Clustering would also improve the accuracy of classification. The input feature set can be clustered using any of the clustering techniques. Research has proved that the classification results are better on clustered feature set.

Table 2. Comparison of classifiers

Data Set	Algorithm	Accuracy	RMSE	FMeasure	Precision	Recall
Breast Data	Decision Tree (J48)	66.04	0.3092	0.662	0.67	0.66
	Naive_Bayes	70.75	0.2946	0.707	0.713	0.708
	Multilayer Perceptron	64.15	0.283	0.647	0.657	0.642
	SVM	60.38	0.334	0.548	0.547	0.604
	KNN	71.7	0.2987	0.716	0.719	0.717
VetrebralColumn	Decision Tree (J48)	81.6	0.3742	0.812	0.812	0.816
	Naive_Bayes	77.74	0.4315	0.784	0.821	0.777
	Multilayer Perceptron	84.52	0.3257	0.842	0.842	0.845
	SVM	78.71	0.4614	0.77	0.786	0.787
	KNN	81.61	0.4273	0.819	0.824	0.816
EEG Eye State	Decision Tree (J48)	84.5	0.3778	0.845	0.845	0.845
	Naive_Bayes	46.77	0.7017	0.388	0.519	0.468
	Multilayer Perceptron	54.81	0.4977	0.536	0.539	0.548
	SVM	55.13	0.6699	0.392	0.753	0.551
	KNN	83.65	0.4043	0.836	0.836	0.837

FUTURE RESEARCH DIRECTIONS

Research work can be carried out three major ways. First way in which the research can continue further is improve the preprocessing techniques such as feature extraction and feature selection. Preprocessing techniques can be used to enhance the quality of the images before classification. Optimization techniques can be incorporated to retrieve the best features. The second way to further extend research in this area is to apply post processing techniques. The classifier model generated can be optimized to improve the accuracy further. Third way is to concentrate on the classification techniques used. Optimized classifiers can be used to improve the results. Similarly one classifier cannot be the best in all cases. Hence an ensemble of classifiers can be used to moderate the error caused by one classifier with another classifier which could perform better for those samples. Deep learning is also another recent area which can be employed to medical image classification. In the future deep learning can be combined with optimization techniques to improve the accuracy of classification.

CONCLUSION

Medical image classification is used in diagnosis of different types of fatal diseases possible in human organs. Feature extraction is the first step in the process of medical image classification. Geometric, color, texture features are extracted. Feature selection is used to select the most relevant features from the feature set. The relevant feature set is given as input to the classifier. The input feature set would be divided into training set and test set. The classifier would generate a model and the model is validated. If the accuracy is acceptable the model is applied to the new data. Various classification techniques such as decision tree, naive bayes, ANN, CNN, SVM, K-NN are discussed. Recently CNN is specifically used with image classification and improves accuracy. Various measures are used to estimate the performance of the classifiers.

REFERENCES

Ahmed, S. N., Osama, A. H., & Ahmed, H. K. (in press). A decision support system for Acute Leukaemia classification based on digital microscopic images. *Alexandria Engineering Journal.*

Andrés, G.-F., Ángel, F.-S., Oscar, C.-N., & Cornelio, Y. M. (2017). A machine learning approach to medical image classification: Detecting age-related macular degeneration in fundus images. *Computers & Electrical Engineering*, 1–12.

Bolun, C., Ling, C., & Yixin, C. (2013). Efficient ant colony optimization for image feature selection. *Signal Processing*, *93*(6), 1566–1576. doi:10.1016/j.sigpro.2012.10.022

Djaafar, Z., & Fouad, B. A. (2018). A cooperative swarm intelligence algorithm based on quantum-inspired and rough sets for feature selection. *Computers & Industrial Engineering*, *115*, 26–36. doi:10.1016/j.cie.2017.10.025

Geert, L., Thijs, K., Babak, E. B., Arnaud, A. A., Francesco, C., Mohsen, G., ... Clara, I. S. (2017). A survey on deep learning in medical image analysis. *Medical Image Analysis*, *42*, 60–88. doi:10.1016/j.media.2017.07.005 PMID:28778026

Geethu, M. M., & Monica, S. (2018). MRI based medical image analysis: Survey on brain tumor grade classification. *Biomedical Signal Processing and Control*, *39*, 139–161. doi:10.1016/j.bspc.2017.07.007

Han, J., & Kamber, M. (2011). *Data mining: Concepts and techniques* (3rd ed.). Burlington, MA: Elsevier.

Ivan, S., Ilya, I., & Andrey, F. (2016). New Approaches to Parallelization in Filters Aggregation Based Feature Selection Algorithms. *Procedia Computer Science, 101*, 45–52. doi:10.1016/j.procs.2016.11.007

Jefferson, T. O., Huei, D. L., Newton, S., Claudio, S. R. C., & Feng, C. W. (in press). Prototype System for Feature Extraction, Classification and Study of Medical Images. *Expert Systems with Applications*.

Lichman, M. (2013). *UCI Machine Learning Repository*. Irvine, CA: University of California, School of Information and Computer Science.

Majdi, M., & Seyedali, M. (2018). Whale optimization approaches for wrapper feature selection. *Applied Soft Computing*, *62*, 441–453. doi:10.1016/j.asoc.2017.11.006

Manizheh, G., & Mohammad-Reza, F. (2016). Feature selection using Forest optimization Algorithm. *Pattern Recognition*, *60*, 121–129. doi:10.1016/j.patcog.2016.05.012

Mark, S. N., & Alberto, S. A. (2008). *Feature Extraction and Image Processing* (2nd ed.). Elsevier.

Olga, D., Herbert, E., Anton, L., Michael, M., Daria, M., Roman, K., & Sergey, K. (in press). The classification of endoscopy images with persistent homology. *Pattern Recognition Letters*.

Rattanawadee, P., & Anongnart, S. (2015). Wrapper Feature Subset Selection for Dimension Reduction Based on Ensemble Learning Algorithm. *Procedia Computer Science*, *72*, 162–169. doi:10.1016/j.procs.2015.12.117

Ruijie, Z., Jian, S., Fushan, W., Xiong, L., & Arun, K. S. (in press). Medical image classification based on multi-scale non-negative sparse coding. *Artificial Intelligence in Medicine*.

Sergei, K. (2007). Using hard and soft models for classification of medical images. *Chemometrics and Intelligent Laboratory Systems*, *88*(1), 100–106. doi:10.1016/j.chemolab.2006.08.012

Sharif, M. S., Qahwaji, R., Ipsona, S., & Brahma, A. (2015). Medical image classification based on artificial intelligence approaches: A practical study on normal and abnormal confocal corneal images. *Applied Soft Computing*, *36*, 269–282. doi:10.1016/j.asoc.2015.07.019

Tanvi, G., Tapan, K. G., Gupta, R. K., & Panigrahi, B. K. (in press). Classification of patients with tumor using MR FLAIR images. *Pattern Recognition Letters*.

Witten, I. H., Frank, E., & Hall, M. A. (2011). *Data mining: Practical machine learning tools and techniques*. Burlington, MA: Morgan Kaufmann.

Yang, S., Weidong, C., Heng, H., Yun, Z., Yue, W., & David, D. (in press). FengLocality-constrained Subcluster Representation Ensemble for Lung Image Classification. *Medical Image Analysis*.

ADDITIONAL READING

Ashnil, K., Jinman, K., & David, L. (2017). An Ensemble of Fine-Tuned Convolutional Neural Networks for Medical Image Classification. *IEEE Journal of Biomedical and Health Informatics*, *21*(1), 31–40. doi:10.1109/JBHI.2016.2635663 PMID:28114041

Bankman, I. N. (Ed.). (2008). *Handbook of Medical Image Processing and Analysis* (2nd ed.). Elsevier.

Costaridou, L. (Ed.). (2005). *Medical Image Analysis Methods*. CRC Press. doi:10.1201/9780203500453

Dhawan, A. P. (2011). *Medical Image Analysis* (2nd ed.). Wiley-IEEE Press. doi:10.1002/9780470918548

Saima, A. L., & Rosziati, I. (2013). A Framework for Medical Images Classification Using Soft Set. *Procedia Technology*, *11*, 548–556. doi:10.1016/j.protcy.2013.12.227

Umbaugh, S. E., Wei, Y.-S., & Zuke, M. (1997). Feature extraction in image analysis. A program for facilitating data reduction in medical image classification. *IEEE Engineering in Medicine and Biology Magazine*, *16*(4), 62–73. doi:10.1109/51.603650 PMID:9241522

KEY TERMS AND DEFINITIONS

Classification: A supervised learning process used to predict the class label of a data instance. Training set is used to generate a model and it can be used to predict the class label of test data. An efficient model would be used to classify the new data.

Clustering: Clustering is a unsupervised learning technique used to group the data based on similarity of the data. The class/target of the data is not available and the algorithm itself will group the data into classes or groups.

Convolution Neural Network: This is a variant of ANN and consists of different types of hidden layers named as convolution layer, pooling layer. This network is more suitable to handle images and video. Original image is convoluted as it goes deeper in the network and at the last layer activation function can be used to produce a single class as output.

Feature Selection: The feature set of an image may contain irrelevant or redundant features. These features would hinder the performance of the classifier. The process of selecting the most relevant features from the given feature set is called feature selection.

Feature Set: It is the collection of features that are the internal characteristics of an image and are extracted using feature extraction techniques.

Forward Selection: This feature selection method starts with a empty set of features and at iteration it adds the best features to the resultant set. This is continued in a step by step manner by selecting the best features in every iteration.

Overfitting: The classifier accuracy would be extra ordinary when the test data and the training data are overlapping. But when the model is applied to a new data it will fail to show acceptable accuracy. This condition is called as overfitting.

Chapter 4
The Fundamentals of Medical Image Restoration

Kirti Raj Bhatele
Rustamji Institute of Technology, India

Devanshu Tiwari
Rajiv Gandhi Proudyogiki Vishwavidyalaya, India

ABSTRACT

This chapter simply encapsulates the basics of image restoration, various noise models, and degradation model including some blur and image restoration filters. The mining of high resolution information from the low-resolution images is a very vital task in several applications of digital image processing. In recent times, a lot of research work has been carried out in this field in order to improve the resolution of real medical images especially when the given images are corrupted with some kind of noise. The displayed images are the result of the various stages that might cause imperfections in the digital images, for instance the so-called imaging and capturing process can itself degrade the original scene. The imperfections present in the image need to be studied and analyzed if the noise present in the images is not modelled properly. There are different types of degradations which are considered such as noise, geometrical degradations, imperfections (due to improper illumination and color), and blur. Blurring in the images is generally caused by the relative motion between the camera and the original object being captured or due to poor focusing of an optical system. In the production of aerial photographs for remote sensing purposes, blurs are introduced by the atmospheric turbulence, aberrations in the optical system, and relative motion between the camera and the ground. Apart from the blurring effect, noise also creates imperfections in the images that corrupt the images under analysis. The noise may be introduced by several factors (e.g., medium, recording or capturing system, or by the quantization process). Due to this noise or blur present in the images, resolution needs to be improved and the image is to be restored from the geometrically warped, blurred, and noisy images.

DOI: 10.4018/978-1-5225-5876-7.ch004

INTRODUCTION

Normally images are generated to record or display vital information. Due to imperfections within the imaging and capturing process, however, the recorded photo always represents a degraded version of the authentic scene. The undoing of these imperfections is vital to among the subsequent photograph processing obligations. There exists a wide range of different degradations that want to be taken into account, masking as an instance noise, geometrical degradations (pin cushion distortion), illumination and coloration imperfections (beneath/over-exposure, saturation), and blur. Blurring is a form of bandwidth discount of a great photo because of the imperfect photo formation method. it is able to be as a result of relative motion between the digital camera and the unique scene, or with the aid of an optical system that is out of consciousness. Generally, the Blurs are introduced in the aerial photos which are produced for faraway sensing purposes due to the aberrations within the optical machine, atmospheric turbulence and relative motion among the dig cam and the floor. Such blurring isn't limited to optical photos, as an instance electron micrographs are corrupted with the aid of spherical aberrations of the electron lenses, and CT scans suffer from X-ray scatter. Similarly, to those blurring outcomes, noise usually corrupts any recorded image. Noise may be delivered by using the medium thru which the image is created (random absorption or scatter effects), with the aid of the recording medium (sensor noise), through size mistakes because of the constrained accuracy of the recording gadget, and by using quantization of the statistics for virtual storage. The field of image recuperation (now and again known as image deblurring or image deconvolution) is involved with the reconstruction or estimation of the uncorrupted photo from a blurred and noisy one. Basically, it attempts to carry out an operation at the picture that is the inverse of the imperfections within the picture formation gadget. Inside the use of image recuperation strategies, the traits of the degrading gadget and the noise are assumed to be known a priori. In realistic situations, however, one won't be able to reap these facts immediately from the image formation technique. The objective of blur identification is to predict the attributes of the imperfect imaging system from the discovered degraded images itself previous to the healing technique. The aggregate of image restoration and blur identification is frequently referred to as blind photo Deconvolution (Acharya & Ray, 2005).

GENERAL DEGRADATION MODEL

Image restoration is the process employed to "compensate for" or "undo" defects which degrade an image. Image Degradation occurs in many forms such as motion blur, noise, and camera mis focus. Especially in cases like motion blur, it is possible to come up with a very good estimate of the actual blurring function and "undo" the blur to restore the original image. In cases where the image is corrupted by noise, the best we may hope to do is to compensate for the degradation it caused. A general block diagram of a degradation model is shown in Figure 1.

Where *g* is the corrupted image obtained by passing the original image *f* through a low pass filter (blurring function) *b* and adding noise to it.

Degradation Model for Continuous Function

If an image f(x,y) is to be convolved with the two-dimensional impulse function δ(x,y), then it can be expressed as:

$$f(x,y)=\int_{-\infty}^{\infty}\int_{-\infty}^{\infty} f(x,y)\delta(x-x_0, y-y_0)dxdy \quad (1)$$

Using dummy variables α and β, we can represent

$$f(x,y)=\int_{-\infty}^{\infty}\int_{-\infty}^{\infty} f(\alpha,\beta)\delta(x-a,y-\beta)d\alpha d\beta \quad (2)$$

Now,

$$g(x,y)=H[f(x,y)]+w(x,y) \quad (3)$$

and

$$H=[\int_{-\infty}^{\infty}\int_{-\infty}^{\infty} f(\alpha,\beta)\delta(x-\alpha,y-\beta)d\alpha d\beta]+w(x,y) \quad (4)$$

Using H as linear operator, we can write

$$g(x,y)=\int_{-\infty}^{\infty}\int_{-\infty}^{\infty} H[f(\alpha,\beta)\delta(x-\alpha,y-\beta)d\alpha d\beta]+w(x,y) \quad (5)$$

As we know that f (α,β) is independent of x and y and hence, by applying the homogeneity property, the Equation can be expressed as:

Figure 1. Block diagram of a degradation model

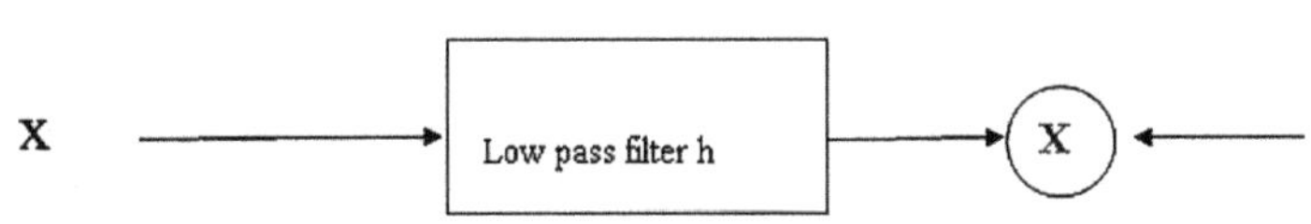

$$g(x,y)=\int^{\infty}_{-\infty}\int^{\infty}_{-\infty} f(\alpha,\beta)H[\delta(x-\alpha,y-\beta)d\alpha d\beta]+w(x,y) \tag{6}$$

When

$h(x,\alpha,y,\beta) = H[\delta(x-\alpha,y-\beta)]$

Then,

$$g(x,y)=\int^{\infty}_{-\infty}\int^{\infty}_{-\infty} f(\alpha,\beta)h(x,\alpha,y,\beta)d\alpha d\beta]+w(x,y) \tag{7}$$

The equation for degradation model for continuous image function f(x,y).

Degradation Model for Discrete Function

Due to wide use of digital signals in various computer-based applications, it is very important to formulate a discrete signal degradation model. Let two functions be f(x) and h(x) sampled uniformly to form arrays of dimensions A and B respectively (Dash, Ratnakar, Sa, Pankaj Kumar & Majhi, Banshidhar, 2011).

The discrete signal is in the range 0, 1, 2............(A-1) for f(x) and h(x) be in the range 0,1,2,.....(B-1) Avoiding any overlapping between the individual periods requires a common period M >=A+B-1 and for individual function f(x) and h(x), they are represented as $f_e(x)$ and $h_e(x)$ is given as

$$g_e(x)=\Sigma_{m=0}^{m-1} f_e(m)h_e(x-m) \tag{8}$$

for m = 0,1,2,....M-1.

ESTIMATION OF DEGRADATION FUNCTION

Degradation function may be estimated in mainly three important ways. This can be achieved using mathematical modeling, observation or experimentation. This degradation function is utilized during image restoration also termed as blind restoration method. The function required to be estimated for any given restoration image. If the observed image is expressed as g(x,y) and the constructed image is represented as f'(x,y),then neglecting the effect of noise, H can be estimated as:

$$H(u,v)=G(u,v)/F'(x,y) \tag{9}$$

where H(u,v), G(u,v) and F'(u,v) are the Fourier transformation of h(x,y), g(x,y) and f'(x,y) respectively.

NOISE MODELS

During the image acquisition and transmission of digital images, the noise does get incorporated largely. In the acquisition of an image, a variety of factors such as Environmental conditions, Light levels (low light conditions require high gain amplification) Sensor temperature (higher temp implies more amplification noise) does have an effect over the performance of imaging sensors. The images also get corrupted due to interference in the channel for instance lightning or other Atmospheric disturbances during the transmission of images. Altogether a different model has to be opted each time that accurately regenerate the spatial characteristics of the noise depending on the specific noise source (Gonzalez & Woods, 2008).

Gaussian Noise

The Gaussian noise models due to its mathematical tractability in both the frequency and spatial field are used regularly in practice. The following equation given below simply presents the Probability density function (PDF) of a Gaussian random variable z:

$$PG(Z) = \frac{1}{\sqrt{2\pi\sigma}} e^{\frac{-(-z-\mu)2}{2\sigma^2}} \tag{10}$$

In this equation, π means the mean value, the grey level is represented by z and σ represents the standard deviation. As the application of the Gaussian model is so handy that it is commonly used in scenarios where they are applicable at best (Gonzalez & Woods, 2008).

Rayleigh Noise

The Rayleigh noise PDF (Probability Density Function) is defined by

$$PR(z) = \begin{cases} \frac{2}{b}(z-a)e^{-\frac{(z-a)^2}{b}} & for\ z \geq a \\ 0 & for\ z \leq a \end{cases} \tag{11}$$

where the variance and mean are given by (also see Figure 2)

$$\mu = a + \sqrt{\pi b / 4}$$

$$\sigma^2 = \frac{b(4-\pi)}{4}$$

As the shape is skewed of the Rayleigh density function, so it is very useful for approximating histograms (skewed).

Erlang Noise

The Erlang noise PDF (Probability density function) is represented by the equation 12 given below

$$PR(z) = \begin{cases} \frac{a^b z^{b-1}}{(b-1)!} e^{-az} & \text{for } z \geq 0 \\ 0 & \text{for } z \leq 0 \end{cases} \quad (12)$$

where b is a positive integer and a>0,

The variance and mean are given by (also see Figure 3)

$$\mu = \frac{b}{a}$$

$$\sigma^2 = \frac{b}{a^2}$$

Figure 2. Rayleigh probability density function

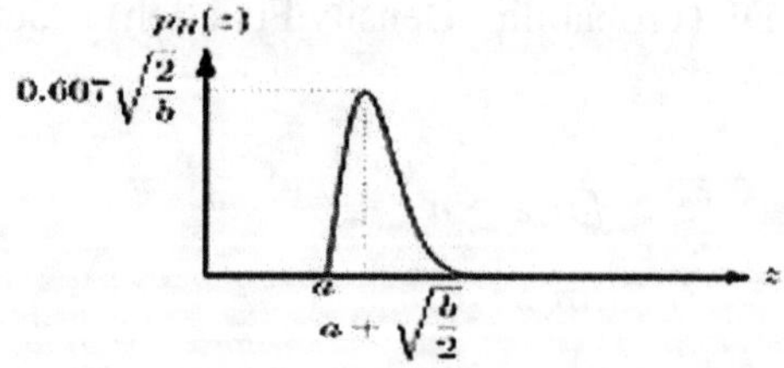

Figure 3. Erlang probability density function

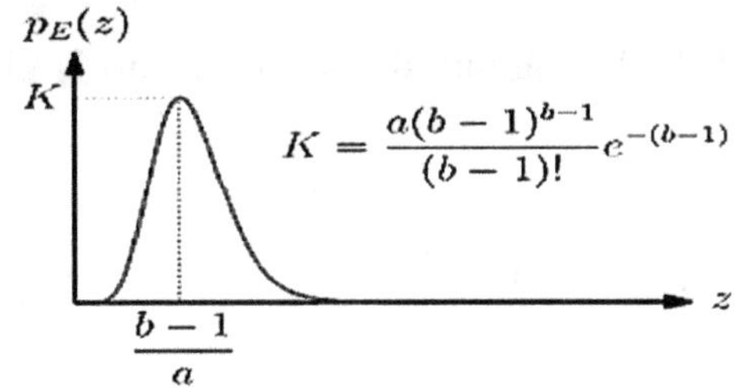

Exponential Noise

The Exponential noise PDF (Probability density function) is given by the equation given below

$$Pexp(z) = \begin{cases} ae^{-az} & for\ z \geq 0 \\ 0 & for\ z \leq 0 \end{cases} \tag{13}$$

where a>0.

The variance and mean of the density function are

$$\mu = \frac{1}{a}$$

$$\sigma^2 = \frac{1}{a^2}$$

A special case of the Erlang noise model with b = 1 is the exponential noise model shown in Figure 4.

Figure 4. The probability density function of Exponential noise

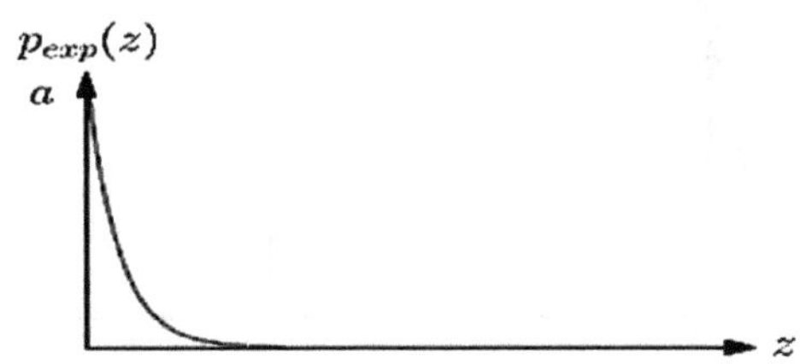

Uniform Noise

The Uniform noise PDF (Probability density function) is given by the equation given below

$$PU(z) = \begin{cases} \dfrac{1}{b-a} & for\, a \le z \le b \\ 0 & for\, otherwise \end{cases} \quad (14)$$

The variance and mean of the density function are (also see Figure 5)

$$\mu = \frac{a+b}{2}$$

$$\sigma^2 = \frac{(b-a)^2}{12}$$

Impulse (Salt and Pepper) Noise

The bipolar impulse noise model PDF (Probability density function) is given by the equation given below

$$\text{P I (z)} = \begin{cases} P_a & for\, z = a \\ P_b & for\, z = b \\ 0 & otherwise \end{cases} \quad (15)$$

Figure 5. The probability density function of Uniform noise

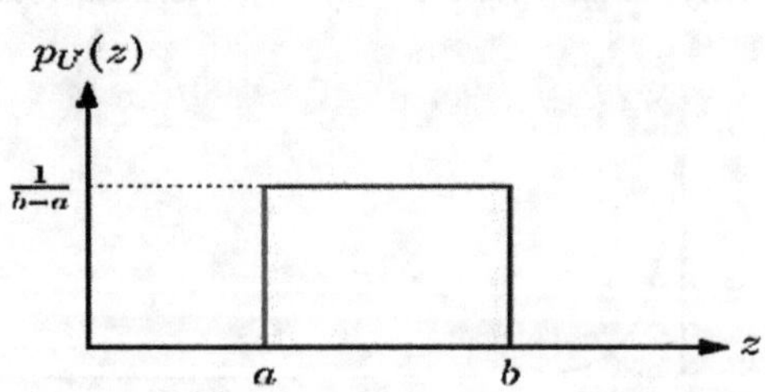

The grey-level b appears as a light dot (salt) in the image only if If b *is greater than a.* On the other hand, a will appear as pepper (dark dot). The PDF (Probability density function) is called unipolar only if either $P_a = 0$ or $P_b = 0$. Because impulse corruption is generally large compared to the signal strength, the assumption is usually that a and b are converted into digit as saturated values thus white (salt) and black (pepper) (see Figure 6).

One of the useful means for approximating a broad range of noise corruption situations found in practice is presented by the noise models above. For an instance: The source of the noise (Gaussian)in images is mostly because of the sensor noise induced due to the high temperature and electronic circuit noise or illumination. The Noise model which is Rayleigh noise model is actually utilized to exemplify the noise phenomena in range images thus the Exponential and Erlang noise models find their application in Laser imaging. Mostly the Impulse noise occurs in scenarios where high transients (faulty switching) take place (Fan & Nagy, 2010).

FILTERS AND IMAGE QUALITY

The various Filters used for filtering the noise are the median filter; max filter, min filter and linear average filter etc. are preferably employed for the restoration of the pixels by using the local information from the neighborhood of that pixel. These types of filters are known as the local filters. When the filters perform restoration of each pixel by simply using information from the entire image is called global filters. The ultimate source of Blurring in images is due to the optical restrictions within an imaging device, which has a point spread function (PSF). A blurred image of a single point source of light is the PSF and its additive noise power spectrum simply covers the whole frequency domain equally. Some parameters based on statistics such as Peak Signal – to Noise Ratio (PSNR) and Mean Squared Error (MSE) play a very important role in restoring Images and assessing their quality.

Figure 6. The probability density function of bipolar impulse noise

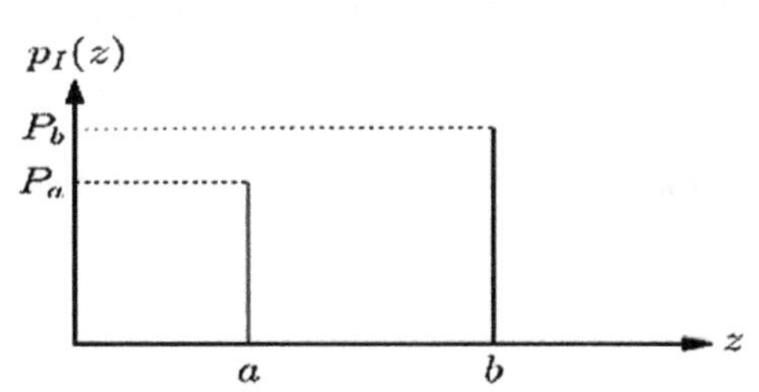

In order to measure the image quality for the same given image simply the results are compared because one image with inferior relative error may look not better as compare to another image with superior relative error. The filter performance greatly replies on the signal-to-noise ratio of the output and an objective parameter (PSNR) are used here which is defined as:

$$PSNR\ (dB)=10log_{10}(255^2/MSE) \quad (16)$$

And MSE is defined as

$$MSE=1/MN\Sigma_{X=1}^{M}\ \Sigma_{Y=1}^{N}\ [f(x,y)]=f'(x,y)]^2 \quad (17)$$

Occasionally for the purpose of performance evaluation, an improved signal-to-noise ratio (ISNR) is also used. This improved signal-to-noise ratio (ISNR) simply comes out with the improved SNR values especially with regard to the corrupt image by the restoration filter.

BLUR MODEL

The convolution of an ideal image with a 2D point spread function (PSF) can be modeled as blurring of images. Normally if a point source or single intensity point is present in a image then this is recorded as a spread-out intensity pattern. Eventually at every spatial location, the image is blurred in the same way and because of the local blurs or rotational blurs; the PSFs do not follow this.

The blurring of images is a spatial process of continuous type. As the algorithms of restoration and identification are at all times based on the discrete images (spatially), the blur models are expressed in continuous forms followed by discrete or sampled functions. The assumed sampling rate is to be just enough in order to reduce the aliasing errors. Any blur model PSF d(x,y) should satisfy the following constraints:

1. d (x,y) takes on positive values only.
2. The point spread function d(x,y) is also real-valued for real-valued images,.
3. The imperfections in the image formation process are modeled as passive operations.

For spatially continuous blurs, the PSF should satisfy the following conditions:

$$\int_{\infty}^{\infty} d\left(x,y\right)dxdy = 1 \tag{18}$$

And for spatially discrete blurs,

$$\sum_{n1=0}^{N-1}\sum_{n2=0}^{m-1} d\left(x,y\right) = 1 \tag{19}$$

If no any blur is apparent, then the spatially continuous PSF can be modeled as a Dirac delta function as under:

$$d\left(x,y\right) = \delta\left(x,y\right) \tag{20}$$

And the spatially discrete PSF as a unit pulse given as follows

$$d(x,y) = \delta(x,y) = \begin{pmatrix} 2 & if\ x = y = 0 \\ 0 & elsewhere \end{pmatrix} \tag{21}$$

The amount of spreading in continuous image is smaller than the sampling grid used in getting the discrete image.

Motion Blur

The motion blur of different types can be distinguished on the basis of the relative motion between the scene and the recording device. This relative motion may be in the form of a rotation, translation, sudden change of scale or some combinations of these motions. If the sight is to be pictured, then it converts relative to the capturing device at a steady velocity 'v' relative to an angle of $\varnothing$ radians along the horizontal axis throughout the interval of exposure (0, $t_{exposure}$). In terms of length of motion defined as l, the PSF is given as follows:

$$d\left(x,y;l,\varnothing\right) = \begin{pmatrix} 1/l & if\ \sqrt{a^2+b^2} = -\tan\varnothing \\ 0 & elsewhere \end{pmatrix} \tag{22}$$

MEDICAL IMAGE RESTORATION

The phenomenon, which deals with the restoration of medical images, corrupted with imperfections termed as Medical image restoration. Let's assume that the captured image be represented by g(x, y) and the linear restoration filter point spread function is denoted by h(x,y), then the restored image is represented as

$$f(x,y)= h(x,y)* g(x,y) \tag{23}$$

This can be expressed in spectral domain as

$$F(u,v) = H(u,v)G(u,v) \tag{24}$$

Improvement in the quality of the restored image i.e. recorded blurred image is measured with the help of SNR, i.e., signal-to-noise ratio after the application of image restoration to the images. This parameter is defined as

$$SNR_s = 10\log_{10}\left(\frac{Varianceoftheidealimagef(x,y)}{Varianceofthedifferenceimageg(x,y) - f(x,y)}\right) dB$$

The restored image SNR is defined as

$$SNR_{f'} = 10\log_{10}\left(\frac{Varianceoftheidealimagef(x,y)}{Varianceofthedifferenceimagef'(x,y) - f(x,y)}\right) dB$$

The SNR improvement is measured as

$$\Delta SNR = SNR_{f'} - SNR_s$$

$$= 10\log_{10}\left(\frac{Varianceoftheidealimageg(x,y) - f(x,y)}{Varianceofthedifferenceimagef'(x,y) - f(x,y)}\right) dB$$

Inverse Filter

An Inverse filter can be defined as a linear filter whose point spread function h_{uv} (x,y) is the inverse of the blurring function (x,y) as follows:

$$h\left(inv\right)\left(x,y\right)*d\left(x,y\right)=\sum_{k1=0}^{N-1}\sum_{k2=0}^{M-1}hinv\left(k1,k2\right)d\left(x-k1,y-k2\right)=\delta\left(x,y\right) \tag{25}$$

Even though, it is very complex to design and in above equation which is the spectral counterpart shows the solution to the problem related to the design as follows:

$$H_{inv}\ (u,v) = 1/D\ (u,v) \tag{26}$$

The blur PSF as a priori knowledge is the only required information for the implementation of this filter.

BLUR IDENTIFICATION

The PSF can be analyzed and even without a given knowledge of PSF, Image restoration can be achieved especially when the object distance, object motion and camera motion are known. The blur identification procedure will estimate the length and direction of the motion if the blur is due to the motion.

The point spread function d(x,y) as a small set of coefficients within a given finite support can be explained with the help of Blur models. This will allow the estimation of PSF coefficients. The Blur PSF values can be modeled with help of different sizes square matrix for example 6*6 or 3*3. The nine or thirty-six PSF coefficients is required for the blur identification respectively (Iyer & Gogawale, 2006).

Spectral Blur Estimation

The blurs can be categorized as the motion and out-of-focus blur possessing spectral zeros. The structure of zeros patterns can be used to predict the type and degree of blur within these two classes. The Fourier transform of restoration filter function G(u,v) consist of special zeros of PSF.

The computation of two dimensional Cepstrum of image g(x,y) is another method of identifying motion blur. The inverse Fourier transform of the logarithm of |G(u,v)| is the Cepstrum.

$$g'(x,y)=F^{-1}\{Log\ |G(u,v)|\} \tag{27}$$

Where F^{-1} is the inverse Fourier transform operator.

The g'(x, y) has got a large spike at a distance L^m as the origin, if the noise is not considered. Around the centre of the image, these spikes quite visible as bright spots.

Blur Estimation Using Maximum Likelihood

The individual coefficient of the point spread function are very difficult to estimate, in case PSF does not have spectral zero properties or out-of-focus blur cannot be assumed or if the blur motion. By using the maximum likelihood estimation of blur is particularly used for the unknown coefficient above mentioned problem is resolved. If stochastic knowledge is not available especially about the parameter to be estimated then in this case, a popular method of parameter estimation is the maximum likelihood estimation. This method initiates with the assumption that the image is ideal that eventually can be described with the two dimensional model of autoregressive whose parameter are variance σ_x^2 of white noise and prediction coefficient $a_{ij,..}$ As both the image model noise v (x, y) and the observation noise w(x,y) are assumed as Gaussian distribution (Jayaraman, Esakkirajan. & Veerakima). Then, the observed image log-likelihood function can be formulated with the given image model and blur parameters as follows:

$$L(\varnothing) = -\sum_U \sum_V \log p(u,v) + \frac{|G(u,v)|^2}{P(u,v)} \tag{28}$$

where $\varnothing$ is the set of parameter to be estimated as

$$\varnothing = \{aij, {\sigma_v}^2, (x,y), {\sigma^2}_w\} \tag{29}$$

And P (u,v) is defined as

$$P(u,v) = {\sigma_v}^2 \frac{|D(u,v)|^2}{|1 - A(u,v)|^2} + {\sigma^2}_w \tag{30}$$

where A(u,v) is the discrete 2D Fourier transforms of $a_{ij.}$

The ultimate purpose of the maximum likelihood blur estimation method is to come across the values for the parameters a_{ij}, σ_v^2, $d(x, y)$, σ_w^2, that can enhance the log-likelihood function $L(\theta)$. But this method of maximum likelihood suffers with the problems that need non trivial solutions; the function of log-likelihood has many local maxima and is highly non-linear which in turn make optimization very hard to perform. Various approach exist to optimize $L(\theta)$ for a given reasonable initial estimate of θ. There are two important steps involve in this method which are follows:

- **E-Step (Expectation Step):** A restore image $f'\in_x(x,y)$ is computed for a given estimate of the parameter θ by using wiener restoration filter whose calculation of power spectrum can be made with the help of given image model parameters such as a_{ij}, and σ_v^2.
- **M-Step (Maximization Step):** The restoration of image is carried out in the Expectation step and a new estimate of θ can be computed. Hence the restored image $f'\in_x(x,y)$ the image model parameter a_{ij} and σ_v^2 can be estimated directly as

$$g(x,y) \approx d(x,y) * f_e^{'}(x,y) \tag{31}$$

The maximum likelihood method procedure is illustrated with the help of the Figure 7.

SUPER RESOLUTION METHOD

The method which is used to restore the high resolution images from the interpolated low resolution noisy observations is known as the Super resolution method. The Super resolution method primarily based on the estimation of the accurate sub pixel

Figure 7. The method of Maximum Likelihood blurs identification

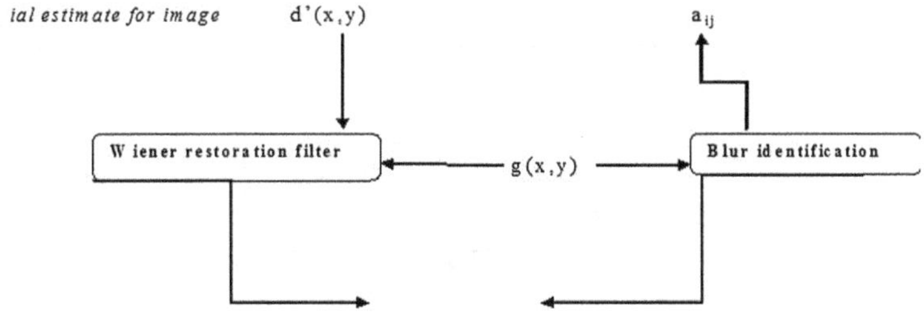

motion. This method is categorised broadly into two types- spatial domain techniques and frequency domain techniques (Farsiu, Robinson, Elad, & Milanfar). Generally for performing the low resolution image enhancement, it's the Bilinear or bicubic interpolation processes are used. The process of restoration is illustrated in Figure 8.

The image restoration method consists of three stages which are image registration, image fusion and image de-blurring. In order to find out the geometric transformation between two or more views of the same scene, image registration is used. In between the points in one image and the points in second image, a unique association is found and both the points of the images represent the same physical point in the scene. This fusion play a important role in the extraction of information acquired in several domains and is employed to combine the multi-temporal, complimentary multisensory and multi-view information into one new image. A number of fusion applications exist especially for medical imaging in order to evaluate the CT, MRI and PET images.

Richardson-Lucy Method

An algorithm was developed specially to restore the blurred and noisy images efficiently are the Richardson-Lucy Algorithm. The Richardson-Lucy method was devised specially for the data comprising of countable events, discrete, which follow a Poisson distribution. The likelihood of performing convolution in between the

Figure 8. Image Restoration process for super resolution

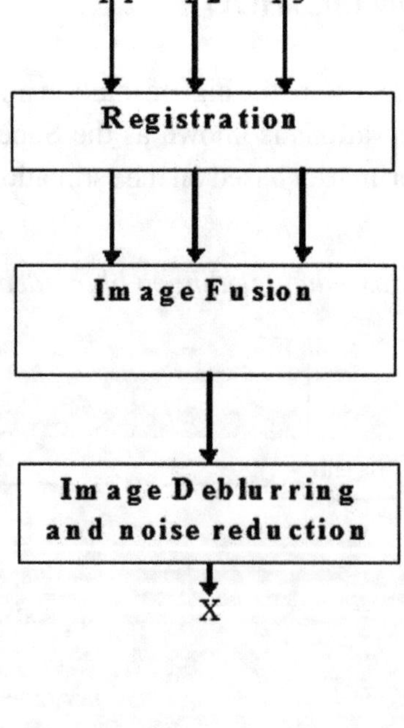

resulting image along with the PSF is maximizes by this method (Jain, 2005). By using the multiplicative corrections, the non-linear maximum likelihood function is minimized iteratively which is given below:

$$f'_{k+1}(x,y)=f'_k(x,y)[h(-x,-y)*(g(x,y)\,/\,h(x,y)*f'(x,y))] \tag{32}$$

In it, the symbol '*' represents the convolution and f' is used to estimate of the degraded image.

A noise amplification problem is the only limitation of Richardson-Lucy algorithm. The degradation model in the frequency domain can be written as

$$G(u,v)=F(u,v)\,H(u,v) + N(u,v) \tag{33}$$

If the PSF is known and assuming the noise component is to be negligible or zero, then

$$F(u,v)=G(u,v)/H(u,v) \tag{34}$$

In order to minimize the error function, the stochastic least mean square filtering operation is used which is expressed as:

$$e^2=min\ E[\ \{f(x,y)-f'(x,y)\}^2] \tag{35}$$

APPLICATIONS OF IMAGE RESTORATION

Image restoration is important in various applications. Some of the major applications are briefly explained below:

1. **Medical Imaging:** In the field of medical imaging and its application for instance computed tomography (CT) and magnetic resonance imaging (MRI), as the acquisition of multiple images is possible while the resolution quality is limited. Thus, the phenomenon of image restoration helps in enhancing the accuracy of surgeon.
2. **Satellite Imaging:** Primarily remote sensing (one of the Satellite imaging -based applications) are very significant applications when it comes to the analysis of data related to remotely sensed images and satellite images. In order to improve the resolution of the captured satellite images through low cost satellite system, Multispectral image restoration can be applied.

CONCLUSION

Generally, in this chapter the concepts related to image restoration are discussed briefly. As Image restoration is a process used for restoring the original images which are corrupted and in which imperfections are analysed. Image enhancement and Image restoration are not at all the same thing because certain features of the image are emphasised, thereby making the image more pleasing to the observer using image enhancement. The exact image modelling plays a key role in the effective image restoration which finds an approximation as close as possible in some measure to the original image from a blurred and noisy image. This chapter also illustrate the degradation function which can be estimated in three different ways namely experimentation, observation and mathematical modelling. This chapter also discuss about different types of noise models. The presented noise models above provide a useful tool for approximating a broad range of noise corruption situations found in practice. For example: Gaussian noise arises in images due to sensor noise caused by poor illumination and/or high temperature and electronic circuit noise. The Rayleigh noise model is used to characterise noise phenomena in range images Exponential and Erlang noise models find their application in Laser imaging. Impulse noise takes place in situations where high transients (faulty switching) occur. Filters including median filter, linear average filter, max filter and min filter, etc. are used to restore the pixels that use information from the local neighbourhood of pixels. These filters are referred to as local filters. The filters using information from the entire image to restore each pixel are called global filters. The last section of the chapter is dedicated to the blurring of images which is modelled as convolution of an ideal image with a 2D point spread function. When the ideal image f(x,y) consists of a single intensity point or point source, this is recorded as a spread out intensity pattern. Lastly the chapter discuss the Super resolution method which is used to restore the high resolution images from the interpolated low resolution noisy observations. This method depends on the accurate sub pixel motion estimation. Super resolution restoration method is broadly categorised into two types- Frequency domain techniques and spatial domain techniques. Finally the image restoration is very useful in medical imaging such as computed tomography and Magnetic resonance imaging (MRI). Since the acquisition of multiple images is possible while the resolution quality is limited.

REFERENCES

Acharya & Ray. (2005). *Image processing: Principles and Applications*. Wiley-Inter Science.

Choras, R. S. (2007). Image feature Extraction techniques and their applications for CBIR and Biometrics system. *International Journal of Biology and Biomedical Engineering, 1*(1), 231-238.

Dash, R., Sa, P. K., & Majhi, B. (2011). *Spatial Variant Deblurring of Images*, International Journal of Computational Vision and Robotics. *Inderscience Publishers, 2*(1), 80–88.

Fan, Y. W., & Nagy, J. G. (2010). Synthetic boundary conditions for image blurring. *Linear Algebra and Its Applications, 434*(11), 2244–2268. doi:10.1016/j.laa.2009.12.021

Farsiu, S., Robinson, D., Elad, M., & Milanfar, P. (2004). Advances and Challenges in Super resolution. *International Journal of Imaging Systems and Technology, 14*(2), 47–57. doi:10.1002/ima.20007

Gonzalez, R., & Woods, R. (2008). *Digital image processing* (3rd cd.). Prentice Hall of India.

Gonzalez, R. C., & Woods, R. E. (2002). *Digital Image processing* (2nd ed.). Prentice Hall of India.

Iyer, S., & Gogawale, S. V. (2006). *Image enhancemement and restoration techniques in digital image processing*. Computer Society of India Communications.

Jain, A.K. (2005). *Fundamentals of Digital image Processing* (4th ed.). Pearson Education.

Jayaraman, S., Esakkirajan, S., & Veerakima, T. (n.d.). *Digital Image Processing* (3rd ed.). Tata McGraw Hill Education Private Limited.

Lokhande, R., Arya, K.V., & Gupta, P. (2006). Identification of parameters and restoration of motion blurred images. *Proceedings of the 2006 ACM Symposium on Applied Computing, 9*, 301-305.

Chapter 5
Optimal Feature Selection and Extraction for Eye Disease Diagnosis

Alli P.
Velammal College of Engineering and Technology, India

S. K. Somasundaram
PSNA College of Engineering and Technology, India

ABSTRACT

Ophthalmologists utilize retinal fundus images of humans for the detection, diagnosis, and prediction of many eye diseases. Automatic scrutiny of fundus images are foremost apprehension for ophthalmologists and investigators. The manual recognition of blood vessels is most deceptive because the blood vessels in a fundus image are multifaceted and with low contrast. Unearthing of blood vessels proffers information on pathological transformation and can smooth the progress of rating diseases severity or mechanically diagnosing the diseases. The manual recognition method turns out to be annoying. Consequently, the automatic recognition of blood vessels is also more significant. For extracting the vessel in fundus images unswerving and habitual methods are obligatory. The proposed methodology is designed to effectively diagnose the eye disease by performing feature extraction succeeded by feature selection and to improve the performance factors such as feature extraction ratio, feature selection time, sensitivity, and specificity when compared to the state-of-art methods.

DOI: 10.4018/978-1-5225-5876-7.ch005

INTRODUCTION

Insulin resistance or its deficiency may result various complication such as diabetic mellitus (DM), Diabetic Retinopathy (DR). The DR is a diabetic eye disease, where damage occurs in the retina due to diabetes. The Retina of the human eye gets damaged owing to change in the blood vessels inside the eye. DR affects up to 80% of all diabetic patients and also usually it affects both the eyes. The fundus image of an eye gives the internal structure of the eye including the normal features like macula, fovea, blood vessels, optic disc, etc. and abnormal features like microaneurysms, hemorrhages, Hard and Soft exudates, etc. Programmed analysis of fundus images turned out to be a concern for the investigators and ophthalmologists to diagnose DR at an early stage and prevent vision loss for the patient.

DR can be classified on the damage to blood vessels as: Non-proliferative DR (NPDR) and Proliferative DR (PDR). NPDR is caused by damaged blood vessels in the retina which begins to leak addition fluid and small quantity of blood in to the internal parts of the eye. PDR Occurs when there is not enough flow of blood due to the close of blood vessels inside the retina. To supply blood, the retina automatically corrects itself by developing new blood vessels, known as neovascularization. The new blood vessels are abnormal and don't supply the retina with proper blood flow.

Ophthalmologists utilize Retinal Fundus images of humans for the detection diagnosis and prediction of many eye diseases. Automatic scrutiny of Fundus images are foremost apprehension for ophthalmologists and investigators. Most of the hemorrhage based Fundus image recognition has principally categorized the hemorrhages and microaneurysm into a cluster. The widespread technique used for recognition of hemorrhages is morphological method, which is used for mining image features by grouping of various techniques.

The manual recognition of blood vessels is most deceptive because the blood vessels in a Fundus image are multifaceted and with low contrast. Unearthing of blood vessels proffers information on pathological transformation and can smooth the progress of rating diseases severity or mechanically diagnosing the diseases. The manual recognition method turns out to be annoying. Consequently, the automatic recognition of blood vessels is also more significant. For extracting the vessel in fundus images unswerving and habitual methods are obligatory. The proposed methodology effectively diagnose DR diseases and improves the performance factors such as extraction feature ratio, feature selection time, sensitivity and specificity

RELATED WORKS

All eye blood vessels congregate at the Optic Disc (OD) whose detection also plays an imperative role in diagnosing the eye diseases. Existing template-based methodology (Aquino et al., 2010) uses Circular Hough Transform and edge detection techniques to segment the OD. An Optic Disc containing sub-image is wheedled out and its surrounding region are chosen but it does not automatically localize the selected features. An optimally comfortable morphological operator is used for exudates detection on diabetic retinopathy patients and low-contrast images (Sopharak et al., 2008). These mechanically detected exudates are validated by associating with expert ophthalmologists hand-drawn ground-truths but do not insert more detailed features to the system.

Exudates based diabetic macular edema detection in Fundus images (Giancardo et al., 2012) does not employ machine learning methods to categorize candidate exudates into true positives and false positives. Macular edema detection require extensive ground truth segmentations by experts which is problematic to attain and also fails to create a competitive diabetic retinopathy selection system to transparently diagnose the disease state. Combining algorithms (Qureshi et al., 2012) for automatic detection of optic disc and macula in Fundus images is used to discover the macula center. Combining algorithm arise issue in improving the sensitivity of tasks, such as the detection of the optic disc and blood vessels, and also fails to localize faint and small exudates.

The creation of 3D models helps visualizing interpretation and might serve up for perfunctory models (Manivannan et al., 2017). 3D models of Fundus images have become increasingly popular, providing more or less accurate reconstructions of volumes, spatial distribution, orientation and size of images. A set of features based on morphology (Rossant et al., 2011) and intensity are measured on each region-grown object. The assessment of these feature candidates are graded as either a factual or a spurious object.

Fast OD localization techniques (Mahfouz & Fahmy, 2010) experience from unfeasible-high computation times. Directionality of the retinal vessels and intensity profile image features is used but accuracy reduced in image feature extraction. Automatic Retinal Lesion Detection as combines feature information contained within the images in a framework and effortlessly extendible to diverse types of retinal lesions. Development of an automatic Diabetic Retinopathy (DR) screening system not makes the grade to notice the presence of many abnormalities related to DR.

Automatic Retinal Lesion Detection method (ARLD) (Acharya, 2013; Rocha et al., 2012) combines feature information contained within the images in a framework and effortlessly extendible to diverse types of retinal lesion. The method uses a training set where ophthalmic specialists have marked regions of interest within the retinal image that contain the lesion. The DR-related lesion detection is able to learn images containing lesion and detect retinal lesion automatically. The decision-support approach requires pinpointing the location of each lesion to allow the specialist to evaluate the image for diagnosis.

An Ensemble-based framework (Antal & Hadju, 2010; Lazar & Hadju, 2013) that ascertains microaneurysms which relies on a set of pairs, from which a search algorithm selects an optimal combination. An exhaustive quantitative analysis is also given to prove the superiority of over individual algorithms. Candidate extractors were obtained for the original images without any preprocessing. The Candidate extraction is accomplished by grayscale diameter closing and proved to efficient in ascertaining microaneurysms.

The distribution and variability of vessels around each image point are estimated using the concept of entropy of vascular directions in combining vascular and intensity information method (Medonc et al., 2013). The use of the entropy map for evaluating the quality of the vascular segmentation and deciding on the criteria for estimating the localization of the disc are particularly vital. Initial OD position is validated if all other local maxima of entropy occurring indifferent image locations (Goatman et al., 2011). Final post-processing phase is applied to restricted region around the estimated position of the disc, in order to get the final OD location.

To replace the human graders an Automated Diabetic Retinopathy Image Assessment Systems (ADRIAS) (Tufail et al., 2017) was introduced. Manually graded retinal images were processed by 3 ARIAS: iGradingM, Retmarker, and EyeArt. Discrepancies between ARIAS and human graded results were noted for observations. The sensitivity and the specificity factors are greatly improved.

Rejection-based strategy (Ram et al, 2011) aims very early clutter labeling, which is beneficial to the overall detection. This methodology uses images acquired in different settings with different cameras. It facilitates the progressive rejection of clutter responses and gives prime importance to clutter rejection rather than signal microaneurysms detection. The responses classified as clutter is removed from further consideration and retain the remaining responses as putative targets.

The Optical Coherence Tomography (OCT) method (Botto de Barros Garcia et al., 2017) bestow a swift and non-instrument method to appraise retinal structures at a minuscule stage. The various concepts for the diabetic retinopathy diagnosis using OCT were discussed. OCT provides in-depth details about the retinal image which in turn makes it more efficient method in detecting eye related diseases.

The existing methods not succeeded in recognizing all eye pathologies like microaneurysms, hemorrhages, neovascularization, etc. The present methods unable to separate pathologies from small vessels in retinal fundus image and does not employ machine learning methods to pigeonhole candidate exudates into diabetic retinopathy. Also there is a scope for the improvement of performance factors such as sensitivity, specificity, classification accuracy and ranking efficiency.

PROPOSED METHODOLOGY

The proposed method is organized to effectively diagnose the eye disease by performing feature extraction succeeded by feature selection and to improve the performance factors such as extraction ratio, feature selection time, sensitivity and specificity.

A Mathematical Transformation based Feature Extraction (MTFE) is employed to perform effective feature extraction process. Mathematical transformation is a vital tool in extraction, filtering and segmentation in medical images. The morphological gradient which is the difference between dilation and erosion of the images is recorded to extract the images from retinal fundus images. Subsequently, a feature clustering algorithm is applied to extract most salient features including pathologies from the retinal images. From the extracted image, the pathological features are selected based on feature clustering algorithm.

After developing feature extraction framework, a Deep Learning based Feature Selection (DLFS) procedure is developed. Deep learning is a modern machine learning methodology which employs a manifold of compound layers of processing units for feature extraction and transformation. The most important attribute of deep learning is its capability to extrapolate new features from an inadequate set of features in a training set. The ability of deep learning to manipulate unlabeled features helps Ophthalmologists to minimize time in diagnosing the disease. In turn it allows the Ophthalmologist to analyze with more complex feature sets when compared to many other machine learning tools.

The deep learning procedure effectively selects pathologies and classifies them without any expert intervention. The determination product is able to localize weak and tiny exudates. The high accuracy of this procedure on retinal fundus images shows much fruitful result for developing sensible computerized eye disease diagnosis system. The Figure 1 illustrates the architecture diagram for the proposed methodology.

Figure 1. The architecture diagram for the proposed methodology

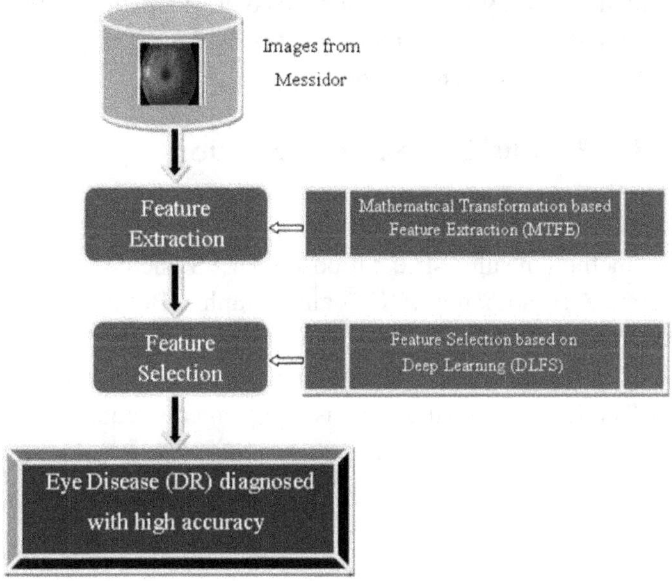

RESULTS AND DISCUSSIONS

The proposed methodology is implemented in MATLAB environment using Messidor database. The Messidor database is a public database widely used as benchmark for computer abetted judgements of diabetic retinopathy. The 1200 eye fundus color images of the posterior pole for the Messidor database were assimilated by 3 ophthalmologic departments using a color video 3CCD camera with a 45 degree field of view. The images were captured using 8 bits per color plane at 1440*960, 2240*1488 or 2304*1536 pixels. 800 images out of 1200 images were acquired with pupil dilation and 400 without dilation. The 1200 images are packaged in 3 sets, one per ophthalmologic department. Each set is alienated into 4 zipped sub sets each holding 100 images.

Experimental Results by Feature Extraction

By using Messidor database, the proposed method results are compared with existing method results. The proposed MTFE method is compared with Automated Diabetic Retinopathy Image Assessment Software (ADRIAS) (Tufail et al., 2017), Optical Coherence Tomography (OCT) angiography (Botto de Barros Garcia et al., 2017) and Gray Level and Moment Invariant Based Features & NN method (GLMIFNN) (Marin et al., 2011).

The Figure 2 shows that proposed MTFE method for feature extraction improves the feature extraction ratio by 5-7% compared to ADRAIS method, 10-12% compared to OCT method and 8-12% compared to GLMIFNN method. The comparison of feature extraction ratio is shown in Table 1.

Experimental Results by Feature Selection

By using Messidor database, the proposed DLFS method results are compared with existing method results. The proposed DLFS method is compared with Optical Coherence Tomography (OCT) angiography (Botto de Barros Garcia et al., 2017), Multi-Scale Retinal Vessel Segmentation (MSRVS) method (Nayebifar & Moghaddam, 2013), and Fuzzy Histon Segmentation (FHS) method (Mookiah et al., 2013b). The feature selection time is represented in eqn. (1)

$$\text{The feature selection time} = \sum_{i=1}^{n} f_i^T \left(FT\right) \quad (1)$$

where f_i^T refers to the features, f_i selected in Time (T) and FI refers to the feature selected from Fundus Image (FI). The time (T) is measures in terms of milliseconds (ms).

The Figure 3 shows the proposed DLFS method for feature selection decreases the feature selection time by 2-4% compared to OCT method, 3-6% compared to

Table 1. Tabulation of feature extraction ratio

No. of Images	Feature Extraction Ratio			
	MTFE Method	ADRIAS Method	OCT Method	GLMIFNN Method
10	85	83	83	82
20	87	84	83	83
30	88	86	85	84
40	90	89	86	85
50	92	90	89	88
60	93	92	90	90
70	94	93	92	91
80	95	94	93	92
90	95	94	93	92
100	96	95	94	93

Figure 2. Comparison of Feature extraction ratio

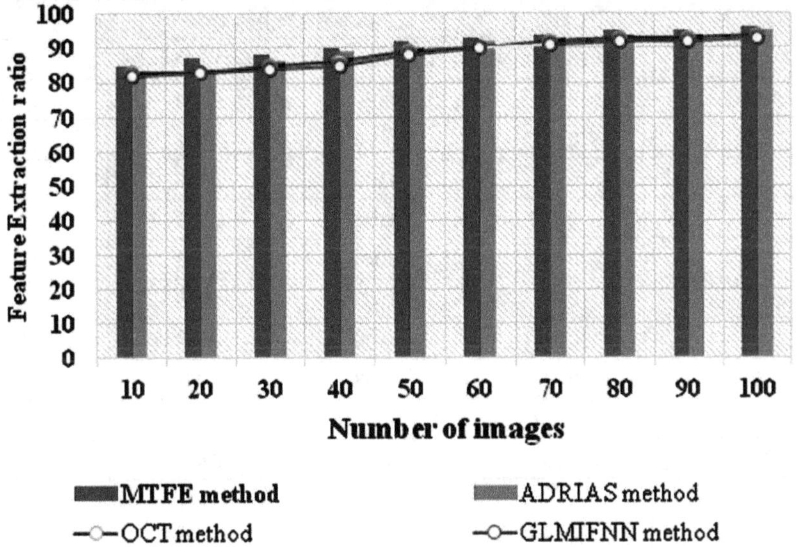

MSRVS method and 5-8% compared to FHS method. The comparison of feature selection time is shown in the Table 2.

Experimental Results for Sensitivity and Specificity

By using Messidor database, the proposed DFS method results are compared with existing method results. The proposed DLFS method is compared with Optical Coherence Tomography (OCT) angiography (Botto de Barros Garcia et al., 2017) method and Automated Diabetic Retinopathy Image Assessment Software (ADRAIS) (Tufail et al., 2017) method. The sensitivity and specificity is measured in terms of % using eqn. (2) and eqn. (3)

$$\text{Sensitivity} = \frac{TP}{TP + FN} * 100 \tag{2}$$

where True Positive (TP) refers to the number of DR diseases whereas False Negative (FN) refers to undetected DR diseases

$$\text{Specificity} = \frac{TN}{TN + FP} * 100 \tag{3}$$

Table 2. Tabulation of feature selection time (ms)

No. of Images	Feature Selection Time			
	DLFS Method	OCT Method	MSRVS Method	FHS Method
10	0.028	0.030	0.033	0.035
20	0.031	0.032	0.035	0.038
30	0.034	0.033	0.037	0.041
40	0.035	0.038	0.040	0.043
50	0.037	0.040	0.043	0.046
60	0.038	0.042	0.045	0.049
70	0.041	0.044	0.048	0.052
80	0.044	0.048	0.051	0.055
90	0.047	0.051	0.053	0.059
100	0.049	0.052	0.056	0.061

Figure 3. Comparison of feature selection time

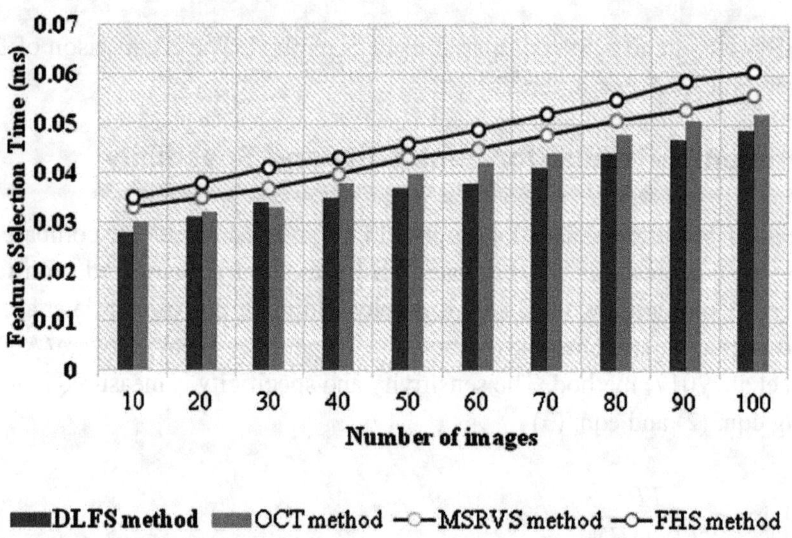

where True Negative (TN) refer to the number of correctly identified non diabetic retinopathy diseases whereas False Positive (FP) represents the number of wrongly identified non diabetic retinopathy diseases.

Figure 4 shows the proposed DLFS method improves the sensitivity and specificity by 5 – 8% compared to OCT method and 8 – 10% compared to ADRIAS method. The comparison of Sensitivity and Specificity is shown in the Table 3.

Table 3. Tabulation of sensitivity and specificity

No. of Images	Sensitivity (%)			Specificity (%)		
	DLFS Method	OCT Method	ADRIAS Method	DLFS Method	OCT Method	ADRIAS Method
10	80	78	77	82	81	81
20	83	80	80	84	83	82
30	84	82	81	84	83	83
40	86	84	81	85	85	84
50	87	86	83	86	85	85
60	89	88	85	87	86	86
70	91	89	87	88	87	86
80	94	91	90	90	88	87
90	95	93	92	91	89	89
100	95	94	94	92	91	90

Figure 4. Comparison of Sensitivity and Specificity. (a) Measure of Sensitivity (b) Measure of Specificity

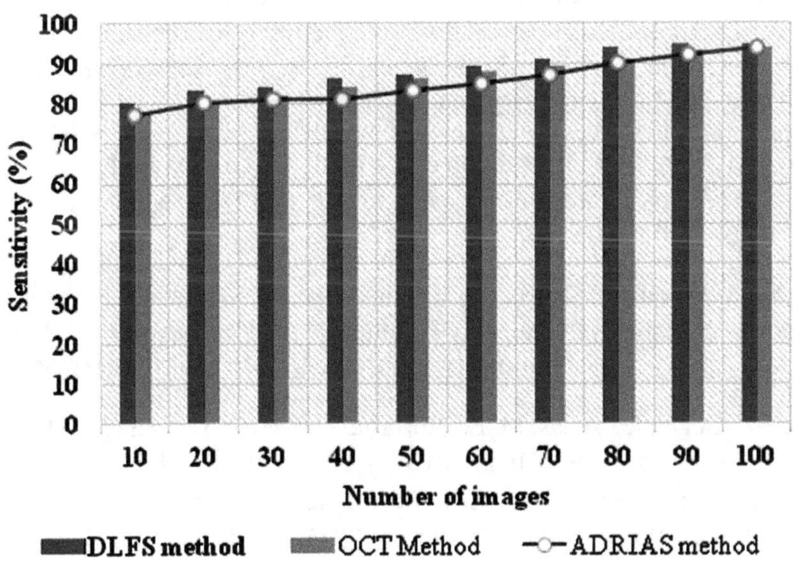

CONCLUSION

The mathematical transformation based Feature Extraction (MTFE) method is used to implement feature extraction. A feature clustering technique is applied to extract the features along with the pathologies from the retinal fundus image of the human eye. After feature extraction model is framed, a Deep Learning based Feature Selection (DLFS) procedure is devised. This DLFS method accurately selects pathologies without any human assistance. After a series of experimental results with the proposed methods, the performance factors such as feature extraction ratio, feature selection time, Sensitivity, and Specificity are improved significantly.

REFERENCES

Acharya, U. R., Faust, O., Kadri, N. A., Suri, J. S., & Yu, W. (2013). Automated identification of normal and diabetes heart rate signals using nonlinear measures. *Computers in Biology and Medicine*, *43*(10), 1523–1529. doi:10.1016/j.compbiomed.2013.05.024 PMID:24034744

Adnan Tufail, F. R. C. O. (2017). Automated Diabetic Retinopathy Image Assessment Software: Diagnostic Accuracy and Cost-Effectiveness Compared with Human Graders. *American Academy of Ophthalmology*, *124*(3), 343–351. doi:10.1016/j.ophtha.2016.11.014 PMID:28024825

Ahmed, E. (2010). Fast Localization of the Optic Disc Using Projection of Image Features. *IEEE Transactions on Image Processing*, *19*(12), 3285–3289. doi:10.1109/TIP.2010.2052280 PMID:20550999

Antal, B., & Hajdu, A. (2010). An Ensemble-Based System for Microaneurysm Detection and Diabetic Retinopathy Grading. *IEEE Transactions on Biomedical Engineering*, *59*(6), 1720–1726. doi:10.1109/TBME.2012.2193126 PMID:22481810

Aquino, A., Gegúndez-Arias, M. E., & Marín, D. (2010). Detecting the Optic Disc Boundary in Digital Fundus Images Using Morphological, Edge Detection, and Feature Extraction Techniques. *IEEE Transactions on Medical Imaging*, *29*(11), 1860–1869. doi:10.1109/TMI.2010.2053042 PMID:20562037

Giancardo, Meriaudeau, Karnowski, Li, Garg, Tobin Jr., & Chaum. (2012). Exudate-based diabetic macular edema detection in fundus images using publicly available datasets. *Medical Image Analysis*, *16*(1), 216–226. PMID:21865074

Goatman, K. A., Fleming, A. D., Philip, S., Williams, G. J., Olson, J. A., & Sharp, P. F. (2011). Detection of new vessels on the optic disc using retinal photographs. *IEEE Transactions on Medical Imaging*, *30*(4), 972–979. doi:10.1109/TMI.2010.2099236 PMID:21156389

Lazar, I., & Hajdu, A. (2013). Retinal microaneurysm detection through local rotating cross-section profile analysis. *IEEE Transactions on Medical Imaging*, *32*(2), 400–407. doi:10.1109/TMI.2012.2228665 PMID:23192523

Manivannan, S., Cobb, C., Burgess, S., & Trucco, E. (2017). Sub-category classifiers for multiple-instance learning and its application to retinal nerve fiber layer visibility classification. *IEEE Transactions on Medical Imaging*, *36*(5), 1140–1150. doi:10.1109/TMI.2017.2653623 PMID:28092529

Marin, D., Aquino, A., Gegundez-Arias, M. E., & Bravo, J. M. (2011). A new supervised method for blood vessel segmentation in retinal images by using gray-level and moment invariants-based features. *IEEE Transactions on Medical Imaging*, *30*(1), 146–158. doi:10.1109/TMI.2010.2064333 PMID:20699207

Mauricio Botto de Barros Garcia, J., Leonardo Cruvinel Isaac, D., & Avila, M. (2017). Diabetic retinopathy and OCT angiography: Clinical findings and future perspectives. *International Journal of Retina and Vitreous*, *3*(14), 1–10. PMID:28078103

Mendonc, Sousaa, Mendonc¸ & Campilhoa. (2013). Automatic localization of the optic disc by combining vascular and intensity information. *Computerized Medical Imaging and Graphics*, *37*(5–6), 409–417. PMID:23726437

Mookiah, M. R. K., Acharya, U. R., Chua, C. K., Min, L. C., Ng, E. Y. K., Mushrif, M. M., & Laude, A. (2013b). Automated detection of optic disk in retinal fundus images using intuitionistic fuzzy histon segmentation. *Proceedings of the Institution of Mechanical Engineers, Part H.*, *227*(1), 37–49. doi:10.1177/0954411912458740 PMID:23516954

Mookiah, M. R. K., Acharya, U. R., Martis, R. J., Chua, C. K., Min, L. C., Ng, E. Y. K., & Laude, A. (2013a). Evolutionary algorithm based classifier parameter tuning for automatic diabetic retinopathy grading: A hybrid feature extraction approach. *Knowledge-Based Systems*, *39*(0), 9–22. doi:10.1016/j.knosys.2012.09.008

Nayebifar, B., & Moghaddam, H. A. (2013). A novel method for retinal vessel tracking using particle filters. *Computers in Biology and Medicine*, *43*(5), 541–548. doi:10.1016/j.compbiomed.2013.01.016 PMID:23434235

Qureshi, Kovacs, Harangi, Nagy, Peto, & Hajdu. (2012). Combining algorithms for automatic detection of optic disc and macula in fundus images. *Computer Vision and Image Understanding, 116*(1), 138-145.

Ram, K., Joshi, G. D., & Sivaswamy, J. (2011). A Successive Clutter-Rejection-Based Approach for Early Detection of Diabetic Retinopathy. *IEEE Transactions on Biomedical Engineering*, *58*(3), 664–673. doi:10.1109/TBME.2010.2096223 PMID:21134810

Rocha, A., Carvalho, T., Jelinek, H. F., Goldenstein, S., & Wainer, J. (2012). Points of Interest and Visual Dictionaries for Automatic Retinal Lesion Detection. *IEEE Transactions on Biomedical Engineering*, *59*(8), 2244–2253. doi:10.1109/TBME.2012.2201717 PMID:22665502

Rossant, F., Badellino, M., Chavillon, A., Bloch, I., & Paques, M. (2011). A morphological approach for vessel segmentation in eye fundus images, with quantitative evaluation. *Journal of Medical Imaging and Health Informatics.*, *1*(1), 42–49. doi:10.1166/jmihi.2011.1006

Sopharak, Uyyanonvara, & Barmanb, & Williamson. (2008). Automatic detection of diabetic retinopathy exudates from non-dilated retinal images using mathematical morphology methods. *Computerized Medical Imaging and Graphics*, *32*(8), 720–727. PMID:18930631

Section 3

Medical Image Segmentation for Improved Clinical Diagnosis

Chapter 6
Certain Investigation Titles on the Segmentation of Colon and Removal of Opacified Fluid for Virtual Colonoscopy

Gayathri Devi Krishnamoorthy
Dr. N. G. P. Institute of Technology, India

Kishore B.
Dr. Mahalingam College of Engineering and Technology, India

ABSTRACT

Colorectal cancer (CRC) is a most important type of cancer that can be detected by virtual colonoscopy (VC) in the colon or rectum, and it is the major cause of death prevailing in the world. The CAD technique requires the segmentation of the colon to be accurate and can be implemented by two approaches. The first approach focuses on the segmentation of lungs in the computed tomography (CT) images downloaded from The Cancer Imaging Archive (TCIA) using clustering approach. The second method focused on the automatic segmentation of colon, removal of opacified fluid and bowels for all the slices in a dataset in a sequential order using MATLAB. The second approach requires more computational time, and hence, in order to reduce, the semiautomatic segmentation of colon was implemented in 3D seeded region growing and fuzzy clustering approach in MEVISLAB software. The approaches were implemented in multiple datasets and the accuracy were verified with manual segmentation by radiologist, and the importance of removing opacified fluid were shown for improving the accuracy of colon segments.

DOI: 10.4018/978-1-5225-5876-7.ch006

INTRODUCTION

Colorectal Cancer (CRC) is a type of cancerous growth that develops in the colon or in the rectum, as shown in Figure 1. The Gastrointestinal (GI) system composed of colon and rectum are important parts of the digestive system. The probability of the occurrence of the cancer in the small intestine (bowels) is minimal when compared to the large intestine (colon), a muscular tube approximately 5 feet long in the region or in the rectum. The structure of the colon is comprised of four portions,

1. Ascending colon is located between a pouch called the cecum where the undigested food enters and the transverse colon. This branch of colon will extend upwards and terminate at a right colic flexure on the right side of the abdomen as shown in the Figure 1.
2. The transverse colon which is the longest part will bend downwards as it traverses from right to left for a short distance and it will bend upwards to form a U shaped curve. This part of the curve will finish below the spleen to form another flexure called splenic or left colic flexure.
3. The above section will be continued by the descending colon. As its name implies, this segment will descend from the splenic flexure to the lower level on the left side.
4. The fourth part is called the sigmoid colon for the reason that this segment will be of "S" shape; the sigmoid colon joins the rectum, which in turn will connect to the anus.

Figure 1. Detailed Anatomy of the colon and rectum

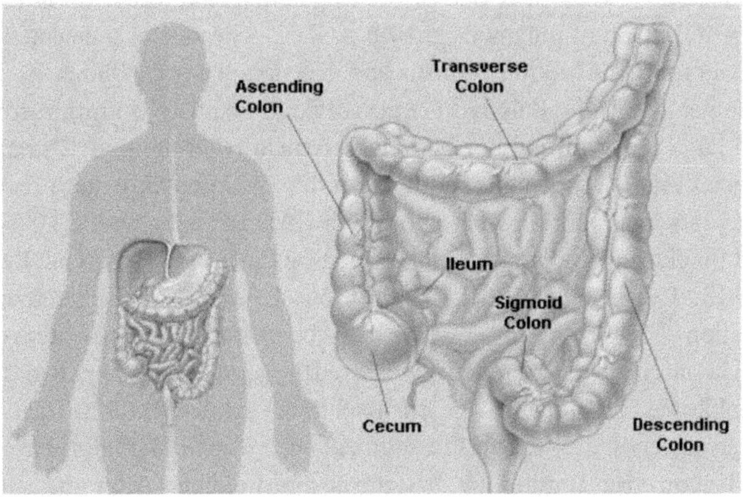

Different radiological procedures and imaging modalities widely used to identify CRC are computed tomography (CT), virtual computed tomography colonoscopy, endorectal ultrasound, and magnetic resonance imaging (MRI).Among these techniques CT has been preferred due to following reasons:

- CT is a preferred examination technique for investigation of abdominal organs for elderly patients even if they have an implanted medical device of any kind.
- It causes less pain for the complete assessment of the large bowels and small bowels where air or carbon dioxide is injected in the rectum via thin catheter. It is accurate, non-invasive, less sensitive to patient movement, fast and simple.
- The results of this screening technique can be diagnosed by an experienced radiologist with very high accuracy so the patients can be guided for further treatment and this technique eliminates the need for additional diagnostic procedures such as needle biopsies, exploratory surgery and surgical biopsy.
- If a large growth is identified during colonoscopy, then CT colonography (CTC) can be recommended on the same day for a detailed analysis of the colon.
- The cost of CTC is significantly when compared to other investigation techniques.

CAD TECHNIQUES TO INVESTIGATE THE POLYP (GROWTH) IN CTC

The segmentation of colon is one of the imperative step in the CAD techniques for the identification of polyps or growth in CTC. The size of a detected polyp is a significant norm for future diagnosis and decision making (John & Bond, 2000; Richardson et al., 2011). Polyps were classified as small ($\leq$ 5 mm), medium (6-9 mm) and large ($\geq$10 mm).Polyp size measurement from 6mm to 10 mm is to be considered. CAD is fundamentally based on highly complex pattern recognition. In recent years a number of prototype Colon CAD schemes with CTC have been proposed for detecting polyps to reduce the False Positive (FP) polyps (Bevilacqua et al., 2013; Bernal et al., 2012).The various CAD schemes that requires the segmentation of colon to be accurate are listed below for the identification of polyps

Yoshida and Nappi (2001) initially measured the geometric features to differentiate polyps, folds and colonic walls at each voxel in the extracted colon. The connected component analysis was applied to segment the suspicious region based on the measured geometric features by hysteresis thresholding. After that, the polyp candidates were detected by finding the voxels with low curvedness values and high shape index by means of hysteresis thresholding. At last, they proposed a fuzzy clustering to the candidates to segment polyp. However, their algorithm were used for identifying only small number of polyps, hence the accuracy of the detection of all size of polyps could not be commented.

An automated system to identify colonic polyps of varying size which have irregular shape and curvature is presented in Yao et al. (2004). This method is based on a formation of knowledge-guided intensity adjustment, FCM clustering and deformable models. The proposed approach is compared with the manual segmentation to evaluate the performance of the proposed segmentation approach in terms of accuracy. The method is observed to remove 30% of FP detections.

Bogoni et al. (2005) have proposed a method for the identification of medium sized polyp's ≥ 6 mm by modifying feature extraction phase in the classical polyp detection scheme by implementing the wrapper method for feature selection, in which the classifier decides which features are useful. The method was validated on 150 datasets, in which 88 cases were allotted for training and 62 cases were used for testing. A total of 53 unique polyps were identified in training dataset in which 19 polyps were small with a size less than 6 mm, 25 polyps with medium size ranging from 6–9 mm and 9 large polyps (10–20 mm) with an average sensitivity of 81.1%.The training set identified 39 unique polyps among which 18 were small, 11 mid-size and 10 large size polyps with a sensitivity of 82.1%.This method have failed to handle the sources such as stools and faecal material which may produce False Positive(FP).

Hong, Qiu, and rie Kaufman., (2006) have overcome the above disadvantage by applying digital cleansing technique for removal of stools in the colon to reduce the FP. This was implemented by first segmenting and digital cleansing the colon acquired using CT from abdominal data set by partial volume segmentation algorithm. A region growing based segmentation algorithm is used to extract a topologically simple segmentation of the colon lumen. The 3D colon surface that is generated will be mapped to a 2D rectangle and this mapping simplifies our polyp detection problem from 3D to 2D. A 2D image is generated using volumetric ray-casting algorithm and the K-L transformation matrix is applied where the pixels classified belonging to a polyp are colored in red whose diameter is larger than 5 mm. The red regions in this 2D image are highly suspicious for being polyps, indicating that the physicians should observe these areas in the 3D view very carefully.

Yao and Summers (2007) has explained the segmentation of colonic polyps on haustral folds in the walls of the colon. This approach is based on a combination of 3D knowledge-guided intensity tuning, fuzzy clustering and adaptive deformable model. A dual-distance algorithm is presented by the author to detect the fold region. Then a counter force is proposed in the model evolution to improve the over-segmentation problem that frequently occurs to polyps on haustral folds. The experiment was done on 395 patients with 83 polyps. The results were evaluated against manual measurement.

Shahbazi et al. (2008) presented and extended a set of algorithms, characteristically depending on morphological operators, for the purpose of automatic colonic polyp discovery implemented to CT scans. The input noisy images are enhanced by means of Morphological Image Cleaning (MIC) scheme. Subsequently, the colon wall is fragmented through region growing subjected to morphological grassfire process. With the intention of detecting polyp candidates, a novel Automatic Morphological Polyp Detection (AMPD) scheme is formulated. Candidate features are separated as polyps and non-polyps performing a new Template Matching Algorithm (TMA) which depends on Euclidean distance searching.

Chowdhury et al. (2008) proposed a polyp detection method for the identification of polyps larger than 10 mm .The experimental results indicate that the technique achieved 100% sensitivity with 3.38 FP/dataset when applied to low dose real patient data while the other categories of polyps have lesser sensitivity. This involves automatic colon segmentation by estimating the volume/length of the connected component to discriminate the bowels and the colon. The second main component is to extract the polyp candidate surface followed by the extraction of the features that comprises of the standard deviation of the various parameters that can discriminate polyps and fold. This similar type of colon segmentation was also proposed by Berta et al. (2009).

Sundaram et al. (2008) approached in a different way by applying Smoothed Shape Operators(SSO) to identify the polyps. The colon data is represented in the form of mesh surface, and computation is performed on this surface and hence the curvature of the polyps that is estimated will be stable and not affected by the nearby tissues in the CT image. The output of the SSO operates is in the form of patches. Every computation is presented on the surface, not in the voxel grid. The data that has been represented in the form of mesh can be unfolded by finite element to revert back to colon. All of these patches are displayed in a new approach called patch view so that it can be checked by the radiologist and if any FP is present it can be discarded. The disadvantage in the method proposed was the complexity involved in detecting the polyps.

Chen et al. (2008) implemented a CAD system that is based on anisotropic 3D surface evolution representation for discovering protrusion shape based colonic polyp on the rounded surface. The significant characteristic of the proposed method is that it can detect protrusion with both convex and concave shapes. In accordance with gaussian and mean curvature flows, the scheme deforms the convex or concave surface in anticipating that the second principal curvature will lead to zero. The diffusion directions are varied to avoid convex surfaces from converting into concave shapes.

The deformation meadow quantitatively computes the quantity of protrudeness. This scheme has been analysed by synthetic phantoms and real colon datasets.

Li et al. (2009) presented a multiobjective Genetic Algorithm (GA) approach to optimize a CAD system for detecting colonic polyps. The sequential classifier is used in CTC CAD to detect the initial level of polyp in the surface of colon. This classifier uses a threshold on curvature-based features to cluster doubtful colon surface regions into polyp candidates. Though, several number of medium-sized polyps, 6-9 mm in diameter, were left out in the initial detection process. To solve this issues, GA is proposed by developing the Pareto front of the Pareto optimal set.

Zhu et al. (2009) proposed a CAD scheme to detect colonic polyps in CTC images without any human intervention. Primarily, a thick colon wall illustration, that is, a Volumetric Mucosa (VM) with many voxels wide generally, was segmented from CTC images with the assistance of partial-volume image segmentation technique. Depending on this VM, a level set-based adaptive convolution method was used for estimating the first and second-order spatial derivatives more accurately to start the geometric analysis.

Ravesteijn et al. (2010) introduced a low-complex CAD system that considered all the difficulties that a classifier will face to classify the polyps. Hence this system focussed on candidate extraction and a simple low complex logistic classifier. The extracted candidates from the candidate extraction stage are ordered by a linear logistic classifier which classifies in accordance with only three features: The mean internal intensity, protrusion of the colon wall and a feature to remove detections on the rectal enema tube. The ordering of the features were performed by regression analysis to estimate the performance which were analysed by Free-Response Receiver Operating Characteristics (FROC) curves.

Grigorescu et al. (2010) developed an algorithm for the automatic detection and segmentation of polyps larger than 10 mm in diameter. This paper modifies the segmentation phase in the classical polyp detection scheme by evaluating the LH histogram which separates the fat and muscle density in CTC data. It focuses mainly on the tissue separation surrounding the colon lumen and finds the appropriate region for poly detection. The first stage removes the image noise and the small food remnants by using the intensity information. The next stage is to group the location that passed the above stage based on the proximity of closeness to each other. After segmentation and performing morphological operation to remove the small connection between muscles like structure, the diameter of the segmented region is calculated if it has a diameter greater than 50 mm it is to be considered as a larger polyp.

The polyp detection system developed by Fiori et al. (2011) identifies small polyps that is greater than 3 mm in diameter, flat polyps and polyps greater than 6 mm in diameter. Small polyps are normally ignored by the radiologist because only a small percentage of those polyps turn into malignant (Winawer & Zauber, 2002). This paper segment the colon from the abdominal volume in the CT by proposing a probability map for three classes of interest air, liquid and interface, the union of these three classes forms the inside of the colon. The curvature-based surface motions with suitable modification is implemented to smoothen the colon surface and to remove the noise after segmentation step. Feature Extraction extracts 6 geometric features by considering the shape of neighborhood area of the polyp in addition to polyp intrinsic geometry and structure. In addition to feature extraction 5 texture feature entropy, energy, contrast, sumMean, and homogeneity are also extracted to aid the classification and extraction of polyps.

Lee et al. (2011) presented a method for the identification of polyps (3-6 mm) by producing a numerical phantom. The filtering procedure begins with 3-D Gaussian filtering, followed by a Hessian matrix computation and its eigen decomposition. This phantom is used for the evaluation of effectiveness of the volumetric structural features such as Gaussian Kernel GK, Suppression Threshold ST and Volume Threshold VT to discriminate basic structures in the colon. The former two are parameters of the blob-likeness filter and the third was used for candidate detection.

Yonghua Xu et al. (2012) introduced a Structure-Analysis Electronic Cleansing (SAEC) with in CTC to evaluate the feasibility and sensitivity, also in detecting colorectal flat lesions. They proposed a scheme for the polyp identification by registration techniques in which registration of the segmented colon images in both prone and supine position will be employed for the identification of the polyp. Bernal et al. (2012) developed a CAD scheme for the detection and segmentation of polyps in colonoscopy videos. McKenna et al. (2012) proposed a hybrid approach where the minimal knowledge persons whose is not trained well for identification of polyps can identify polyps using distributed human intelligence.

Amin and Wee-chung (2013) implemented a method which combines FCM clustering and level set scheme for image segmentation. In this approach, primarily Chan and Vese's level set technique and Bayes classifier in accordance with mixture of density models are employed to discover a prior membership value for every pixel. Subsequently, a Supervised Kernel based Fuzzy C-Means clustering (SKFCM) scheme support by preceding membership values is expanded for segmentation. The working of this scheme has been analysed through high-throughput fluorescence microscopy colon cancer cell images, which are commonly utilized for the purpose of investigation of several normal and neoplastic process.

Bevilacqua (2013) have proposed three new different approaches for the identification of polyps by supervised artificial neural network approach. Initially separate the dataset and employed the vector element of 7 X 7 X 7 volumes which is obtained by scanning the lumen border. The second technique separated the dataset into four classes based on the shape and the position of the polyp. It is based on analysis of 2D slices using a 2D ANN. In the third case implementation of 3D ANN have been made based on the density values of the cubes where polyp is located. The disadvantage were that it were implemented with limited dataset. The segmentation of desired region were performed by removing the background region using standard region growing techniques and the colon region were segmented by assigning seeds internal to the colon and by generating mask.

Hampshire (2013) have proposed a method for the extraction of the colon from abdominal CT images acquired in both the supine and prone position. This paper focuses on matching the haustral fold detection that will be present in the borders of the colon for both the supine and prone position .

Kainz et al.(2017) discussed an approach to segment and classify using deep convolution neural networks.Two classifiers were used to segment the glands,t he first classifier will separate the glands from background and the second for identifying the structures that separates the gland. The colorectal cancer section were identified as benign or malignant in several datasets

Thus the above literature reveals that for the identification of polyps in CAD scheme, the following approaches were applied for the segmentation of colon

- Multistage procedure: Removal of air region around the body, Segmentation of Lungs and Colon reconstruction using anatomical knowledge and volume/ length (V/L) analysis.
- Region Growing subjected to morphological grassfire process.
- Creation of binary image S1 by the concept of thresholding with a value ≤ 700HU, Removal of lungs by negative mask of a 3-D seeded region-filling, Creation of binary image S2 from S1 and morphological dilation operation is performed.
- Confidence connected Region Growing Technique. If needed multiple seed points to segment collapsed colon.
- A pre-processing stage for dealing with the air and liquid composition of the colon volume, Second stage that consists of smoothing the pre-processed image and obtaining the final colon surface by thresholding the smoothed volume.
- Deformation model approach
- Anatomy-based extraction (ABE) and Colon-based analysis (CBA).
- Iterative Partial Volume Segmentation algorithm followed by dilation and erosion
- Combination of Fuzzy C-Means clustering (FCM) and level set scheme.

This paper focusses on the segmentation of colon in three approaches

1. Segmentation of large intestine using Clustering approach
2. Automatic segmentation of colon and the removal of Bowels using Neural network approach
3. Semi automatic segmentation of colon and the removal of opacified fluid using 3D Seeded region growing approach

COLERECTAL CANCER

The growth of CRC will ranges for a period from 10 to 20 years in which some of them may be noncancerous growths termed as polyp that will lie on the inner layers of the colon or rectum which is called as adenomatous polyp or adenoma. Adenomas will develop in glandular cells, which generate mucus to lubricate the colorectum (Naishadham et al., 2011). All the adenomas growth have the chance of growing into stages of cancer, but only less than 10% may develop into invasive cancer. This will occur only if the size of the growth increases (Pickhardt et al., 2013). Cancer that develops in glandular cells is called adenocarcinoma, and most of the colorectal cancers (about 96%) are adenocarcinomas.

Stages of Colorectal Cancer

The cancer will develop on the inner lining of the wall of large intestine as shown in Figure 2. The cancers developed into the wall may invade the nearby blood cells via lymph vessels that are thin channels which carries the cellular waste and fluid. There is a probability that cancer cells will invade the adjacent lymph nodes that will have bean-shaped structures. Cancerous cells will also spread to the liver or lungs through blood vessels, or it can be spread into the pelvis and abdominal cavity to other organs and tissues, for instance the peritoneum (membrane lining the abdomen) and ovary. The spread of cancer cells to other of the body is called metastasis.

The amount of cancer that has invaded the other organs at the time of diagnosis is called as staging. This decides the treatment and in assessing prognosis (prediction of disease results) that should be given. The two most common staging systems are the Malignant Tumours (TNM) system, commonly used in clinical settings, and the Surveillance, Epidemiology, and End Results (SEER) summary staging system, used for very descriptive and statistical analysis of tumor registry data. The stages of colorectal cancer through SEER summary staging system is illustrated below under four categories.

- **In situ:** Cancers that have not initiated to overrun the wall of the colon or rectum

Figure 2. Colorectal cancer growth

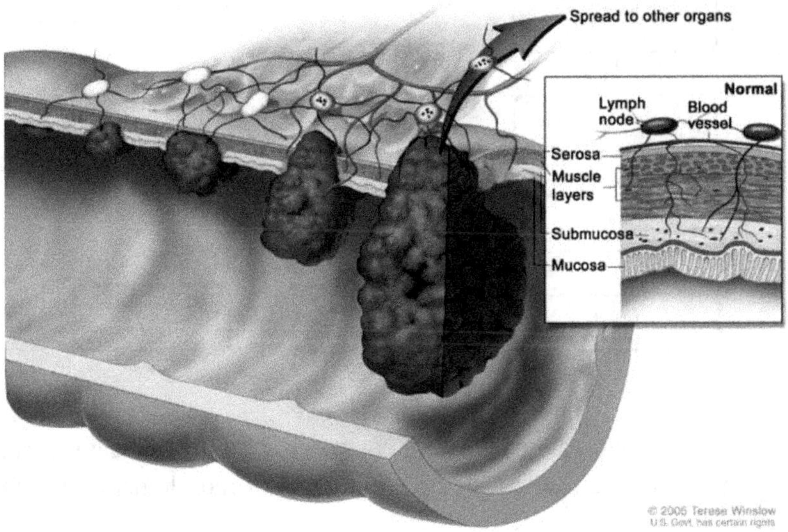

- **Local:** Cancers that have grown into the wall of the colon or rectum, but have not expanded through the wall to invade close to tissues.
- **Regional:** Cancers that have spread all the way through the wall of the colon or rectum and have invaded close by tissue, or that have spread to nearby lymph nodes.
- **Distant:** Cancers that have spread to several other parts of the body, such as the liver or lung.

AN APPROACH ON THE SEGMENTATION OF LARGE INTESTINE AND REMOVAL OF LUNGS USING CLUSTERING APPROACH

The flow diagram of the implementation is shown in the Figure 3 (Devi et al., 2014). The datasets of the abdominal CT image in DICOM format of size 512 X 512 downloaded from TCIA link (Cancer Imaging Archives, 2017) were considered for the segmentation of large intestine. The number of axial slices in a dataset varied from 200 to 450. The Intensity based Clustering and FCM clustering approaches were used which initiates the grouping of pixels with similar characteristics into clusters. The connected component analysis was implemented for different neighbourhood connectivity. Then 8 neighbourhood connectivity were preferred for segmenting the colon segments by separating the background which consist of lungs. The segmented

Figure 3. Framework for the segmentation of colon

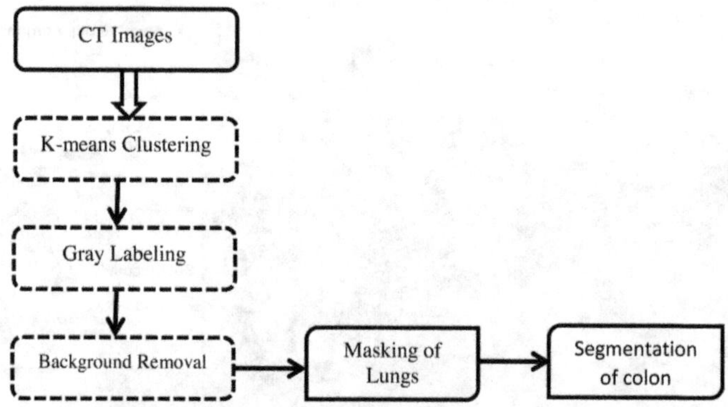

results of the implemented method were compared with the manual segmentation colon structures that were segmented with the help of radiologist using ITK snap software.

The sample axial slice of a dataset is shown in the Figure 4(a). Thus the background, lungs and colon have nearly equal Hounsfield value (HU) that lies in the range of -950 to -1200 HU. Thus the clustering techniques segment both colon and non-colon segments (lungs, background and small intestine).The clustering techniques requires the initialization of centroid [0 150 255], 0 for black, 255 for white and a intermediate value 150.The reason of initializing with three centroids was that the organ of interest in this research is colon segments which are black in color covers the range from 0 to 150 and the non-colon segments (bones, soft tissue) covers the range from 150 to 255.

Thus the clustered segments shown in Figure 4(b) are uniquely labelled by the method of connected component analysis using 8 neighborhood connectivity. The labelled output is shown in Figure 4(c). Thus all the surrounding pixels are analysed with respect to centre pixels for labelling process.

The desired colon segment can be extracted by masking the lungs as shown in the Figure 5 below and the corresponding 3D rendered output is shown in the Figure 6.

SECOND APPROACH: AUTOMATIC SEGMENTATION OF COLON BY THE REMOVAL OF LUNGS AND OPACIFIED FLUID USING CASCADE FEED FORWARD NEURAL NETWORK

The Second approach segments the large intestine from the CT images as shown in the framework given in the Figure 7 (Devi et al., 2015). The abdominal organs in each axial slice will consist of background, large intestine (colon), small

Figure 4. (a) Input Axial Slice b) Clustered Image c) labeling of Gray images

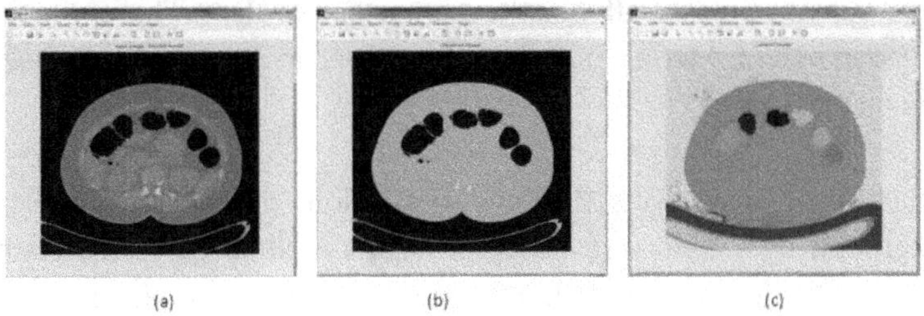

Figure 5. The Top row shows different slices of a particular dataset and the bottom row shows the corresponding segmented output by Fuzzy C means algorithm

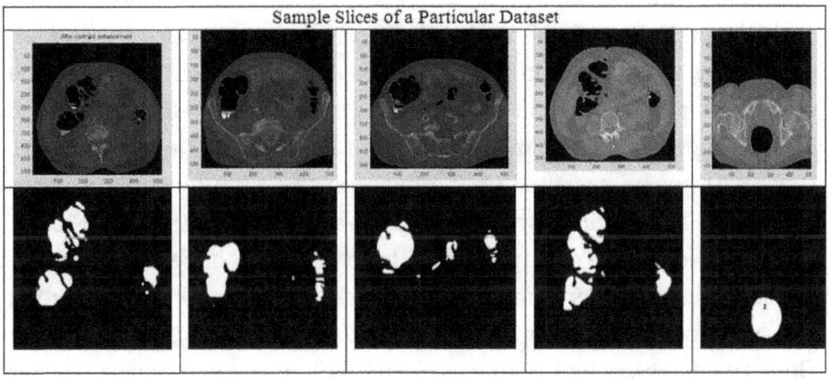

Figure 6. 3D rendering of all the segmented 315 slices

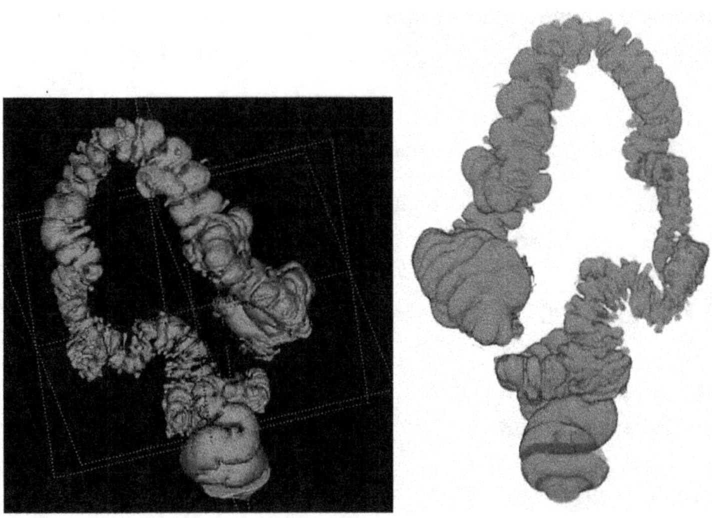

intestine, opacified fluid, rectum, lungs and noise. Rectum and colon categories are considered as positive class. All the others are negative class. This entire framework implemented in MATLAB acts individually on each axial slice in a dataset as given in the sequence below

1. Extraction of air packets that includes colon, lungs, small noises and the background by Otsu's thresholding. Otsu's method performs segmentation by means of automatic thresholding and reduces the image from gray scale to binary form. The Foreground will be estranged from the surroundings by removing the air portions outside the body of the subject
2. The extraction of lungs is initiated with connected component analysis by approaching with 8 neighborhood connectivity. The estimation of features associated with the shape of the organs such as area will be analyzed, since they varies from slice to slice and will reduce in a descending portion for consecutive slices. The maximum numbers of connected region (L) that an axial slice can have for the extraction of lungs are 18, since as the colon segments start originating there will be more number of CC. For L>18, the above narrated steps will not be executed as the occurrence of the lung segments will be minimum. The Figure 8 shows the removal of lungs for a sample axial slice.
3. The extraction of the opacified fluid filled parts inside the colon are implemented using cascade feed forward neural network. The networks are already trained to handle the Partial Volume Effect (PVE) which consists of air filled region, fluid filled region and boundaries (AFB) which interconnect the air-fluid indicated by the blue line as shown in Figure 9. The white opacified fluid and the bone region will have an intensity value at the higher end and it will vary from 55000 to 63000.The one possible solution to locate the liquid region, the adjacent existence of both interface and fluid region. The intensity value that can be assigned for training the network are listed below:

A = 0 to 10000

```
// for intensity values from 0 to 10000 it is considered as
region of colon filled with air;
```

P/M = 30000 to 55000

```
// for intensity values from 10000 to 55000 it is considered as
either muscles or a PVE;
```

M = 10000 to 55000

```
//for intensity value from 10000 to 55000 it is considered as
muscles;
```

HI = 55000 to 63000

```
//for intensity values from 55000 to 65000 it is considered as
either bones or liquid.
```

4. The steps 6 and 7 are mainly focused on removing the tiny hole as shown in the Figure 10. The Figure 10(b) is the output after otsu's thresholding(D_0) and Figure 10(c) is the output after the removal of lungs (D_1) which has introduced some tiny holes. Thus the outputs are in binary form where 0 represents black and 1 represent white. The AND operation performed between D_0 and D_1 ensure that output is high only if the particular segment is present in both D_0 and D_1 as shown in the Figure 10(d). Thus this figure clearly illustrates both bowel (small intestine) and colon are black in color and there is a reduction in the number of tiny holes.
5. The removal of bowels is performed by Slice Difference Removal method (SLDR) method. This method evaluates by taking the difference between two consecutive slices or it is equivalent to performing an XOR operation between the formerly segmented slice and the present slice. The former slice output were considered here as reference for the removal of bowels, in view of the fact that there will be continuity existing between two slices. An XOR operation will produce a binary output of zero (black) in areas of colon as similar areas exist. An output of high in areas of bowels as shown in the Figure 11(b). Taking the negative of the processed output will produce only the colon segments and remove the bowels as shown in Figure 11(c). This output will undergo an XOR operation with the next consecutive slice and all the slices of a dataset will be processed for the removal of bowels. The opacified fluid that were extracted as shown in the Figure 11(a) for the sample slice in Figure 10(a) will be combined with the colon segment. The outputs for two slices of a dataset are shown in Figure 12. The Slice No 185 has clearly shown the removal of bowels and the output is matching with the ground truth. The slice no 277 has emphasized on the removal of bowels and the concatenation of fluid with the colon. The 3D rendered output of all the slices for the sample datasets before and after the framework are shown in Figure 13.

Figure 7. The overview of the proposed method

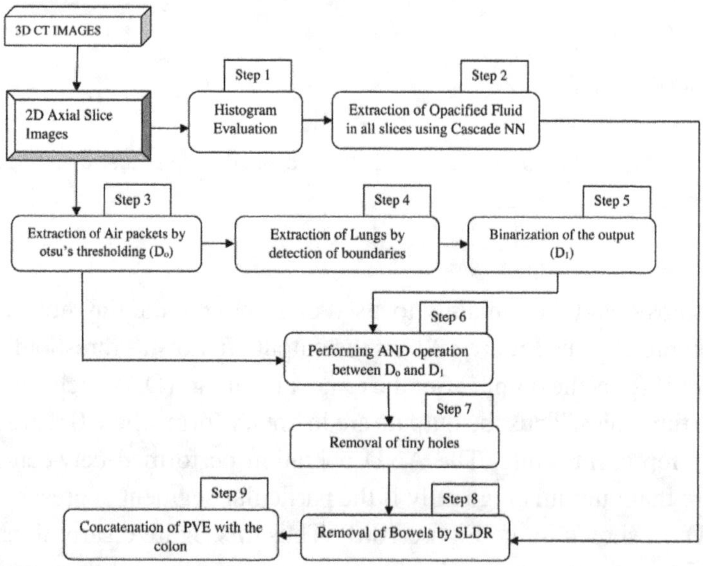

Figure 8. Extraction of Lungs

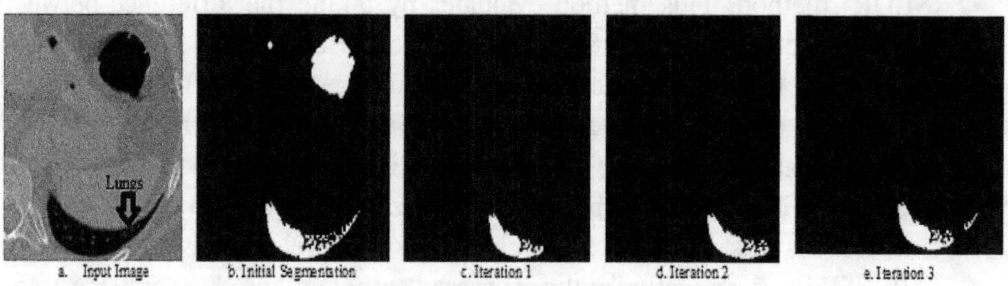

THIRD APPROACH-THE SEMI AUTOMATIC SEGMENTATION OF COLON AND THE REMOVAL OF OPACIFIED FLUID USING 3D SEEDED REGION GROWING

The second approach requires more computational time to produce the output as the operation will be performed from slice to slice. Hence to overcome the above disadvantage, third approach shown in Figure 14 were implemented in MEVISLAB

This approach is executed in the following steps

Figure 9. CT Axial slice with partial volume effect

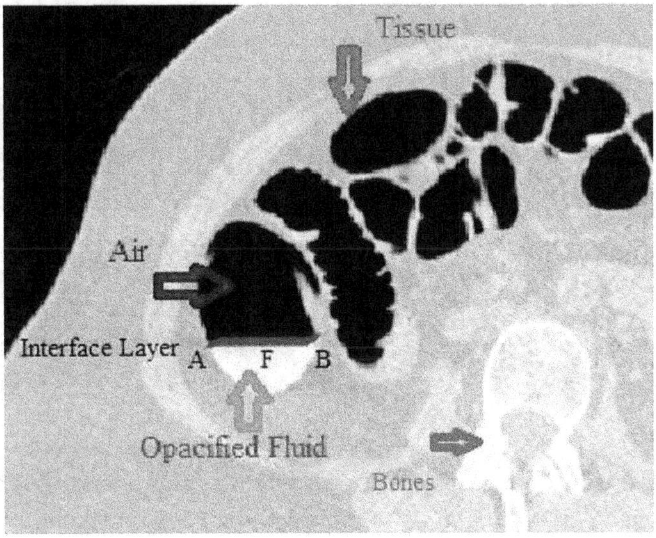

Figure 10. a) Input- Axial Slice b) Output-D_0 c) Output-D_1 d) Out F= And(D_0, D1)

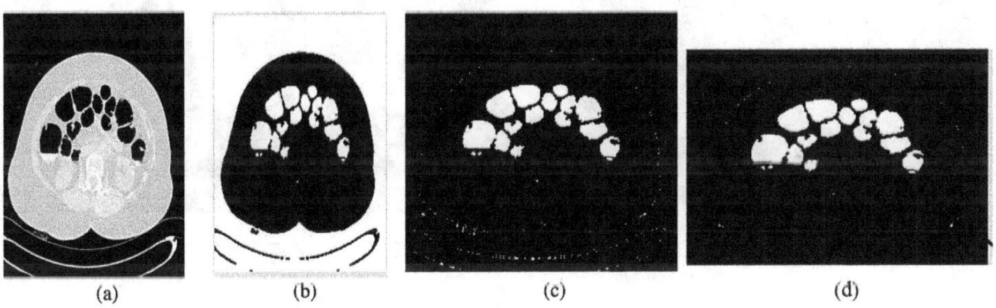

Figure 11. a) Removal Of opacified Fluid b)Removal of Bowels c) Output of SLDR

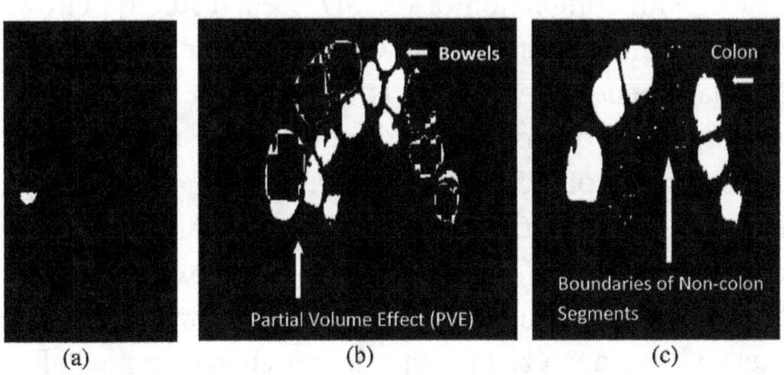

Figure 12. Output of Sample Axial slices of Dataset (No of slices: 629)

Sample slice Number	Input Image	D0	Ground Truth	Difference	Output
185	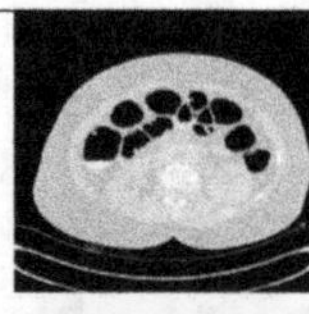	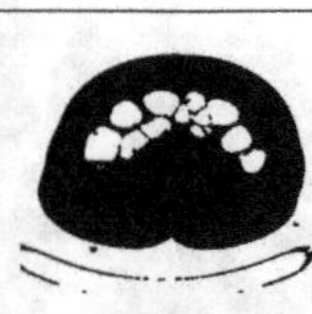	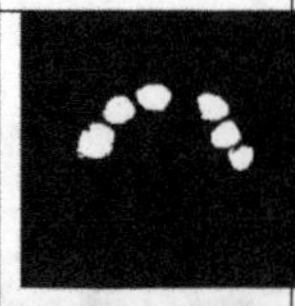	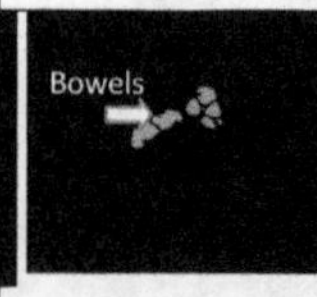	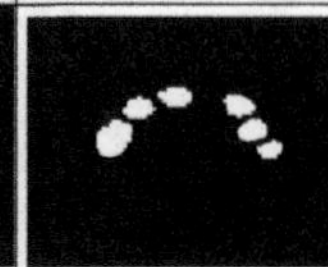
277	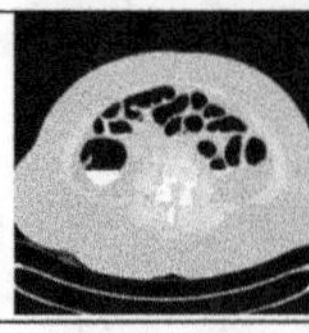	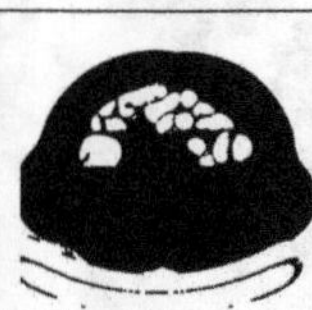	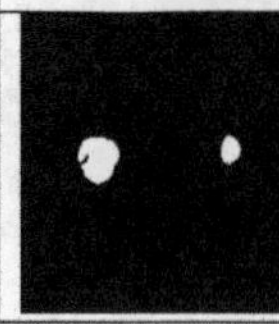	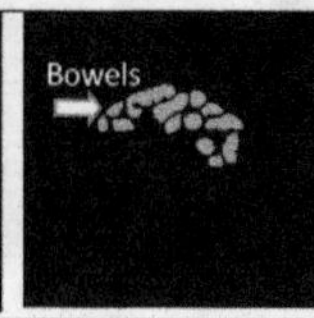	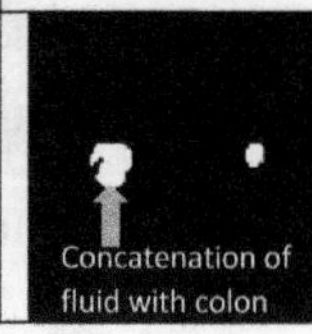

Figure 13. (a) Output of dataset 1 before the removal of bowels (b): Output of dataset 1 after the segmentation (c)Output of dataset 2 after the segmentation

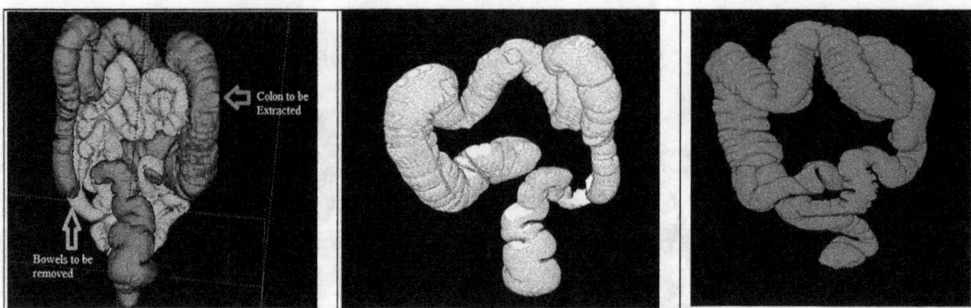

Step 1: The distribution of the intensity values of the voxels in a particular dataset can be known from the histogram plot.

Step 2: The successful completion of the 3D Seeded Region Growing (3DSRG) requires the assignment of the following parameter as shown in the Figure 16

- The placement of seed point is indicated by a small red square in the rectum portion based on the prior literatures surveyed. The voxel has an intensity value of -954 Hounsfield Unit(HU)
- Assignment of 3D-6 Neighbourhood relation which will check the 4 adjacent neighbours surrounding the seed voxel, one pixel in the above slice and one pixel in the below slice as shown in the Figure 15. These pixels will be analyzed for the similar characteristics of the seed point. If it matches that corresponding voxel will be added to that seed point and the region starts growing.

Figure 14. Framework for the third approach

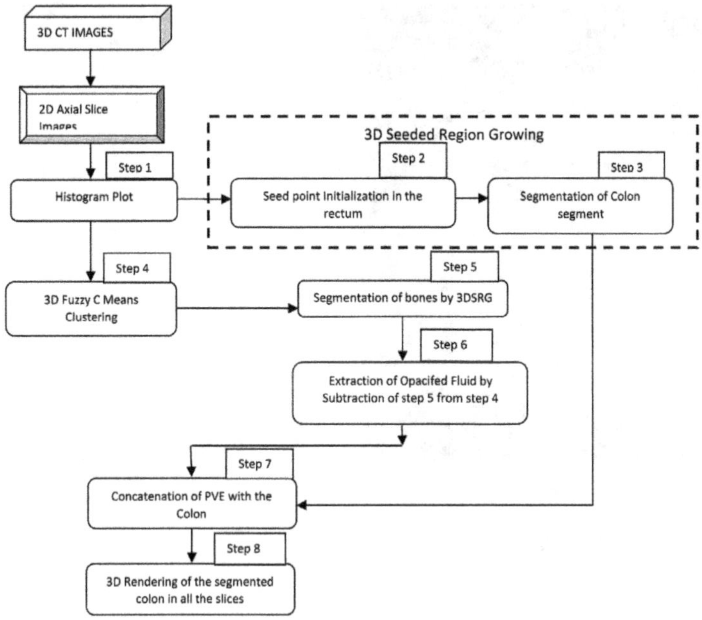

Figure 15. Illustration of 3D 6-Connected Neighbour Connectivity

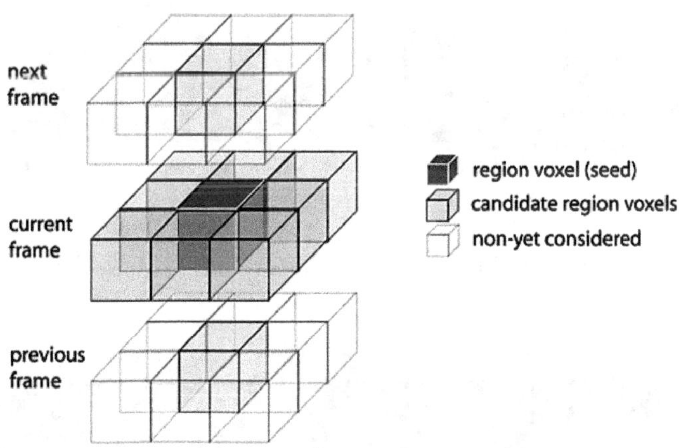

This algorithm starts adding the nighbouring pixel based on the seed point characteristics, 3D 6- neighborhood connectivity and will automatically vary within 5% of the step size of the assigned threshold. The output that is produced is shown in the Figure 17 for the sample dataset 1 that has been explained earlier before and after the removal of bowels.

Figure 16. Implementation of 3D SDRG for the extraction of colon

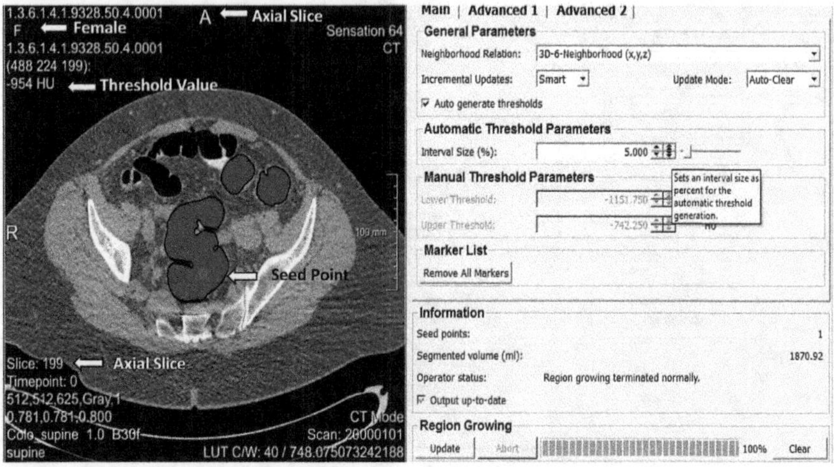

Figure 17. Segmentation of Colon

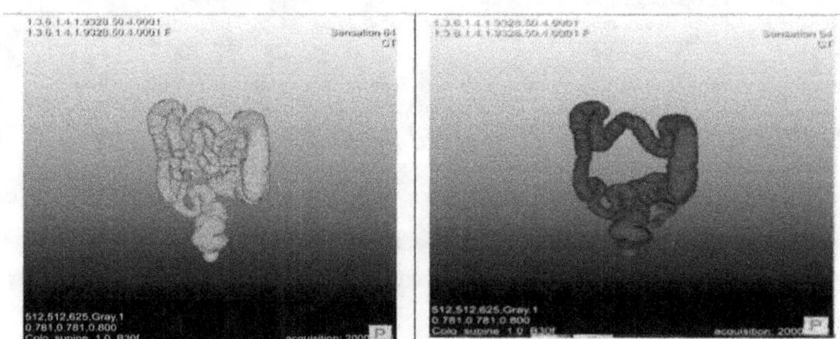

Before the removal of bowels	*After the removal of bowels*

Figure 18. a) Input Image, b) Removal of Bones and Opacified Fluid, c) Removal of Opacified Fluid

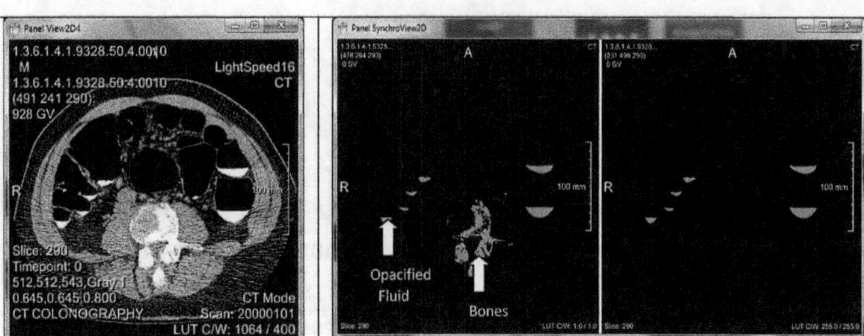

a) Input Image	*b) Removal of Bones and Opacified Fluid*	*c) Removal of Opacified Fluid*

Step 3: Fuzzy connectedness approach clusters both the bones and the opacified fluid as both has the same intensity as shown in Figure 18(b). Three parameters that are to be set for fuzzy clustering approach are classes, fuzziness and σ(epsilon). The class values were assigned to 2 which separates the slice into two division, bones and the opacified fluid have white values and all other segments have black value. The second parameter ∅ is related with membership values of the classification that can range from 1 to ∞. The assignment of high values will result in misclassification and the value assigned was 3.5. The epsilon value or the stopping criteria assigned were 0.427. The output of 3D fuzzy clustering which contain both bone and opacified fluid are shown in Figure 18(b).The bones were separated using 3DSDRG by assigning 26–neighbourhood connectivity and the resulting figure is subtracted from Figure 18(b).The Final figure shown in Figure 18(c) has opacified fluid only.

Step 4: Concatenation of the extracted PVE region from step 3 is added with the segmented air packets in step 2 to get the final output as shown in the Figure 19. The volume rendered output of the Figure 20 clearly reveals that by the concatenation of the opacified fluid with colon segments, the accuracy in the segmentation has been improved by the inclusion of haustral folds and by the addition of the missing segments.

Figure 19. Concatenation of opacified fluid with colon segments

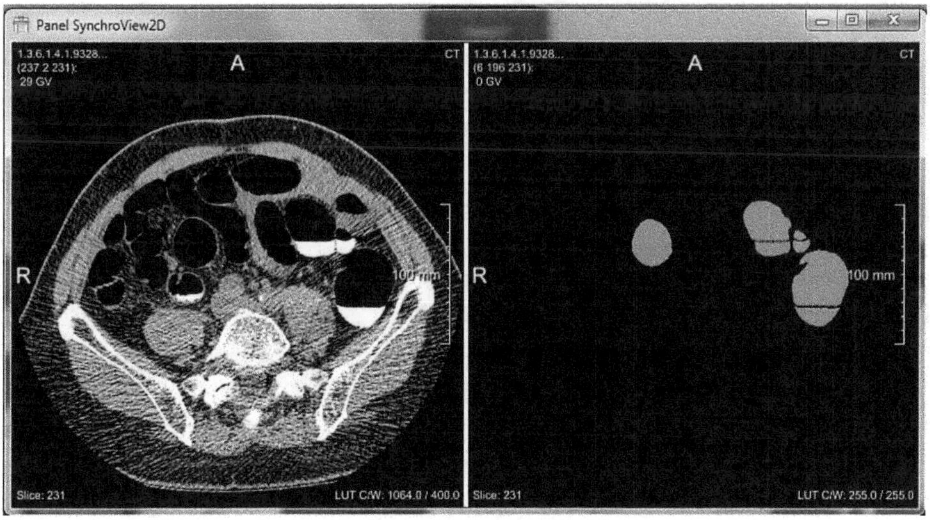

Figure 20. (a): 3D rendered output of dataset before the removal of opacified fluid (b): 3D rendered output of dataset after the concatenation of the opacified fluid with the colon

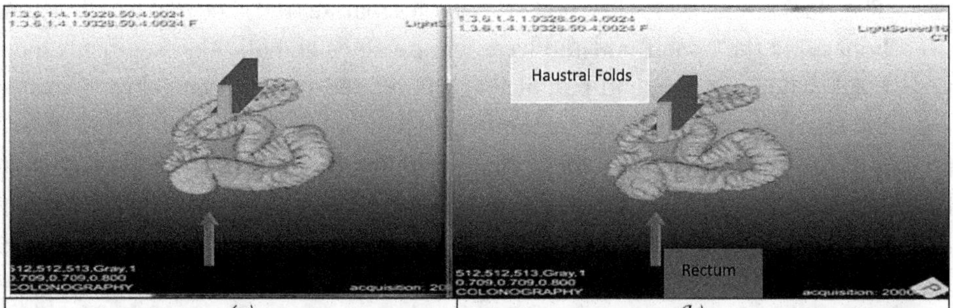

(a) (b)

Table 1. Comparison of the approaches

Approach	Techniques Used	Remarks
First approach: Segmentation of large intestine and removal of lungs using Clustering approach	Intensity based clustering and FCM clustering methods	To segment the colon and the focus was on the removal of bowel
Second approach: Automatic segmentation of colon by the removal of lungs and opacified fluid using cascade feed forward neural network	Otsu thresholding: the identification of colon and bowels Boundary detection algorithm - removal of lung cascade feedforward neural network trained with Bayesian Regulation Algorithm - Extraction of Opacified fluid which SLice Difference Removal (SLDR) method- Removal of Bowels	Advantage: Automatic Method Disadvantage: More Computational Time
Third Approach: The semi automatic segmentation of colon and the removal of opacified fluid using 3D seeded region growing	3D seeded region growing – Removal of colon Fuzzy connectedness approach - Removal of opacified fluid	Advantage: Reduced Computational Time Disadvantage: Semiautomatic Method

CONCLUSION

Thus three different approaches discussed for the segmentation of the colon are shown in Table 1.

The first approach focused on the removal of lungs. The second approach was an automatic approach in which both the removal of lungs and opacified fluid were shown. The third approach foussed on reducing the computational time of the second approach, which will produce an output within a fraction of seconds, but it was an semiautomatic approach. Thus all the above approaches were compared with manual segmentation by the radiologist to verify the segmentation results. Thus the third approach can be extended in future to identify the interface layer.

REFERENCES

Bernal, J., Sánchez, J., & Vilarino, F. (2012). Towards automatic polyp detection with a polyp appearance model. *Pattern Recognition*, *45*(9), 3166–3182. doi:10.1016/j.patcog.2012.03.002

Bernal, J., Sánchez, J., & Vilarino, F. (2012). Towards automatic polyp detection with a polyp appearance model. *Pattern Recognition*, *45*(9), 3166–3182. doi:10.1016/j.patcog.2012.03.002

Bevilacqua, V. (2013). Three-dimensional virtual colonoscopy for automatic polyps detection by artificial neural network approach: New tests on an enlarged cohort of polyps. *Neurocomputing*, *116*, 62–75. doi:10.1016/j.neucom.2012.03.026

Bevilacqua, V. (2013). Three-dimensional virtual colonoscopy for automatic polyps detection by artificial neural network approach: New tests on an enlarged cohort of polyps. *Neurocomputing*, *116*, 62–75. doi:10.1016/j.neucom.2012.03.026

Bogoni, L. (n.d.). CAD for Colonography: A tool to address a growing need. *British Journal of Radiology*.

Bond, J. H. (2000). Polyp guideline: Diagnosis, treatment, and surveillance for patients with colorectal polyps. *The American Journal of Gastroenterology*, *95*(11), 3053–3063. doi:10.1111/j.1572-0241.2000.03434.x PMID:11095318

Cancer Imaging Archives. (2017). *TCIA Collections*. Retrieved from http://cancerimagingarchive.net

Centers for Disease Control and Prevention (CDC). (2011). Vital signs: Colorectal cancer screening, incidence, and mortality--United States, 2002-2010. *MMWR. Morbidity and Mortality Weekly Report*, *60*(26), 884. PMID:21734636

Chen, D., Abdelmunim, H., Farag, A. A., Falk, R., & Dryden, G. (2008, September). Segmentation of colon tissue in ct colonography using adaptive level sets method. In MICCAI 2008 workshop: computational and visualization challenges in the new era of virtual colonoscopy (pp. 108-115). Academic Press.

Chowdhury, T. A., Whelan, P. F., & Ghita, O. (2008). A fully automatic CAD-CTC system based on curvature analysis for standard and low-dose CT data. *IEEE Transactions on Biomedical Engineering*, *55*(3), 888–901. doi:10.1109/TBME.2007.909506 PMID:18334380

Fiori, M., Musé, P., & Sapiro, G. (2011). *A complete system for polyps flagging in virtual colonoscopy*. Academic Press.

Gayathri Devi, K., & Radhakrishnan, R. (2014). A Comparative Study on the Automatic Segmentation of Colon in CT Colonography Using K- Means And Fuzzy C-Means Clustering. *Australian Journal of Basic and Applied Sciences*, *8*(9), 422–432.

Gayathri Devi, K., & Radhakrishnan, R. (2015). Automatic segmentation of colon in 3D CT images and removal of opacified fluid using cascade feed forward neural network. *Computational and mathematical methods in medicine.*

Gharipour, A., & Liew, A. W. C. (2013, July). Colon cell image segmentation based on level set and kernel-based fuzzy clustering. In *International Conference on Intelligent Computing* (pp. 120-129). Springer. 10.1007/978-3-642-39482-9_14

Grigorescu, S. E., Nevo, S. T., Liedenbaum, M. H., Truyen, R., Stoker, J., Van Vliet, L. J., & Vos, F. M. (2010). Automated detection and segmentation of large lesions in CT Colonography. *IEEE Transactions on Biomedical Engineering*, *57*(3), 675–684. doi:10.1109/TBME.2009.2035632 PMID:19884071

Hampshire, T., Roth, H. R., Helbren, E., Plumb, A., Boone, D., Slabaugh, G., & Hawkes, D. J. (2013). Endoluminal surface registration for CT colonography using haustral fold matching. *Medical Image Analysis*, *17*(8), 946–958. doi:10.1016/j.media.2013.04.006 PMID:23845949

Hong, W., Gu, X., Qiu, F., Jin, M., & Kaufman, A. (2006, June). Conformal virtual colon flattening. In *Proceedings of the 2006 ACM symposium on Solid and physical modeling* (pp. 85-93). ACM. 10.1145/1128888.1128901

Huang, A., Li, J., Summers, R. M., Petrick, N., & Hara, A. K. (2010). Improving polyp detection algorithms for CT colonography: Pareto front approach. *Pattern Recognition Letters*, *31*(11), 1461–1469. doi:10.1016/j.patrec.2010.03.013 PMID:20548966

Kainz, P., Pfeiffer, M., & Urschler, M. (2017). Segmentation and classification of colon glands with deep convolutional neural networks and total variation regularization. *PeerJ*, *5*, e3874. doi:10.7717/peerj.3874 PMID:29018612

Lee, J. G., Kim, J. H., Kim, S. H., Park, H. S., & Choi, B. I. (2011). A straightforward approach to computer-aided polyp detection using a polyp-specific volumetric feature in CT colonography. *Computers in Biology and Medicine*, *41*(9), 790–801. doi:10.1016/j.compbiomed.2011.06.015 PMID:21762887

McKenna, M. T., Wang, S., Nguyen, T. B., Burns, J. E., Petrick, N., & Summers, R. M. (2012). Strategies for improved interpretation of computer-aided detections for CT colonography utilizing distributed human intelligence. *Medical Image Analysis*, *16*(6), 1280–1292. doi:10.1016/j.media.2012.04.007 PMID:22705287

Naishadham, D., Lansdorp-Vogelaar, I., Siegel, R., Cokkinides, V., & Jemal, A. (2011). State disparities in colorectal cancer mortality patterns in the United States. *Cancer Epidemiology, Biomarkers & Prevention*, *20*(7), 1296–1302. doi:10.1158/1055-9965.EPI-11-0250 PMID:21737410

Pickhardt, P. J., Kim, D. H., Pooler, B. D., Hinshaw, J. L., Barlow, D., Jensen, D., ... Cash, B. D. (2013). Assessment of volumetric growth rates of small colorectal polyps with CT colonography: A longitudinal study of natural history. *The Lancet Oncology*, *14*(8), 711–720. doi:10.1016/S1470-2045(13)70216-X PMID:23746988

Shahbazi, M., Sattari, M., & Ghazic, M. (2008). Automatic polyp detection from CT colonography using mathematical morphology. In *Proceedings of the 21st ISPRS Congress* (pp. 823-828). Academic Press.

Sundaram, P., Zomorodian, A., Beaulieu, C., & Napel, S. (2008). Colon polyp detection using smoothed shape operators: Preliminary results. *Medical Image Analysis*, *12*(2), 99–119. doi:10.1016/j.media.2007.08.001 PMID:17910934

Van Ravesteijn, V. F., Van Wijk, C., Vos, F. M., Truyen, R., Peters, J. F., Stoker, J., & Van Vliet, L. J. (2010). Computer-aided detection of polyps in CT colonography using logistic regression. *IEEE Transactions on Medical Imaging*, *29*(1), 120–131. doi:10.1109/TMI.2009.2028576 PMID:19666332

Winawer, S. J., & Zauber, A. G. (2002). The advanced adenoma as the primary target of screening. *Gastrointestinal Endoscopy Clinics*, *12*(1), 1–9. doi:10.1016/S1052-5157(03)00053-9 PMID:11916153

Xu, Y., Cai, W., Nappi, J., & Yoshida, H. (2012). Fecal-tagging CT colonography with structure-analysis electronic cleansing for detection of colorectal flat lesions. *European Journal of Radiology*, *81*(8), 1712–1716. doi:10.1016/j.ejrad.2011.04.051 PMID:21596500

Yao, J., Miller, M., Franaszek, M., & Summers, R. M. (2004). Colonic polyp segmentation in CT colonography-based on fuzzy clustering and deformable models. *IEEE Transactions on Medical Imaging*, *23*(11), 1344–1352. doi:10.1109/TMI.2004.826941 PMID:15554123

Yao, J., & Summers, R. M. (2007, April). Detection and segmentation of colonic polyps on haustral folds. In *Biomedical Imaging: From Nano to Macro, 2007. ISBI 2007. 4th IEEE International Symposium on* (pp. 900-903). IEEE. 10.1109/ISBI.2007.356998

Yoshida, H., & Nappi, J. (2001). Three-dimensional computer-aided diagnosis scheme for detection of colonic polyps. *IEEE Transactions on Medical Imaging*, *20*(12), 1261–1274. doi:10.1109/42.974921 PMID:11811826

Zhu, H., Duan, C., Pickhardt, P., Wang, S., & Liang, Z. (2009). Computer-aided detection of colonic polyps with level set-based adaptive convolution in volumetric mucosa to advance CT colonography toward a screening modality. *Cancer Management and Research*, *1*, 1–13. doi:10.2147/CMAR.S4546 PMID:20428331

Section 4
Study of Compression and Denoising in Clinical Diagnosis

Chapter 7
Medical Data Storage and Compression

Saravanan Chandran
National Institute of Technology Durgapur, India

ABSTRACT

This chapter introduces medical imaging devices and its history. Further, the chapter discusses the history of the DICOM image and DICOM standard. The chapter also discusses image acquisition. Moreover, the chapter discusses the various software used for processing DICOM image. The chapter also discusses the limitations of DICOM and other medical image data formats. The basic structure of the DICOM is described in this chapter. Further, various research articles on medical image processing are discussed.

INTRODUCTION

The diagnosis of a disease plays vital role in the medical field. The digital medical imaging devices, such as X-Ray, Computer Tomography (CT), Magnetic Resonance Imaging (MRI), Ultrasound, Angiography, Mammography, Positron Emission Tomography (PET), Single Photon Emission Computed Tomography (SPECT), Endoscopy, Optical Coherence Tomography, etc. are used nowadays by the physicians for diagnosing myriad diseases. Numerous researchers have been developing various algorithms and models for diagnosing diseases and status or stages of the diseases. Early diagnosis of the diseases and stages of the diseases helps early recovery and avoid casualties. These digital medical imaging devices are assisting the physicians for early diagnosis of the disease and its stage for further treatment.

DOI: 10.4018/978-1-5225-5876-7.ch007

In the 1970s, digital diagnostic imaging devices produces a different digital image formats. Thus, the American College of Radiology (ACR) and the National Electrical Manufactures Association (NEMA) initiated to develop a common standard for digital medical images. In 1983 they introduced a standard to communicate standard digital medical image information, develop picture archiving and communication systems (PACS) that can be interfaced with other medical and hospital systems, creation of diagnostic information databases can be shared with rest of the world for interrogations. The ACR-NEMA started with their first standard publication No. 300-1985 version 1.0, second one No.300-1988 version 2.0 and several updates made in the standards. The copyright of the DICOM standard is hold by the National Electrical Manufacturers Association (NEMA). The DICOM standards Committee partly consists of NEMA members, developed the DICOM standard.

The Digital Imaging and Communications in Medicine (DICOM) is a popularising standard for producing, displaying, storing, processing, sending, retrieving, querying, and printing information in digital medical imaging (DICOM, 2018). The DICOM standard defined a file format and a network communications protocol for data transmission. The TCP/IP is used by the communication protocol for transmitting information from one system to another system. The DICOM capable systems can send and receive DICOM files having image and patient data together in a standard DICOM format.

MEDICAL DATA STORAGE AND COMPRESSION

The patented DICOM standard is built in medical imaging devices such as scanners, servers, workstations, printers, and network hardware from leading medical diagnostic device manufacturers such as Canon Healthcare Solutions, FUJIFILM Medical Systems U.S.A. Inc., GE Healthcare, Hitachi Healthcare Americas, Konica Minolta Medical Imaging USA Inc., Philips, Samsung Medical Devices, Siemens Healthineers, Swissray International Inc., Toshiba America Medical Systems, etc. The various devices support DICOM format clearly states the DICOM classes they support.

The DICOM standard is implemented in variety of devices as few are mentioned below (Wikipedia, 2018).

- PACS (picture archiving and communication systems)
- Image viewers and display stations
- CAD (computer-aided detection/diagnosis systems)
- 3D visualization systems
- Clinical analysis applications
- Image printers

- Film scanners
- Media burners (that export DICOM files onto CDs, DVDs, etc)
- Media importers (that import DICOM files from CDs, DVDs, USBs, etc)
- RIS (radiology information systems)
- VNA (vendor-neutral archives)
- EMR (electronic medical record) systems
- Radiology reporting systems

The DICOM standard has been widely adopted including dentists' and doctors' offices and hospitals. The DICOM standard is applicable in many medicine fields and few are listed below (Wikipedia, 2018).

- Radiology
- Cardiology
- Oncology
- Radiotherapy
- Neurology
- Orthopedics
- Obstetrics
- Gynecology
- Ophthalmology
- Dentistry
- Maxillofacial surgery
- Dermatology
- Pathology
- Clinical trials
- Veterinary medicine

The digital medical imaging analysis report prepared by the novel algorithms and model systems contribute for accurate diagnosis of the disease and stage. The DICOM reserved 104, 2761, 2762, 11112 for TCP or UDP. Several software developed for processing DICOM such as 3DSlicer, GDCM, Ginkgo CADx, MicroDicom, OsiriX, Orthanc, XnView, Invesalius, etc. A major disadvantage of DICOM is too many optional fields this leads to many fields remain empty or with incorrect data.

Thus, several other standards evolved by various research groups to overcome shortage of DICOM, such as Clinical Data Interchange Standards Consortium (CDISC), electronic health record (EHR), or electronic medical record (EMR), eHealth, Electronic Health Record Communication (EN 13606), Fast Healthcare Interoperability Resources (FHIR, pronounced "fire"), Health Level-7 (HL7), openEHR (open electronic health records), Standard Architecture for Healthcare Information Systems (ENV 12967), etc.

The digital image is represented by m x n pixels in a matrix form which are captured by digital cameras. But, the digital medical image is an image captured by electronics medical diagnostic devices in the form of m x n pixels in a matrix form and patient details stored along with the m x n pixels digital image. These digital medical images are classified into Black and White, Greyscale, and Color. The Black and White images are represented by 0s and 1s. The Greyscale images are represented using 8 bits positive integer values ranging from 0 to 255. The Colour images are represented by three Red, Blue, Green Channels and values ranging from 0 to 255 in the case of 8 bit color images. These digital medical images are easy to store, send, receive, analyse, print, process, in digital form in the storage and Internet.

The hospitals started using digital medical diagnosis devices and produces digital information. The hospitals official tasks are automated such as registration of a patient, online appointment fixing, etc. The number of tasks automated is increasing and various standards developed for organizing health records in structured and standard methods. These instant health records can be instantly accessible by authorized users. One of the standards is DICOM standard, consists of DICOM File Meta Information and DICOM Data set. The DICOM data set consists of Patients details, Study details, Equipment details and Image details. The Clinical Data Interchange Standards Consortium (CDISC) developed standards for clinical and non-clinical research processes. There are different phases in the standard, such as planning, data collection, data tabulations, analysis, data exchange, etc. The electronic health record (EHR) or electronic medical record (EMR) is a digitised patient's paper chart provides instant and secure information to authorized users. EHRs can store patient's diagnoses, medical history, medications, immunization dates, treatment plans, radiology images, laboratory test results, and allergies. Evidence based tools can access data to make decisions about patients. Automates and streamlines the workflow. The main objective of the Electronic Health Record Communication (EN 13606) is to define rigorous and stable information architecture for communicating part or all of the electronic health record (EHR). This is to support interoperability of various systems and components. Health Level-7 (HL7) is producing healthcare data exchange and information modeling standards.

Fast Healthcare Interoperability Resources (FHIR, pronounced "fire") is the new specification can be used as a stand-alone data exchange standard and also be used in partnership with existing standards. The openEHR (open electronic health records) is a virtual community working on turning health data from the physical form into electronic form to ensure universal interoperability. The Standard Architecture for Healthcare Information Systems (ENV 12967) provides guidance on the development of modular open information technology systems in the healthcare sector. The standard consists of three parts, enterprise viewpoint, information viewpoint, and computational viewpoint. Thus, there are various standards available for storing medical data consists of patient details, digital medical images, etc. and compression is essential to reduce the number of bytes required to store the data in the electronic storage devices. In the coming section various research articles related to Medical Data and Image Compression available over the Internet are discussed.

Arthritis is one of the common diseases among senior people aged above 50. More than 100 types of arthritis reported mostly due to bone joints of senior people due to overuse or injury. Common joint issues are swelling, stiffness, and pain and mostly of three different categories mild, moderate, and severe.

The magnetic resonance imaging (MRI) visualizes bone, cartilage, and soft tissues, assists the medical practitioner for the diagnosis of chronic and acute joint syndromes. The X-ray or ultrasound technology will not reveal subchondral bone marrow. But, MRI visualises subchondral bone marrow pathologies (Wikipedia, 2018; DIDCOM, 2018). Abuse or damage on arthritis of knee causes pain. The knee pain intensifies by age. Every year approximately 20 million public consulting therapeutic practitioners for arthritis knee pain in the United States. The knee pains are classified in to acute and chronic. The acute knee pain develops quickly and chronic knee pain develops steadily over time. The largest joints in the body are knees. The knee joints are made with the bones of the lower end of the thighbone (femur), the upper end of the shinbone (tibia), and the knee cap (patella). Bands of tissue called ligaments connect the bones in the knee, which allows freedom of movement with certain limitations. The impacts are absorbed by cartilage in the knees cushioning the ends of the bones. In the recent years, pediatrics patients are reported with CNS tumors in the knee bone (DICOM, 2018).

Arthritis generally refers to inflammation of the joints. Osteoarthritis (OA) is a deteriorating joint disease of the bone joints caused by repair and remodelling of concomitant cartilage, subchondral bone sclerosis (increased bone formation around the joint), and osteophyte and bone cyst formation (Extrahop, 2016). Osteoarthritis causes due to wear and tear of cartilage in joints and happens in any joint of the body. The weight-bearing joints of the hips, knees, spine, and fingers, thumb, neck, and large toe are affected by osteoarthritis. Clinical signs and symptoms such as joint pain, effusion, movement limitation, and gait deviations are results of joint changes. These characteristics make OA a particularly weakening disease affected approximately 21 million adults in USA. In addition, fifty percent of Americans aged 65 and above (17 million) reported having OA in any one of the joint (Ababneh et al., 2011). 250 million people approximately reported to have osteoarthritis in the knee in global (Hunter et al., 2011). These facts made OA a serious public health concern and identifying at early stage prevents major damages to the knee joints. Selected research works related to arthritis are discussed in the following section.

The diagnosis based on digital medical imaging for myriad diseases has been grown rapidly. The digital medical imaging augments the medical professionals for accurate diagnosis of the disease and detection of tumors. The Magnetic Resonance Imaging (MRI) visualizes bone, cartilage, and soft tissues, assists the medical practitioner for the better assessment of chronic and acute joint disorders. The X-ray or ultrasound technology are not visualizing the subchondral bone marrow thus, the MRI is more suitable tool for assessing these pathologies.

Injury and abuse of physical structure of the body are the major cause of knee pain. Lack of proper care of the body and lack of regular physical exercise leads to knee joint pain at the old age. Yearly 20 million people consult medical practitioners for treatment to knee pain in the United States. The knees are the largest joints in the body of human. The knee pain is developed suddenly (acute) or gradually over time (chronic). The knee joints are made up of the thighbone (femur), the shinbone (tibia), and the knee cap (patella). The bones are connected by the bands of tissue called ligaments in the knees, which allows mobility, and helps preventing abnormal movements in the joints. Cartilage of the knees absorbs impact by cushioning the ends of the bones. Recently several CNS tumors of the knee bone are reported in group of pediatric patients (Selvanayaki et al., 2013).

Uncontrollably and abnormally cells split into number of units. These split units form a tumour. Bone tumors are noticed in the bones. The tumor grows and become an abnormal tissue. This abnormal tissue can displace healthy tissue. Some tumors are benign and they are not cancerous. There are several cases reported with knee tumor. Normally benign bone tumors will not spread to other parts of the body and are unlikely to be fatal. They can still be dangerous and may require treatment. Benign tumors can grow and could compress healthy bone tissue. Other tumors are malignant, meaning they're cancerous. Malignant bone tumors can cause cancer to spread throughout the body (AARP, n.d.).

DICOM

The American College of Radiology (ACR) and National Electrical Manufacturers Association (NEMA) has developed DICOM standard. They started in the 1980s and released the second version in 1988. The US Army and Air Force first deployed in a large-scale of ACR/NEMA technology in 1992. Loral Aerospace and Siemens Medical Systems deployed the first US military PACS (Picture Archiving and Communications System) with a consortium of companies. The third version of the standard was released during 1993 and the name was changed to "DICOM." They defined new service classes, added network support and introduced the Conformance Statement to establish the basic DICOM communication protocols for query or retrieval, storage and print classes. The DICOM version has been regularly improved since 1993.

Digital Imaging and Communications in Medicine (DICOM) is a renowned standard in the medical field. The DICOM file has provision to store information about patients and relevant details such as, procedures, images, and imaging equipment. DICOM is has Client-Server architecture and hierarchically structured. It has the following parts:

- Format for the File and data
- Protocol for Data interchange
- Architecture for Network protocol

All modern medical imaging systems like Ultrasounds, X-Rays, MRI (Magnetic Resonance Imaging), and CT (Computed Tomography) support DICOM. The DICOM has two vital part one is the file format and another one is the networking protocol. At present most of the medical images are stored in the storage device in DICOM format. Doctors started using computer software applications which supports DICOM format and DICOM Viewers, which helps to view DICOM images for diagnosing the status of the disease from the medical images. DICOM files comprise of medical images as well as patient name, patient ID, gender of the patient, and birth date of the patient, equipment type and settings of the equipment at that moment, and purpose of the study of medical images for the medical treatment.

The DICOM network protocol supported by several medical applications helps to exchange DICOM files which consist of medical images, patient information and other procedure information. The DICOM files are stored in an archive and the DICOM network protocol helps to search in the archive for imaging studies and display imaging studies in the workstation for further evaluation by the medical practitioners. Several advanced network commands are available for following and control the schedule procedures, treatment, report status, sharing imaging devices between doctors depending on the device and doctor's availability, etc.

The DICOM acts as an Interface and has clear definition. Integration of medical systems manufactured by many different vendors using common standard DICOM helps to achieve sharing information in short time across the countries. If the hospital installs a new medical imaging system and further connects it into the network for querying the medical imaging archive, retrieving the images from the archive that were created by other systems and display them. Similarly, other vendor systems can access the new images produced by the new system and view them in their display. Sharing of images in the network not require any changes or modifications to any of the involved system software.

Basic Structures and Concepts in DICOM

1. DICOM Objects are known as the Information Object Definitions (IOD). All real world data like patients, studies, medical devices, images, patient schedule list, a queue to be sent to a printer are objects with defined templates. These are definitions of the information to be exchanged between a Service Class User (SCU) - Client and Service Class Provider (SCP) - Server.
2. A DICOM modality is a property/attribute of the DICOM data object, e.g. CT, MRI, X-rays etc. are the modalities
3. A DICOM Message is composed of a Command Set followed by a conditional Data Set.
4. Command and Data sets are made of Elements.
5. Elements have a Tag, length and value.
6. Tags have group tag and element tag.
7. DICOM applications provide the services required for the data exchange.
8. DICOM Service Element (DIMSE) are used by Application Entities (AE).
9. There are two types of DIMSE Services, Composite DIMSE-C and Normalized DIMSE-N. These support operations and notifications like storage, retrieval, printing etc. on the SOP instances.
10. AEs have Titles (AET). AE has an IP address assigned. AET are case sensitive and unique.
11. Service Object Pairs (SOPs) have an unique ID (UID). SOP Classes are the fundamental unit of DICOM interoperability.

Sending and receiving DICOM images and searching in other medical systems similar to software applications on Internet sending and receiving digital images and like web browser searching and displaying digital images stored on the far away servers.

The expectations from the DICOM standard are different from doctors to doctors and hospital to hospitals. The various countries follow various systems. Thus, still the researchers are working on to develop a standard DICOM for entire world. The DICOM standard cannot be defined as the basic functions of a computer or laptop or printer or scanner. Integration of various vendors' medical equipment is still having issues. Thus, large budget projects for developing medical interface equipment are very much few in numbers.

The most notable achievement of DICOM is the ability of modern imaging equipment to seamlessly collaborate and integrate together in a multi-vendor environment that led to a great advancement in medical imaging.

The DICOM files will have a filename with .dcm extension. The DICOM file contains patient data and medical images as data. The patient data are collected from other systems such as EMR or HER or HIS systems as HL7 data which are tightly coupled with the equipment, procedures, and image data created by the radiology medical imaging devices as DICOM data.

The DICOM protocol is called as a binary Upper Level Protocol (ULP) over TCP/IP. The ports 104, 2761, 2762 and 11112 are used in DICOM based software for network communications. These ports are used to transmit DICOM data, search, integrate, query, print, distribute, store, share, display medical images and patient data from the radiology archival or storage systems (PACS, RIS) to the workstation for the Radiologist to write reports.

MEDICAL DATA AND IMAGE COMPRESSION

Ababneh, Prescott, and Gurcan (2011) has proposed a fully automated and content based system for knee bone segmentation from magnetic resonance images (MRI) (Ababneh et al., 2011). They divided the framework into two phases I and II. Phase I pre-process the image, extracts the feature, and discovers ROI. Phase II constructs graph and segment the bone using morphological operations. They evaluated the performance of the algorithm by block detection rate and measuring accuracy of the segmentation. They conducted several tests with variety of images, such as 3-D stacks of a patient with arbitrary slice number for patients with varying degrees of OA progression.

They used DICOM images publically available in the Internet with OAI dataset (Nevitt et al., 2006) in this research work. They tested the performance of the proposed segmentation scheme with 376 MR images. Those MR images of sagittal T2 map 120 mm FOV are obtained from three Tesla Siemens machines. The image are 25–35 slices per series, slice thickness is 3 mm, 384 x 384 pixel resolutions, pixel spacing is .3125/.3125 mm. The manual segmentation was performed by two trained readers and accuracy of the proposed segmentation scheme was measured and compared with regions obtained manually. They used Dice Similarity Index (DSI) to quantify the region overlap between the automatic and the manual segmentations (Dice, 1945; Zijdenbos et al., 1994). (As cited in Abadneh et al., 2011).

They selected three patient's three volumes of slices for training. In the training data phase, ROI block discovered using features extracted from each slice with two background blocks and four ROI blocks. Ten patient's data sets volumes of slices (3-D) were used to test the performance of proposed segmentation model. For each patient, slice 8 to slice 21, 14 consecutive slices were selected which are representing the slices of the identifiable femur and tibia bone structures. Ten test patients with different KL grades (0–4) were selected for the experiment. Two readers were provided ten patients data with ground truth segmentation masks for testing inter-reader variability. They proposed two phase approach in that the initial phase identified bone areas with a high accuracy 0.99 detection rate. The final segmentation is accurate with a mean DSI value of 0.95 (Abadneh et al., 2011).

Hunter et al. (2011), evolved semi-quantitative scoring methods Magnetic Resonance Imaging Osteoarthritis Knee Score (MOAKS). Their MOAKS instrument refined the scoring of Bone Marrow Lesions (BMLs), cartilage (sub-regional assessment), and the elements of meniscal morphology scoring. They achieved overall accuracy 75%.

Roy and Bandyopadhyay (2012) proposed a fully automatic algorithm for detecting brain tumors using symmetry. The algorithm detected the tumor, segmented the tumor and calculated area of the tumor. They used median filter to remove noise in the pre-processing stage. The segmentation of tumors in MRI was addressed by multi-step approach watershed. Further, morphological operations erode and dilate were applied. The image is converted into binary for detecting binaries and holes. The smaller objects are removed to highlight the tumor object. The edges of the tumor were detected using Sobel edge detection technique. The tumors size was calculated by number of pixels in the tumor region.

Ahirwar (2013) discussed various segmentation techniques, MRI image modalities, classification of MRI region, and performed statistical test. Self-Organizing Map (SOM) and Neuro fuzzy techniques were used to classify the white matter (WM), gray matter (GM), cerebro-spinal fluid (CSF), and tumor. The author used Keith database for the experimentation. The author listed the effectiveness of the scheme in percentage for precision, accuracy, specificity, sensitivity, false positive rate, positive predictive value, likelihood ratio positive, false negative rate, negative predictive value, likelihood ratio negative, and prevalence of disease.

Selvanayaki and Kalugasalam (2013) proposed meta-heuristic methods for segmenting brain tumor in 3D magnetic resonance images. They divided work into two regions, first one is preprocessing. In the preprocessing they used tracking algorithms to suppress artifacts. Further weighted median filter is used to enhance the image. They evaluated the preprocessed image by Peak Signal-to-Noise Ratio (PSNR) and Average Signal-to-Noise Ratio (ASNR). In the Second stage three algorithms Ant Colony Optimization (ACO), Genetic Algorithm (GA) and Particle Swarm Optimization (PSO), was implemented for identifying and segmenting of suspicious region using and their performance was studied. The algorithms were tested on 21 pairs of MRI from real patient‘s brain database and evaluated the performance of the proposed method. The experiment results show that the Particle swarm optimization produces 99.28% accuracy in tumor detection than ACO and GA.

Gensheimer, Hawkins, Ermoian, and Trister (2015) developed an algorithm for analysing various levels of heterogeneity with clinical imaging. Their algorithm segmented the tumor image recursively into increasingly smaller regions. This process continued till the tumor had been divided into single voxels and segmented at multiple scales. At each scale, they measured heterogeneity by comparing each segmented region with the adjacent region. Further, they calculated the difference in signal intensity histograms. They showed that their proposed algorithm was robust to image artifacts and various tumors shapes using digital phantom images. In the MRI of 18 rhabdomyosarcoma patients they measured primary tumor scales of contrast enhancement heterogeneity. The algorithm produced a biologically motivated segmentation of tumor regions and reports the amount of heterogeneity at various distance scales.

Stomp et al., (2015) studied 6673 individual aged from 45 to 65 years deemed overweight or obese self-reported BMI of 27kg/m^2 or above and residing in the greater area of Leiden (west of the Netherlands). They performed MRI studies on a 1.5-T MRI system (Philips) with a dedicated 8-channel knee coil. The parameters echo train length 6, 150–160 mm field of view, and 304 × 512 matrix were identical for the TSE images. They acquired sequences were (1) coronal proton density (PD) (repetition time (TR)/echo time (TE) 2335/35 ms; 3 mm slice thickness; 0.6 mm interslice gap); (2) coronal fat suppressed PD TSE images (TR/TE 2334/35 ms; 3 mm slice thickness; 0.6 mm interslice gap); (3) sagittal PD TSE images (TR/TE 2338/35; 3.5 mm slice thickness; 0.7 mm interslice gap); (4) sagittal frequency selective fat-suppressed T1-weighted 3D gradient echo (GE) sequence (TR/TE 11/5.5; 25° flip angle; 150 mm field of view, 272 × 512 matrix, 2 mm slice thickness with a 1-mm overlap between images; no gap); (5) axial fat suppressed PD (TSE) images (TR/TE 3225/15; 4 mm slice thickness; 0.8 mm interslice gap). Total acquisition time calculated was 30 min.

Hajiaghayi, Groves, Jafarkhani, and Kheradvar (2017) studied, developed and validated a 3-D automated segmentation method for cardiac Magnetic Resonance Images (MRI). Their proposed segmentation algorithm automatically reconstructed cardiac MRI DICOM data into a 3-D model without relying on prior statistical knowledge. Thus, there is no need of training datasets. They employed the method to detect the left ventricular cavity in the York university database. Their experiment shown significant improvement in segmentation performance compared to other manual segmentation and automated methods.

Uligoj, Vaco, Jerbi, Ekoranja, and Vidakovi (2017) presented and evaluated an algorithm for automatic localization of spherical fiducials in CT scans. The results of the algorithm were evaluated with four skilled human operators. The experiment carried out using twelve patient and eight lab phantom CT scans. The localization error of the algorithm was smaller by 49.29% compared with the human readings and compared with intra-modal estimation smaller by 45.91%. The processing time for localization was reduced by 84.96%. Twenty different test samples containing a total of 116 spherical fiducials were experimented and noticed the reliability on successful localization of the fiducial marker was 100%. The developed fully automated and accurate machine vision algorithm performs accurate localization for the robotic system RObotic Neuro-NAvigation (RONNA).

Skripcak et al. (2016), designed a conceptual model of IT solution for radiotherapy research domain. They developed an open source system for medical IT platform. They designed integrating electronic data capture system (EDC), medical image archive (PACS), and patient identity management system (PIDG). They discussed three deployment scenarios, central, virtually hosted or decentralized environment.

Zenteno, Rojas, Chang and Castaneda (2016) assessed the performance of a newly designed portable low cost and network ready ultrasonic imaging device SonicCare. They compared the new device with other two existing commercial devices. They tested the dead zone, spatial measurement calibration, spatial resolution, functional resolution, and dynamic range, while scanning an ATS 539 multipurpose rubber based phantom for experimental quality assurance. They performed tests with clinical image quality on two local and one rural health services facilities. They measured dimensions and image based screening on liver, gallbladder, and kidney. The experimental quality assurance tests revealed a mean measurement error of 4.7% and a coefficient of variability of 5% while the clinical imaging test revealed that the cross-correlation precision against a clinical non-portable device was ±8.5 mm.

Yan et al. (2016) designed a multistage deep learning framework for classification of images and experimented the framework for recognition of various body parts. Their research work focused at: 1) discovering the local regions that are discriminative and non-informative to the image classification problem, and 2) learn an image-level classifier based on these local regions. They introduced two stages of learning schemes for achieving these two tasks. A convolutional neural network (CNN) was introduced in a multi-instance learning approach for extracting the most discriminative and non-informative local patches from the training slices. Further, the images were classified using the pre-learned CNN boosted with the local patches. The learned and boosted CNN utilised the discriminative local appearances and produced accurate classification than other techniques. The proposed method automatically discovered the discriminative and non-informative local patches through multi-instance deep learning and there is no requirement for manual annotation. They validated their method on a synthetic dataset and a large scale CT dataset. The experiment results show better performances than state-of-the-art approaches, including the standard deep CNN.

Godinho, Viana-Ferreira, Bastiao Silva, and Costa (2016) developed smart routing mechanism for distributed medical imaging networks. The proposed system has innovative cache system based on splitting and dynamic management of digital imaging and communications in medicine objects. They conducted an experiment successfully on the proposed system using a regional PACS archive. The experimental results show that the proposed system is better than the conventional approaches.

Uligoj, Vaco, Jerbi, Ekoranja, and Vidakovi (2017), presented and evaluated an algorithm for automatic localization of spherical fiducials in CT scans. The approach is unique which combines machine vision algorithms, biomedical image filtration methods, and mathematical estimation methods. The performance of the proposed algorithm was test with the results of the proposed method and skilled human operators. The proposed algorithm reduces the localization error and processing time. The proposed algorithm achieved 100% reliability.

Hajiaghayi, Groves, Jafarkhani, and Kheradvar (2017), developed and validated a fast automatic 3-D segmentation method for cardiac magnetic resonance imaging. The proposed algorithm automatically develops a 3-D model by reconstructing the cardiac MRI DICOM data without any prior statistical knowledge. They used York university database for the experiment. The proposed 3-D active contour method was used for detecting the left ventricular cavity in 33 subjects with heterogeneous heart diseases. They identified papillary muscles and added to the chamber using a convex hull of the left ventricle and interpolation. They segmented the myocardium using similar 3-D segmentation method. The experiment result shows improvement in segmentation performance compared to other automated and manual methods.

CONCLUSION

Automation of medical industry is in high demand. Storing patient information, pathological test results, medical images etc. also part of it. Storing medical information and processing medical data in the computers requires special attention. The computer system and digital electronics system assists the medical experts for easy access to medical information. Thus, various researches progressing in the field of developing novel frameworks, architectures, algorithms, methods, models, etc. This chapter has discussed various research articles discussing about the novel algorithms or methods on medical image applications.

REFERENCES

AARP. (n.d.). *Health Tools*. Retrieved from https://www.aarp.org/health/health_tools.html

Ahirwar, A. (2013). Study of Techniques used for Medical Image Segmentation and Computation of Statistical Test for Region Classification of Brain MRI. *I.J. Information Technology and Computer Science*, *5*(5), 44–53. doi:10.5815/ijitcs.2013.05.06

Associated Osteonecrosis of the Wrist and Knee in Three Pediatric Patients with Recurrent CNS Tumors. (2013). *Journal of Clinical Oncology*, *31*(2).

DICOM. (2018). Retrieved from Dicom.nema.org

Extrahop. (2016). *An Introduction to DICOM (Digital Imaging and Communications in Medicine)*. Retrieved from https://www.extrahop.com/company/blog/2016/introduction-to-dicom-protocol/

Godinho. (2016, January). A Routing Mechanism for Cloud Outsourcing of Medical Imaging Repositories. *IEEE Journal of Biomedical and Health Informatics*, *20*(1).

Hajiaghayi, M., Groves, E. M., Jafarkhani, H., & Kheradvar, A. (2017, January). A 3-D Active Contour Method for Automated Segmentation of the Left Ventricle From Magnetic Resonance Images. *IEEE Transactions on Biomedical Engineering*, *64*(1), 134–144. doi:10.1109/TBME.2016.2542243 PMID:27046887

Hajiaghayi, M., Groves, E. M., Jafarkhani, H., & Kheradvar, A. (2017). A 3-D Active Contour Method for Automated Segmentation of the Left Ventricle From Magnetic Resonance Images. *IEEE Transactions on Biomedical Engineering*, *64*(1), 134–144. doi:10.1109/TBME.2016.2542243 PMID:27046887

Hunter, D. J., Guermazi, A., Lo, G. H., Grainger, A. J., Conaghan, P. G., Boudreau, R. M., & Roemer, F. W. (2011). Evolution of semi-quantitative whole joint assessment of knee OA: MOAKS (MRI Osteoarthritis Knee Score). *Osteoarthritis and Cartilage*, *19*(8), 990–1002. doi:10.1016/j.joca.2011.05.004 PMID:21645627

Michael, F. (2015). Assessing the scale of tumor heterogeneity by complete hierarchical segmentation of MRI. *Physics in Medicine and Biology*, *60*(3), 977–993. doi:10.1088/0031-9155/60/3/977 PMID:25575341

Roy & Bandyopadhyay. (2012). Detection and Quantification of Brain Tumor from MRI of Brain and it's Symmetric Analysis. *International Journal of Information and Communication Technology Research, 2*(6).

Selvanayaki & Kalugasalam. (2013). Intelligent Brain Tumor Tissue Segmentation From Magnetic Resonance Image (MRI) Using Meta Heuristic Algorithms. *Journal of Global Research in Computer Science, 4*(2).

Skripcak, T., Just, U., Simon, M., Buttner, D., Luhr, A., Baumann, M., & Krause, M. (2016, September). Toward Distributed Conduction of Large-Scale Studies in Radiation Therapy and Oncology: Open-Source System Integration Approach. *IEEE Journal of Biomedical and Health Informatics, 20*(5), 1397–1403. doi:10.1109/JBHI.2015.2450833

Stomp, W., Reijnierse, M., Kloppenburg, M., de Mutsert, R., Bovée, J. V. M. G., den Heijer, M., & Bloem, J. L. (2015). Prevalence of cartilaginous tumours as an incidental finding on MRI of the knee. *European Radiology, 25*(12), 3480–3487. doi:10.100700330-015-3764-6 PMID:25994192

Sufyan, Y. (2011). Automatic graph-cut based segmentation of bones from knee magnetic resonance images for osteoarthritis research. *Medical Image Analysis, 15*(4), 438–448. doi:10.1016/j.media.2011.01.007 PMID:21474362

Uligoj, F. (2017). *Automated Marker Localization in the Planning Phase of Robotic Neurosurgery* (Vol. 5). IEEE Access.

Uligoj, F., Vaco, M., Jerbi, B., Ekoranja, B., & Vidakovi, J. (2017). Automated Marker Localization in the Planning Phase of Robotic Neurosurgery. *IEEE Access, 5*, 12265–12274. doi:10.1109/ACCESS.2017.2718621

Wikipedia. (2018). *DICOM*. Retrieved from https://en.wikipedia.org/wiki/DICOM

Yan, Z., Zhan, Y., Peng, Z., & Shu, L. (2016, May). Multi-Instance Deep Learning: Discover Discriminative Local Anatomies for Bodypart Recognition. *IEEE Transactions on Medical Imaging, 35*(5), 1332–1343. doi:10.1109/TMI.2016.2524985

Zenteno, Rojas, Chang, & Castaneda. (2016). SonicCare: Performance of a New Low-Cost and Portable Device for Medical Tele-Ultrasonography on Underserved Areas. *IEEE Latin America Transactions, 14*(7).

Chapter 8
Non-Subsampled Contourlet Transform-Based Effective Denoising of Medical Images:
Denoising of Medical Images Using Contourlet

Karthikeyan P.
Velammal College of Engineering and Technology, India

Vasuki S.
Velammal College of Engineering and Technology, India

Karthik K.
Velammal College of Engineering and Technology, India

ABSTRACT

Noise removal in medical images remains a challenge for the researchers because noise removal introduces artifacts and blurring of the image. Developing medical image denoising algorithm is a difficult operation because a tradeoff between noise reduction and the preservation of actual features of image has to be made in a way that enhances and preserves the diagnostically relevant image content. A special member of the emerging family of multiscale geometric transforms is the contourlet transform which effectively captures the image edges and contours. This overcomes the limitations of the existing method of denoising using wavelet and curvelet. But due to down sampling and up sampling, the contourlet transform is shift-variant. However, shift-invariance is desirable in image analysis applications such as edge detection, contour characterization, and image enhancement. In this chapter, nonsubsampled contourlet transform (shift-invariance transform)-based denoising is presented which more effectively represents edges than contourlet transform.

DOI: 10.4018/978-1-5225-5876-7.ch008

INTRODUCTION

The extraction of features and object recognition of medical images acquired by various imaging modalities plays an essential role in extracting information for diagnosing various diseases. The presence of noise not only produces undesirable visual quality, but also lowers the visibility of low contrast objects. Medical images are usually of low contrast and they are subject to complex type of noise in its acquisition and transmission. All medical images are corrupted by visual noise. The presence of noise gives an image a mottled, grainy, textured, or snowy appearance. This noise can be either image dependent or image independent. It comes from a variety of sources. The diagnosis process would become complex if the image is contaminated with noise. Generally MRI images are affected by Additive White Gaussian Noise (AWGN) and ultrasonography images are affected by speckle noise during image acquisition. So noise removal in medical images plays an essential process for diagnosing the diseases properly (Chan, Law, & Siu, 2003; da Cunha et al., 2006).

In medical images, removal of noise is delicate and difficult task. Noise removal in medical images still remains as a challenge for the researchers because noise removal introduces artifacts and blurring of the image. Developing medical image denoising algorithm is a difficult operation because a tradeoff between noise reduction and preservation of actual features of image has to be made in a way that enhances and preserves the diagnostically relevant image content. A special member of the emerging family of multiscale geometric transform is contourlet transform (Do & Vetterli, 2002). The contourlet transform effectively captures the image edges and contours which are reconstructed using Laplacian pyramid and directional filter bank. This feature overcomes the limitations of the existing method of denoising using wavelet and curvelet. Thresholding is performed on the obtained contourlet coefficients, so that essential information in the image is preserved by removing the noise. But due to downsampling and upsampling, the contourlet transform is shift-variant. However, shift-invariance is desirable in image analysis applications such as edge detection, contour characterization, and image enhancement. This is a major drawback of the existing method which can be eliminated using nonsubsampled contourlet transform based denoising.

In this work, nonsubsampled contourlet transform (NSCT), which is a shift-invariant version of the contourlet transform is presented. The nonsubsampled contourlet transform is based on iterated nonsubsampled filter banks to obtain a shift-invariant directional multiresolution image representation.

The existing denoising algorithms, however tend to attenuate original signal features. In order to overcome this problem, the contourlet transform has been used to suppress noise in digital images. Contourlet based image denoising algorithms generally consist of three steps; (i) Take contourlet transform of the input noisy image (ii) Shrinking a selective part of contourlet coefficients, and (iii) Inverse contourlet transform of the modified coefficients (Kamran et al., 2012; Dengwen & Wengang, 2008). Based on this framework, there are two types of contourlet based noise reduction methods; one is to seek appropriate contourlet basis for higher frequency resolution and the other is to select more appropriate contourlet coefficients to be shrunk i.e., the appropriate thresholding technique to be used is to be chosen.

Multiresolution Transforms

Wavelet Transform

Wavelets are basically mathematical functions which break up the data into different frequency components and each component with a resolution matched to its scale. Wavelets are the better technique to handle the different type of noises which is present in an image. Wavelets, although good at representing point discontinuities, are not good at representing edge discontinuities (Ma, Zie, & Luo, 2009). A comparative study between wavelet coefficient shrinkage filter and several standard speckle filters used for speckle noise suppression, shows that the wavelet-based approach is deployed among the best for speckle removal (Riazifar & Yazdi, 2009). The wavelet decomposition of an image is done as follows: In the first level of decomposition, the image is split into 4 subbands, namely the HH, HL, LH and LL sub bands. The HH sub band gives the diagonal details of the image; the HL sub band gives the horizontal features while the LH subband represents the vertical structures. The LL subband is the low resolution residual consisting of low frequency components, which is further split at higher levels of decomposition.

Curvelet Transform

Curvelets are an appropriate basis for representing images (or other functions) which is smooth apart from singularities along smooth curves, where the curves have bounded curvature, i.e. where objects in the image have a minimum length scale (Tomasi & Manduchi, 1998) This property holds for cartoons, geometrical diagrams, and text. The edges in such images appear increasingly straight when zoomed. Curvelets take advantage of this property, by defining the higher resolution curvelets to be skinnier than the lower resolution curvelets (Hamdi, 2012). However, natural images do not possess this property; they have detail at every scale. Therefore, for natural images, it is preferable to use some sort of directional wavelet transform whose wavelets have the same aspect ratio at every scale. Curvelets provide a representation that is considerably sparser for a reconstructed image than other wavelet transforms. The spatial decomposition of an image using curvelet transform is shown in Figure 1.

Representing 2D Piece Wise Smooth Signal

Consider the wavelet transform of a 2-D piecewise function with a smooth discontinuity curve (Figure 2(a)). Due to the separable construction, 2-D wavelet basis functions have supports on dyadic squares. Consequently, wavelets are good at isolating discontinuity points as only wavelets whose supports overlap with the discontinuity curve generate significant coefficients. However, they are blind to the smoothness of this curve and it is easy to see that there is $O(2^j)$ significant wavelet coefficients at the scale 2^{-j}.

The performance of the wavelet scheme can be improved even when the discontinuity curve is known to be smooth. Simply looking at the wavelet transform in Figure 2(a) suggests that rather treating each significant wavelet coefficient along the discontinuity curve independently, the nearby coefficients can be grouped as their locations are locally correlated (Jiang et al., 2010). The curve scaling relation hints that it is possible to group about $a2^{j/2}$ nearby wavelet basis functions at the scale 2^{-j} into one basis function with a linear structure, so that its width is proportional to its length squared, as shown in Figure 2(b). This grouping operation reduces the number of significant coefficients at the scale 2^{-j} from $O(2^j)$ to $O(2^{j/2})$. Consequently, such a new expansion is superior compared with the wavelet transform in approximating

Figure 1. Spatial Decomposition of a single subband

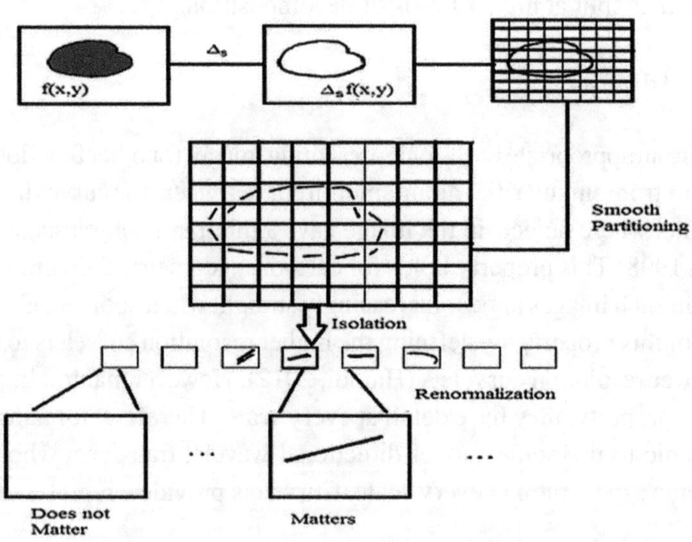

Figure 2. Representing 2D piecewise smooth signals using (a) Wavelet (b) Curvelet

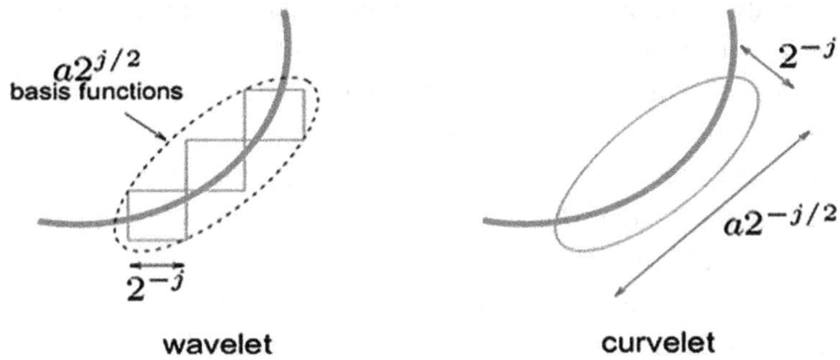

this type of 2-D piecewise smooth functions. This is the primary reason for the success of the curvelet transform.

In order to produce sparse expansions for piecewise smooth images with smooth contours, in addition to localization and multiresolution features, new 2-D schemes should contain basis functions with elongated shapes with different aspect ratios and oriented at different directions.

Moving From Classical Wavelet and Curvelet to Contourlet Transform

The curvelet transform poses several problems when one translates it into the discrete world. First, since it is a block based transform, either the approximated images have blocking effects or an overlapping windows have to be used which increases the redundancy. Secondly, the use of the ridgelet transform, which is defined on a polar coordinate, makes the implementation of the curvelet transform for discrete images on a rectangular coordinate to be very challenging. In, different interpolation approaches were proposed to solve the polar versus rectangular coordinate transform problem, all requiring over complete systems. For example, the discrete implementation of the curvelet transform has a redundancy factor equal to $16J + 1$, where J is the number of multistage levels. This imposes a severe limitation on curvelets in certain applications (Do & Vetterli, 2002).

A special member of the emerging family of multiscale geometric transforms is the contourlet transform which effectively captures the image edges and contours and is constructed using Laplacian pyramid and directional filter bank. The grouping of wavelet coefficients argument in the last section suggests that a sparse image expansion can be obtained by first applying a multiscale transform and then local directional transform to assemble the nearby basis functions at the same scale into linear structures. In essence, a wavelet like transform is used for edge (points) detection, and then a local directional transform for contour segments detection. This approach is similar to the popular Hough transform for line detection in computer vision (Wu & Wu, 2011).

Wavelet transforms have square supports that suitably represent point discontinuities. The new scheme called contourlet transform, representing multi-scaled geometric analysis, contains supports that are elongated and that have multiple directions along the contour (Po & Do, 2006). Comparing wavelet transforms, the multi-scaled geometric analysis contains multi-sets of orientational basis functions, which can efficiently present a smoothly curved contour with fewer coefficients. Hence Contourlet Transform is widely used in denoising medical images to represent the edges without smoothing them.

Non Subsampled Contourlet Transform

The existing method of noise removal is well adapted to point singularities, so it has a problem with orientation selectivity. The contourlet transform based noise removal overcomes the above problems. But due to down sampling and up sampling, the contourlet transform is shift-variant. However, shift-invariance is desirable in image analysis applications such as edge detection, contour characterization, and image enhancement (da Cunha et al., 2006). This is a major drawback of the existing method which can be eliminated by nonsubsampled contourlet transform based denoising method as it effectively represents edges than contourlet transform. In this paper, the nonsubsampled contourlet transform, which is a shift-invariant version of the contourlet transform is presented. The NSCT is built upon iterated nonsubsampled filter banks to obtain a shift-invariant directional multiresolution image representation.

CONTOURLET TRANSFORM

Introduction

Multiscale and time-frequency localization of an image is offered by wavelets. But, wavelets are not effective in representing the images with smooth contours in different directions. Contourlet Transform (CT) addresses this problem by providing two additional properties viz., directionality and anisotropy as shown in Figure 3. The processing using contourlet transform takes two main steps: Laplacian pyramid (LP) decomposition and directional filter bank(DFB). Contourlet transform is a multiscale and directional image representation that uses first a wavelet like structure for edge detection, and then a local directional transform for contour segment detection. A double filter bank structure of the contourlet is shown in Figure 4 for obtaining sparse expansions for typical images having smooth contours. In the double filter bank structure (Chan, Law, & Siu, 2003), Laplacian Pyramid (LP) is used to capture the point discontinuities and then followed by a Directional Filter Bank (DFB), which is used to link these point discontinuities into linear structures.

The band pass images ($d_j[n]$) from the LP are fed into a DFB so that directional information can be captured. The scheme can be iterated on the coarse image ($c_j[n]$). This combination results in a double iterated filter bank structure, named pyramidal directional filter bank (PDFB), which decomposes images into directional subbands at multiple scales as shown in Figure 5.

PDFB: Multiscale Decomposition

One way to achieve a multiscale decomposition is to use a Laplacian pyramid (LP) as introduced by Burt and Adelson. The LP decomposition at each step generates a coarse signal c as sampled low pass version of the original image and the difference signal d as a difference between the original and the prediction, resulting in a band pass image (Figure 6(a)). The process can be iterated on the coarse version. In the reconstruction process, the signal is obtained by simply adding back the difference to the prediction from coarse signal (Figure 6(b)).

The drawback of the Laplacian pyramid is the implicit over sampling. However, in contrast to the critically sampled wavelet scheme, the Laplacian pyramid has the distinguishing feature that each pyramid level generates only one bandpass image (even for multidimensional cases) which does not have scrambled frequencies (Tang, Zhao & Zhao, 2007). This frequency scrambling happens in the wavelet filter bank

Figure 3. Contourlet representation of a Contour

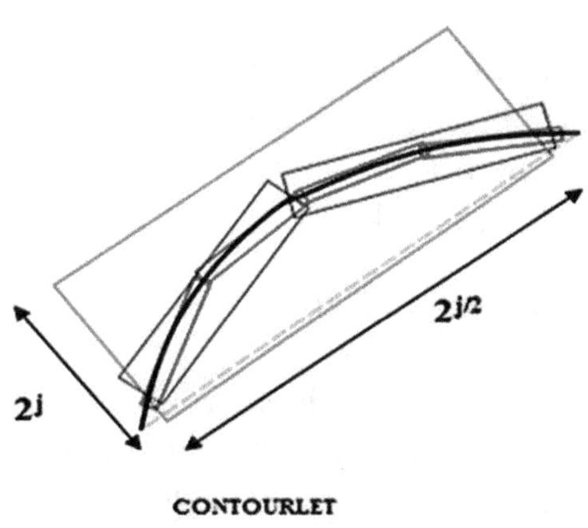

Figure 4. Filter bank structure of Contourlet transform

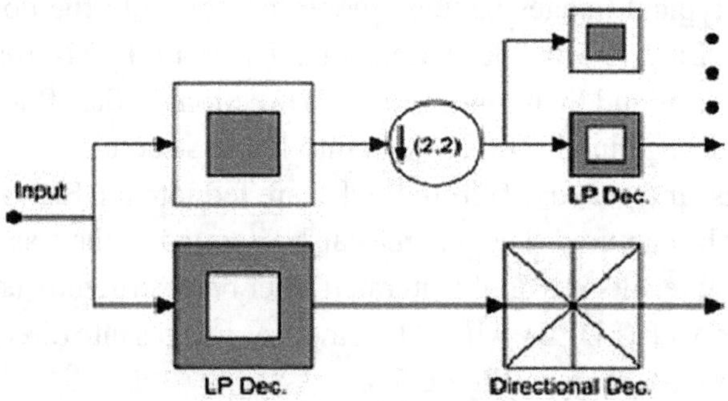

Figure 5. Contourlet decomposition

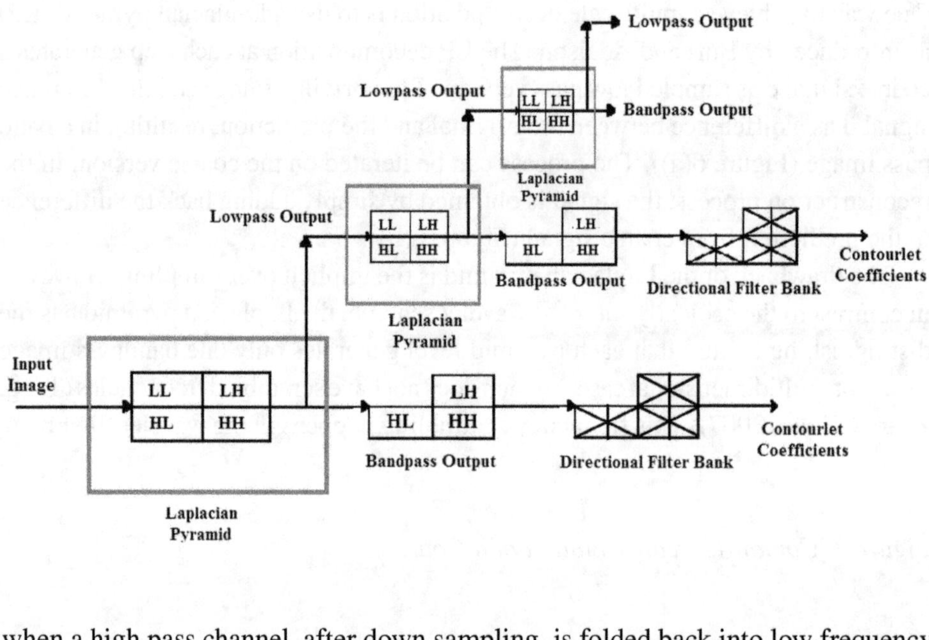

when a high pass channel, after down sampling, is folded back into low frequency band, and thus its spectrum is reflected. In the LP, this effect is avoided by down sampling the low pass channel only. LP with orthogonal filters provides a tight frame with frame bounds equal to 1.

PDFB: Directional Decomposition

To develop efficient or sparse expansions for images having smooth contours, the parabolic scaling relation for curves: width α length^2 is used. The contourlet expansion satisfies the parabolic scaling, by using directional decompositions, where

Figure 6. Laplacian pyramid (a) Decomposition (b) Reconstruction

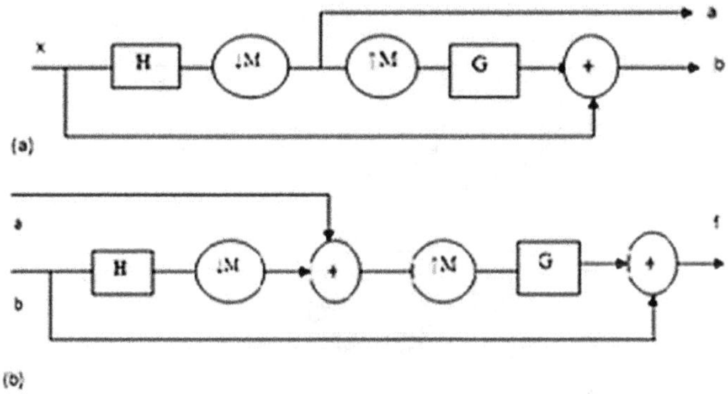

the number of directions is doubled at every other finer scale. DFB is designed to obtain the high frequency content like smooth contours and directional edges. The DFB is implemented using a k-level binary tree decomposition that leads to 2k directional sub bands with wedge shaped frequency partitioning as shown in Figure 7. But, the DFB used in this work is a simplified structure constructed from two building blocks. The first is a two-channel quincunx filter bank with fan filters (Wang et al., 2010; Do & Vetterli, 2003). It divides a 2-D spectrum into two directions, horizontal and vertical. The second is a shearing operator, which amounts to the reordering of image pixels. Due to these two operations, directional information is preserved. This is the desirable characteristic in image denoising to improve edge detection efficiency.

Nonsubsampled Contourlet Transform

The contourlet transform employs Laplacian pyramids for multiscale decomposition, and directional filter banks (DFB) for directional decomposition (Hiremath et al., 2010). To achieve the shift-invariance, the nonsubsampled contourlet transform is built upon nonsubsampled pyramids and nonsubsampled DFB.

Nonsubsampled Pyramids

The nonsubsampled pyramid is entirely different from the counterpart of the contourlet transform, the Laplacian pyramid. The building block of the nonsubsampled pyramid is a two-channel nonsubsampled filter bank as shown in Figure 8(a). A nonsubsampled filter bank has no down-sampling or upsampling, and hence it is shift-invariant (da Cunha et al., 2006). The perfect reconstruction condition is given as

Figure 7. Pyramidal directional decomposition

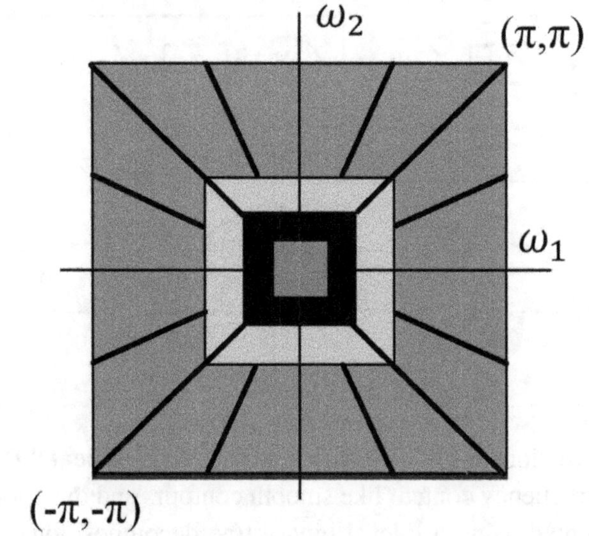

Figure 8. Ideal frequency response of the building block of (a) nonsubsampled pyramid (b) nonsubsampled DFB

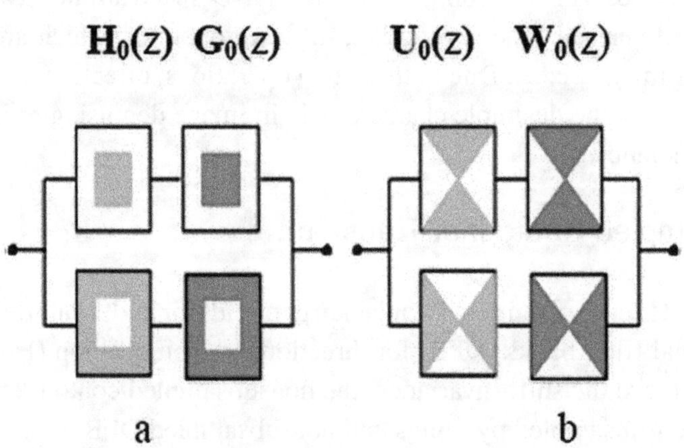

$$H_0(z)G_0(z) + H_1(z)G_1(z) = 1 \quad (1)$$

This condition is much easier to satisfy than the perfect re-construction condition for critically sampled filter banks, and thus allows better filters to be designed. The ideal frequency response of the building block of the nonsubsampled pyramid is given in Figure 8(a). To achieve the multiscale decomposition, nonsubsampled pyramids are constructed using iterated nonsubsampled filter banks (Figure 9) (Hamdi, 2012).

Figure 9. Iteration of two-channeled nonsubsampled filter banks in the analysis part of a nonsubsampled pyramid. For up sampled filters, only effective pass bands within dotted boxes are shown where D0, D1, D2, D3 denotes the decomposed images using the non-subsampled puramidal structure.

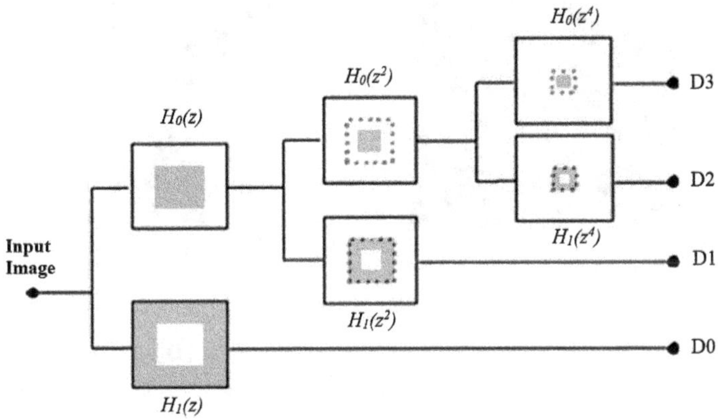

In the next level of processing, all filters are upsampled by 2 in both dimensions. Therefore, they also satisfy the perfect reconstruction condition. Note that filtering with the up sampled filter $H(z^M)$ has the same complexity as filtering with H(z) using the 'a trous' algorithm (Ma, Xie, Luo, 2009). The cascading of the analysis part is shown in Figure 8. The equivalent filters of a k-th level cascading nonsubsampled pyramid are given by

$$H_n^{eq}(z) = \begin{cases} H_1\left(z^{2^{n-1}}\right)\prod_{j=0}^{n-2} H_0\left(z^{2^j}\right) & 1 < n < 2^k \\ \prod_{j=0}^{n-1} H_0\left(z^{2^j}\right) & n = 2^k \end{cases} \quad (2)$$

where z^j stands for $\left[z_1^j, z_2^j\right]$. These filters achieve multiresolution analysis as shown in Figure 10(a).

Nonsubsampled Directional Filter Banks

The nonsubsampled directional filter bank is a shift-invariant version of the critically sampled DFB in the contourlet transform. The building block of a nonsubsampled DFB is also a two-channel nonsubsampled filter bank. However, the ideal frequency response for a nonsubsampled DFB is different as shown in Figure 8(b). To obtain

Figure 10. Frequency divisions of (a) nonsubsampled pyramid (b) non subsampled DFB

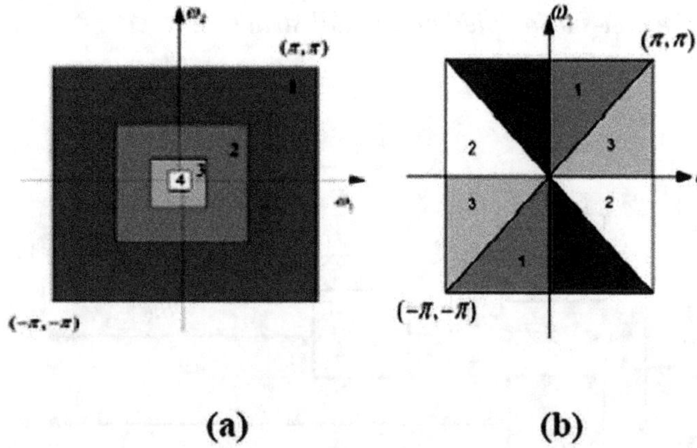

final directional decomposition, nonsubsampled DFB's are iterated. In the next level, all filters are upsampled by a quincunx matrix given by

$$Q = \begin{pmatrix} 1 & 1 \\ 1 & -1 \end{pmatrix} \tag{3}$$

The cascading of the analysis part is shown in Figure 11. Then a four-direction frequency division is obtained as shown in Figure 10(b). The higher level decompositions follow the similar strategy, although they are more complex (Hong bo, 2013).

Figure 11. The analysis part of an iterated nonsubsampled directional filter bank

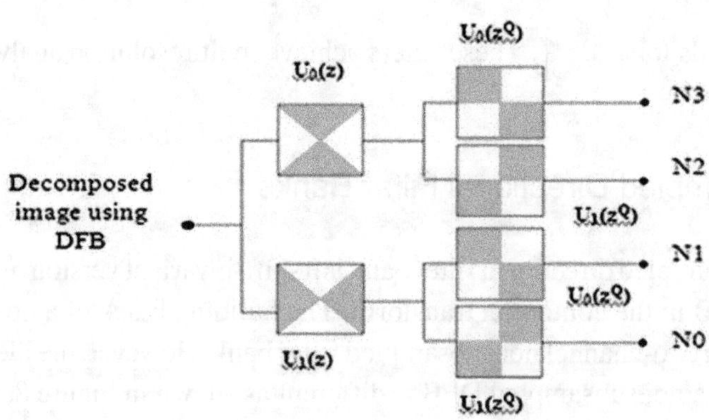

Shift Invariant Contourlet Transform

The nonsubsampled contourlet transform combines Nonsubsampled pyramids and Nonsubsampled DFB's as shown in Figure 12. Nonsubsampled pyramids provide multiscale decomposition and nonsubsampled DFB's provide directional decomposition. This scheme can be iterated repeatedly on the low pass subband outputs of nonsubsampled pyramids (Zhou, Cunda, & Do, 2005).

Figure 12(a) shows the block diagram of NSCT, where a nonsubsampled pyramid split the input into a lowpass subband and a high pass subband. Then a nonsubsampled DFB decomposes the high pass subband into several subbands. The scheme is iterated repeatedly on the low pass subband. Figure 12(b) shows the resulting frequency division where the number of directions is increased with frequency (Hiremath et al., 2010).

Shrinkage and Filtering Techniques

Image Enhancement by Contourlet Transform

Contourlet denoising attempts to remove the noise presents in the gray image while preserving the edge. The common approach to contourlet based denoising is to transform the signal into the contourlet domain, shrink the detail coefficients and transform back to the image domain. A more precise explanation of the contourlet denoising procedure can be given as follows. Assume that the observed data is

$$X(t) = S(t) + N(t) \tag{4}$$

Figure 12. The nonsubsampled contourlet transform: (a) block diagram (b) resulting frequency division

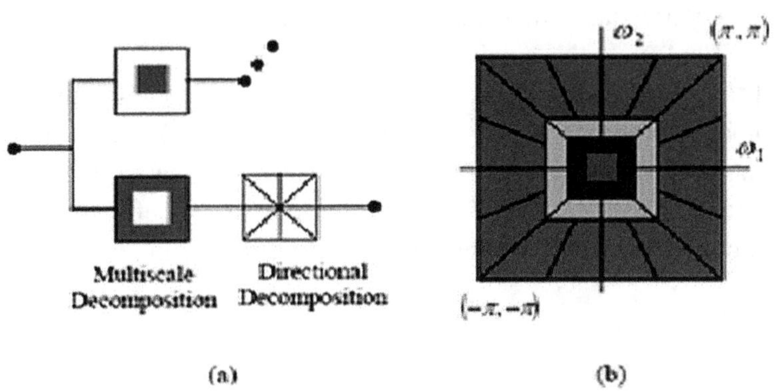

where X is the uncorrupted signal with additive noise. Let C denote the forward and inverse contourlet transform operator, λ denotes the denoising operator with threshold. The aim is to denoise X(t) and recover an estimate of S(t) (Chen & Tian, 2010). The practice of thresholding method for denoising consists of the following three steps:

$$Y = C(X) \tag{5}$$

$$Z = D(Y, \lambda) \tag{6}$$

$$\hat{S}(t) = C^{-1}(Z) \tag{7}$$

The thresholding operator is defined as follows,

$$D(Y,\lambda) = \begin{cases} sign(Y)(|Y| - \lambda) & if |Y| > \lambda \\ 0 & Otherwise \end{cases} \tag{8}$$

An appropriate choice of the threshold value is fundamental to the effectiveness of the described contourlet denoising procedure (Chan, Law, & Siu, 2003; Zhou, Cunha, & Do, 2005). A large threshold might remove important parts of the underlying signal whereas too small threshold retains noise in the reconstruction.

Contourlet Shrinkage Methods

The thresholding approach is sensitive to noise components. In this approach, after taking contourlet transform of the image, small coefficients are dominated by noise, while coefficients with a large absolute value carry more signal information than noise. Replacing the smallest, noisy coefficients by zero and a inverse contourlet transform on the result may lead to a reconstruction with the essential signal characteristics and with less noise (Wang et al., 2010). These methods use a threshold and determine the clean contourlet coefficients based on this threshold. There are three main ways of thresholding the contourlet coefficients, namely the hard thresholding, soft thresholding and adaptive thresholding.

Hard Thresholding

To suppress the noise, the nonlinear transform mentioned in equation 9 is applied to the empirical contourlet coefficients

$$F(x) = x \cdot I(|x| > t) \tag{9}$$

where, t is a certain threshold. The choice of the threshold is a very delicate and important statistical problem. High threshold value leads to a large bias of the estimator. But on the other hand, a small threshold value increases the variance of the smoother. Theoretical calculation yields the following value of the threshold:

$$t = \sqrt{\frac{2\sigma^2 \log(n)}{n}} \tag{10}$$

where n is the length of the input vector and σ^2 is the variance of the noise. The variance of the noise is estimated based on the data. There are two possibilities for choosing a threshold. First it can be done through "eye" using the hard threshold item and entering the desired value of the threshold. In most cases, this threshold value is conservative and therefore a threshold value should be chosen below the offered value. Other possibility is through "automatic" which means the threshold will be chosen as given in equation 7 with the suitably estimated variance (Serief, Barkat, & Bentoutou, 2007).

Soft Thresholding

Hard thresholding is discontinuous. This causes ringing / Gibbs effect in the denoised image. To overcome this, Donoho introduced the soft thresholding method. If the absolute value of a coefficient is less than a threshold λ, then is assumed to be 0, otherwise its value is shrunk by λ. The only difference between the hard and the soft thresholding procedures are in the choice of the nonlinear transform on the empirical wavelet coefficients as shown in Figure 13. For soft thresholding the following nonlinear transform is used (Chen & Tian, 2010):

$$S(x) = sign(x)(|x| - t)I(|x| > t) \tag{11}$$

This removes the discontinuity, but degrades all the other coefficients which tends to blur the image.

Adaptive Thresholding

The threshold T for the contourlet coefficients of noisy image is calculated using Equation 12. If the contourlet coefficients are greater than the threshold, those coefficients are remained unchanged (Hong bo, 2013). If they are less, they are suppressed.

$$T = \frac{3}{4} N \left(\frac{\sigma_n^2}{\sigma_g} \right) \tag{12}$$

Where N is total number of pixels in the image and σ_g is the standard deviation of the noisy image and σ_n^2 is the noise variance in the noisy image at each pixel which is calculated using Mean Absolute Deviation method and is given by

$$\sigma_n^2 = \left(\frac{median\left(c_{i,j}\right)}{0.6745} \right)^2 \tag{13}$$

Figure 13. Comparison of hard and soft thresholding

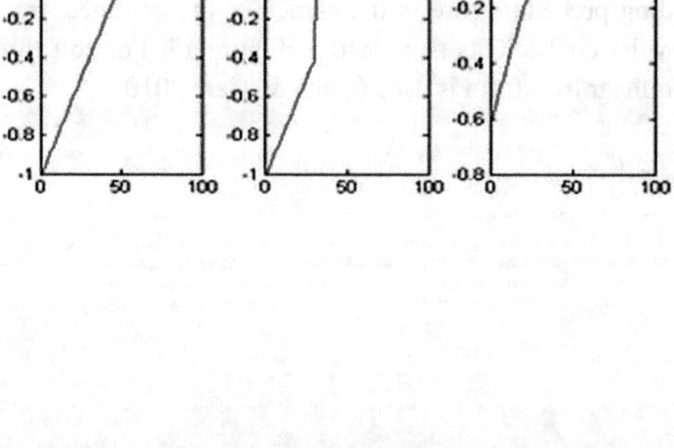

VISU Shrink

This is also called as the universal threshold method. A threshold is given by

$$T = \sigma\sqrt{2\log\left(M\right)} \tag{14}$$

where σ^2 are the noise variance and M is the number of samples. This asymptotically yields a mean square error (MSE) estimate as M tends to infinity. As M increases, threshold value becomes high, which tends to over smoothen the image (Kamran et al., 2012; Dengwen, 2008).

SURE Shrink

This SURE Shrink threshold was developed by Donoho and Johnstone. For each sub-band, the threshold is determined by minimizing Stein's Unbiased Risk Estimate (SURE) for those coefficients. SURE is a method for estimating the loss $\| (\overline{u} - \mu)^2 \|$ in an unbiased fashion, where $\overline{u}$ is the estimated mean and μ is the real mean (Hamdi, 2012; Chen & Tian, 2010).

The threshold is calculated as follows:

$$Sure = \arg\min\left[\sigma^2 - \frac{2\sigma^2}{n}\#\left\{k : abs\left(y_{j,k}\right) < \lambda\right\} + \frac{1}{n}\Sigma\left(\min\left(abs\left(y_{j,k}\right),\lambda\right)^2\right)\right] \tag{15}$$

where n is the number of samples, σ^2 is the noise variance, $y_{j,k}$ are the noisy samples, λ is the threshold and #{k: abs(y_j,k) < λ } indicates the number of samples whose value is less than λ. argmin[f(λ)] indicates the selection of a value for lambda which minimizes the function f (Dengwen & Wengang, 2008). Donoho and Johnstone pointed out that SURE Shrink is automatically smoothness adaptive. This implies that the reconstruction output is smooth wherever the function is smooth and it jumps wherever there is a jump or discontinuity in the function. This method can generate very sparse contourlet coefficients resulting in an inadequate threshold. So, it is suggested that a hybrid approach be used as an alternative (Serief, Barkat, & Bentoutou, 2007).

BAYES Shrink

This method is based on the Bayesian mathematical framework. The contourlet coefficients of a natural image are modeled by a Generalized Gaussian Distribution (GGD). This is used to calculate the threshold using a Bayesian framework (Hiremath et al., 2010).

NEIGH Shrink

VisuShrink is very simple, but its disadvantage is to yield overly smoothed images because the universal threshold T is too large. Just like VisuShrink, Sure Shrink also applies the soft shrinkage rule, but it uses independently chosen thresholds for each sub band through the minimization of the Stein's unbiased Risk estimate (SURE). SURE Shrink performs better than VisuShrink, producing more detailed images. The transformed coefficients in overlapping blocks are thresholded rather than individually or term by term as VisuShrink or Sure Shrink. The basic motivation of block thresholding remains: a coefficient is more likely to contain signal if neighboring coefficients do also. The applied NeighCoeff to image denoising and their method is called Neighshrink (Kamran et al., 2012). Neighshrink outperforms VisuShrink and Sure Shrink. It is well known that increasing the redundancy of contourlet transforms can significantly improve the denoising performances. All detailed scales except the five coarsest scales are thresholded using the universal threshold. Note that this threshold is the same as Donoho's threshold for 1D signal except the replacement of 1D signal with 2D image (Himerath et al., 2010; da Cunha et al, 2006).

VisuShrink does not have any denoising power when the noise level is low. Under such a condition, VisuShrink produces even worse results than the original noisy images. However, Neighshrink performs very well in this case. When the noise level is low, the improvement is large. When the noise level is high, the improvement is low. By studying the denoised images, Neighshrink produces smoother and clearer denoised images. The contourlet coefficients are thresholded by looking at the average value in the neighbourhood window (Dengwen & Wengang, 2008). Conducting this experiment in this paper taking the average of the contourlet coefficients in the neighbourhood window is a natural choice. Unfortunately, it does not provide better performance. Hence these experiments are done using Neighshrink (Po & Do, 2006).

Let $g = \{g_{ij}\}$ will denote the matrix representation of the noisy signal. Then, c=Cg denotes the matrix of contourlet coefficients of the signal under consideration. For every value of c_{ij}, let B_{ij} is a neighbouring window around c_{ij}, c_{ij} denotes the contourlet coefficient to be shrinked. The neighbouring window size can be represented as

L*L, where L is a positive odd number. A 3*3 neighbouring window centered at the contourlet coefficient to be shrinked is shown in Figure 14.

Let

$$S_{ij} = \sum_{(k,l)\in B_{ij}} c_{kl}^2 \tag{16}$$

Omit the corresponding terms in the summation when the above summation has pixel indexes out of the sub-band range. The shrinked coefficient according to the Neighshrink is given by this formula

$$c'_{ij} = c_{ij} c'_{ij} \tag{17}$$

The shrinkage factor β_{ij} can be defined as:

$$B_{ij} = (1 - T^2_{UNI}/Sij^2) \tag{18}$$

Here, the + sign at the end of the formula means to keep the positive value while set it to zero when it is negative and T_{UNI} is the universal threshold, which is defined as

$$T_{UNI} = \sqrt{2\sigma^2 \ln(n)} \tag{19}$$

where 'n' is the length of the signal.

Different coefficient sub-bands are shrinked independently, but the universal threshold T_{UNI} and neighbouring window size L kept unchanged in all sub-bands

*Figure 14. An illustration of the neighbouring window of size 3*3 centered at the coefficient to be shrinked*

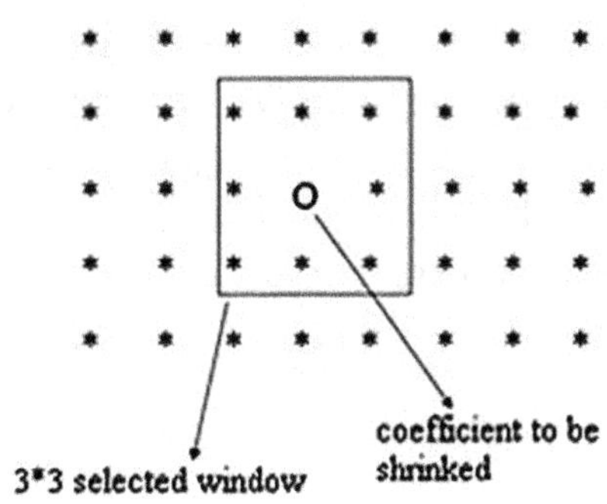

(Chen, Law, & Siu, 2003). The estimated denoised signal $f' = f'_{ij}$ is calculated by taking the inverse contourlet transform of the shrinked contourlet coefficients c'_{ij} i.e. $f' = C^{-1}c'$. In order to determine the modified Neighshrink the optimal threshold and neighbouring window size are calculated as,

(λs,Ls) = argλ,Lmin SURE(ws,λ,L) (20)

Where λ is optimal threshold, L is neighbouring window size, s is sub band and

$$\text{SURE(ws,}\lambda\text{,L)} = \text{Ns} + \Sigma\|\text{gn(wn)}\|22 + 2\ \Sigma\ \frac{\partial g_n}{w_n} \tag{21}$$

$$\text{gn(wn)} = \begin{cases} -\lambda^2 / w_n \\ -w_n \end{cases} \tag{22}$$

Bilateral Filter

Filtering is an important operation of image processing and computer vision. In the broadest sense of the term "filtering", the value of the filtered image at a given location is a function of the values of the input image in a small neighborhood of the same location. For example Gaussian filter computes a weighted average of pixel values in the neighborhood pixel, in which the weights decrease with distance from the neighborhood center. Although formal and quantitative explanations of this weight fall-off can be given, the intuition is that images typically vary slowly over space, so near pixels are likely to have similar values, and it is therefore appropriate to average them together (Tomasi & Manduchi, 1998). The noise values that corrupt these nearby pixels are mutually less correlated than the signal values, so noise is averaged away while the signal is preserved. The assumption is that slow spatial variations fails at edges, which are consequently blurred by linear low-pass filtering. The challenge is to prevent averaging across edges, while still averaging within smooth regions. Many efforts have been devoted to reduce this undesired effect. Bilateral filtering is a simple, non-iterative scheme for edge-preserving smoothing (Ma, Xie, Luo, 2009).

Proposed Contourlet Domain Noise Reduction Algorithm

The algorithm for denoising method based on contourlet transform can be described as follows:

1. Perform contourlet transform to the noisy image; from the decomposition process the coefficients are extracted
2. Estimate the noise variance for each noisy image pixel using equation

$$\sigma_n^2 = \left(\frac{median\left(c_{i,j}\right)}{0.6745} \right)^2 \tag{23}$$

3. The threshold value T for the contourlet coefficients of noisy image is calculated using

$$T = \frac{3}{4} N \left(\frac{\sigma_n^2}{\sigma_g} \right) \tag{24}$$

where N is total number of pixels in the image and σ_g is the standard deviation of the noisy image

4. The contourlet coefficients are compared with the threshold,
    a. If those coefficients are greater than threshold value, they are remained unchanged.
    b. If those coefficients are lesser than threshold value, they are suppressed.
5. Finally all the resultant coefficients are reconstructed by applying inverse contourlet transform, which results in denoised image.

Proposed Denoising Algorithm Using NSCT

Generally, image enhancement methods amplify noises when they amplify weak edges since they cannot distinguish noises from weak edges. In the frequency domain, both weak edges and noises lead to low-value coefficients. The nonsubsampled contourlet transform provides not only multiresolution analysis, but also geometric and directional representation. Therefore, it is easy to distinguish weak edges from noise using NSCT, as weak edges have geometric structures, while noises don't have any geometric structure (Riazifar & Yazdo, 2009; Kamran et al., 2012).

NSCT Decomposition

The nonsubsampled contourlet transform exhibit shift invariance, such that each pixel of the transform subband corresponds to that of the original image in the same location. Therefore, the geometric information can be gathered from pixel by pixel using the NSCT coefficients.

The three classes of pixels: strong edges, weak edges, and noises are observed.

1. First, the strong edges correspond to those pixels with higher coefficient values in all sub-bands.
2. Second, the weak edges correspond to those pixels with low coefficient values in some directional subbands but small value coefficients in other directional subbands within the same scale.
3. Finally, the noises correspond to those pixels with lower coefficient values in all subbands.

Based on these observations, pixels can be classified into three categories by analyzing the distribution of their coefficients in different subbands (da Cunha et al., 2006; Zhou, Cunha, & Do, 2005).

For this purpose, the mean (denoted by mean) and the maximum (denoted by max) magnitude of the coefficients for each pixel is computed and then classified as

$$\begin{cases} Strongedge & if\ mean \geq c\sigma \\ Weakedge & if\ mean < c\sigma, \max \geq c\sigma \\ Noise & if\ mean < c\sigma, \max < c\sigma \end{cases}$$

where c is a parameter ranging from 1 to 5, and σ is the noise standard deviation of the subbands at a specific level. The noise variance of the input image is estimated using the robust median operator and then the noise variance of each subband is computed (Hamdi, 2012).

The goal of image enhancement is to amplify weak edges and to suppress noises. To this end, the NSCT coefficients are modified according to the category of each pixel by a nonlinear mapping function.

Where the above given input x is the original coefficient, and $0 < p < 1$ is the amplifying ratio. This function keeps the coefficients of strong edges, amplifies the coefficients of weak edges, and zeros the coefficients of noises (Do & Vetterli, 2003).

Table 1. Modification of NSCT coefficients

y(x)=	X	Strong edge pixels
	$\max\left(\left(\frac{c\sigma}{\lvert x\rvert}\right)p, 1\right)x$	Weak edge pixel
	0	Noise pixels

Denoising Algorithm

The proposed denoising algorithm is as follows:

1. Decompose the input image using nonsubsampled contourlet decomposition.
2. Here the number of levels of directional subband is 4[n levels=0,3], where in each level there are 2^0, 2^3 directions of decomposition takes place.
3. The output of the directional decomposition image is a cell vector consisting of 4 images, each decomposed in different directions.
4. The strong edges will be in the decomposed image 1-3 whereas the 4th Image is dominated by noisy coefficients.
5. The decomposed image is concatenated to give the resultant decomposed image.
6. Apply Neigh shrink with and without bilateral filter to this decomposed image.
7. Compare the result of both shrinkage methods in terms of PSNR and MSE.

RESULTS AND DISCUSSION

Experiments are conducted to evaluate the performance of the proposed framework. Noisy images are obtained by adding white Gaussian noise to some standard test images. These noisy images are then denoised, using several algorithms and the PSNR results are calculated.

The Peak signal-to-noise ratio (PSNR) and Mean Square Error (MSE) are the two error metrics used to compare image compression quality. PSNR is often used as a quality measurement between the original and compressed image. The higher the PSNR, better the quality of the compressed or reconstructed image. MSE provides the cumulative squared error between the compressed and the original image, whereas PSNR represents a measure of the peak error. The lower the value of MSE, the lower the error.

The denoising techniques compared here are Neigh shrink in Wavelet and contourlet domain with and without using bilateral filter. From the PSNR obtained for different noise level the best technique can be determined.

During NSCT decomposition with n levels from 0 to 3, a cell containing three different images is obtained, which is the outcome at three stages of decomposition. At the first level, the image is decomposed in 2^0directions so that a single highpass is obtained and then the low pass is fed to the next level so that the next image where the image is decomposed in 2^3 directions. Finally the decomposed images at all the stages and after concatenating all the images are shown in Figure 15.

The experiments are conducted on several medical test images of size 256 x 256 and 512 x 512 at different noise levels $\sigma = 2, 5, 10,15$ because the medical images which are highly dominated by noise will not be used for diagnosis purpose. So low noise is added to medical images and the performance of the proposed method is computed. Figure 16 (a) shows the original image. Figure 16 (b) shows noisy image with noise variance $\sigma = 10$. Figure 16 (c) shows the result of the NeighShrink method in thresholding wavelet coefficients with PSNR 33.2622 dB, Figure 16 (d) result of the Bilateral with NeighShrink method providing better PSNR of 35.7021 dB.

Figure 15. NSCT decomposed image

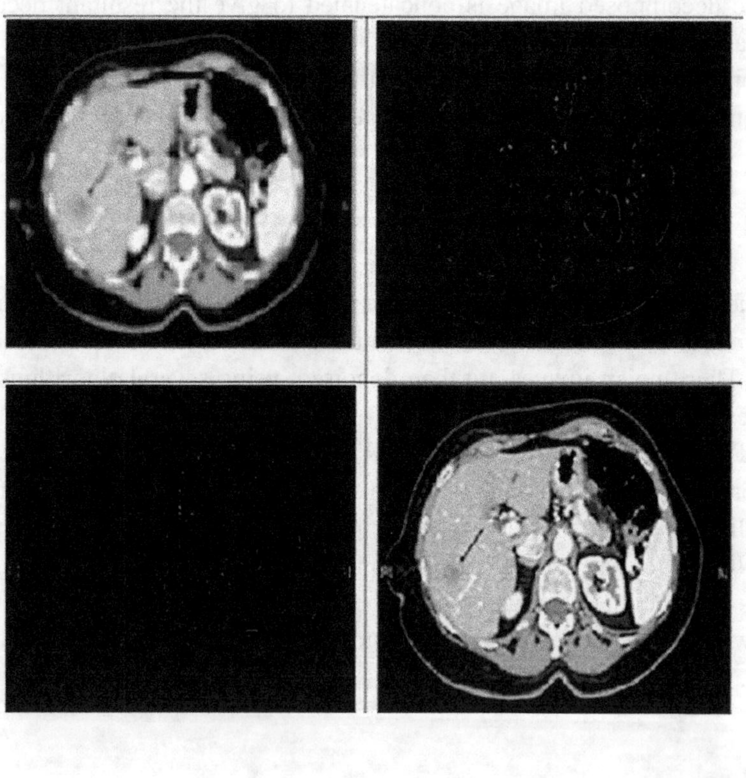

Table 2. PSNR (in dB) comparison of proposed method with existing method

IMAGE	METHOD	σ=2	σ =5	σ =10
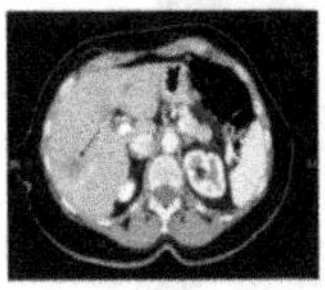	Wavelet with NS	43.5721	36.4693	31.4172
	Wavelet with NSB	44.1745	37.4400	33.0363
	Curvelet with PS	44.2313	37.4502	
	Contourlet with AT			
	NSCT with NS	45.4876	38.5589	36.8280
	NSCT with NSB	**45.5320**	**38.8507**	**37.7303**
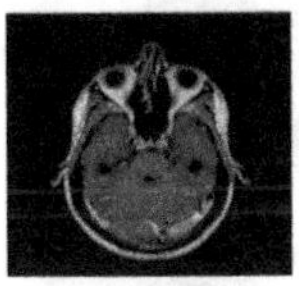	Wavelet with NS	45.9973	39.2867	33.7413
	Wavelet with NSB	46.2420	41.3529	37.6470
	Curvelet with PS			
	Contourlet with AT			
	NSCT with NS	50.1479	44.1588	40.4905
	NSCT with NSB	**50.3329**	**45.2186**	**43.2549**
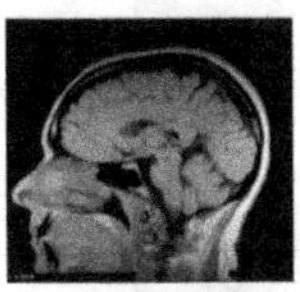	Wavelet with NS	45.5641	39.0557	33.6118
	Wavelet with NSB	45.6996	40.4835	36.8179
	Curvelet with PS			
	Contourlet with AT			
	NSCT with NS	46.0901	44.5388	41.6014
	NSCT with NSB	**46.9656**	**45.1441**	**43.6389**
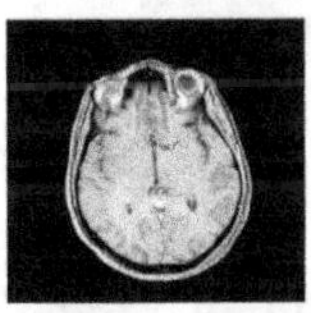	Wavelet with NS	44.2620	37.1504	31.8776
	Wavelet with NSB	44.8130	38.4970	34.0635
	Curvelet with PS			
	Contourlet with AT			
	NSCT with NS	45.1919	40.5443	36.7359
	NSCT with NSB	**45.5675**	**41.2375**	**37.8984**
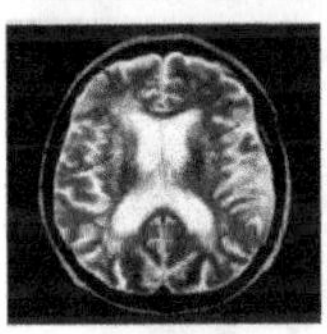	Wavelet with NS	45.1392	38.4802	33.2622
	Wavelet with NSB	45.9079	39.9930	35.7021
	Curvelet with PS			
	Contourlet with AT			
	NSCT with NS	46.1917	41.3264	38.0098
	NSCT with NSB	**46.9674**	**43.0301**	**39.2065**

Figure 17 (a) shows the result of the performance of the NSCT with Neigh shrink which gives a PSNR of 38.0098 dB. Figure 17(b) shows the result of the proposed NeighShrink with bilateral filter in denoising decomposed image using NSCT which gives a higher PSNR of 39.2065 dB when compared with other methods. Here, after three levels of decomposition, three images which are the decomposed original images in different directions are obtained. The first two images have the strong edges, but the last image is dominated by noise so that the third image which is dominated with noise is not considered, while concatenating the images and then the concatenated image is denoised using NeighShrink with and without bilateral filter and the performance are compared in terms of PSNR.

Figure 16. (a) Original image (b) nosiy image (c) result of NeighShrink on wavelet coefficients (d) result of NeighShrink with bilateral on wavelet coefficients

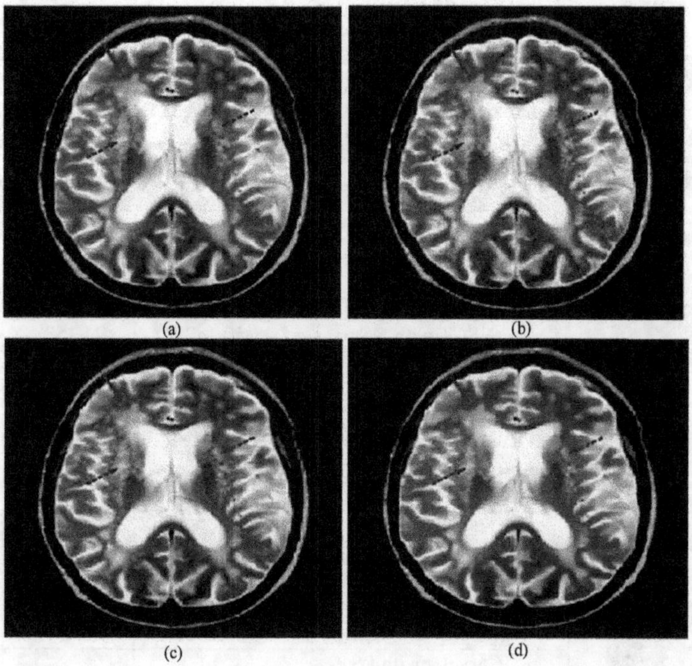

Figure 17. (a) Result of NeighShrink on NSCT coefficients (b) result of NeighShrink with bilateral on NSCT coefficients

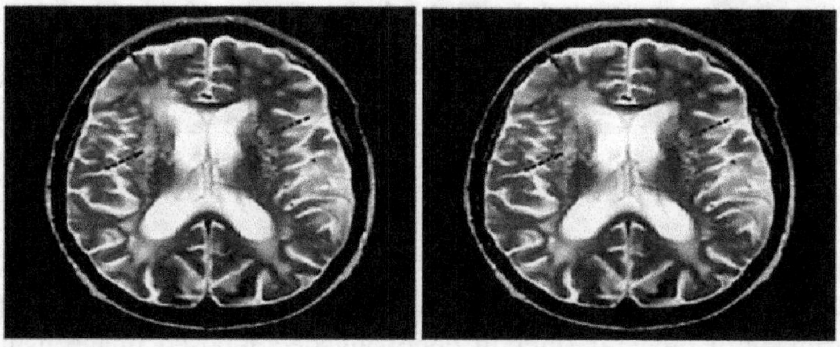

The experimental results showing the PSNR for existing and proposed algorithm are tabulated. Table 2 shows PSNR for existing method and PSNR for proposed method.

NeighShrink plays a vital role in eliminating the noise in edge region. When the noise variance is very much higher, the newly proposed technique which applies the

Bilateral with NeighShrink appears to be a good denoising approach. The PSNR values for the proposed technique are higher than the techniques which already exist in the field. The performance of the proposed method is compared with the existing method in terms of PSNR which shows that the proposed technique outperforms the existing method both visually and in terms of PSNR as shown in Figure 18.

CONCLUSION

In this paper, a powerful method is proposed to address the issue of medical image recovery from its noisy counterpart. It is based on the shift invariant contourlet transform, because shift invariance is desirable in image analysis applications such as edge detection, contour characterization, and image enhancement. The image is adaptively classified into strong and weak edge regions and denoising algorithm is implemented. As a result the contourlet coefficients are modified. Thus noise is eliminated in the edge region. Experiments are conducted and the performance of Neighshrink with and without bilateral filter is compared. The result shows that proposed Neighshrink with bilateral filter effectively removes noise in the NSCT decomposed images significantly. The PSNR value is improved and the edges are preserved better in Neighshrink with bilateral method compared to other methods.

Figure 18. PNSR comparison of the proposed and existing algorithms in Gaussian Noise variation

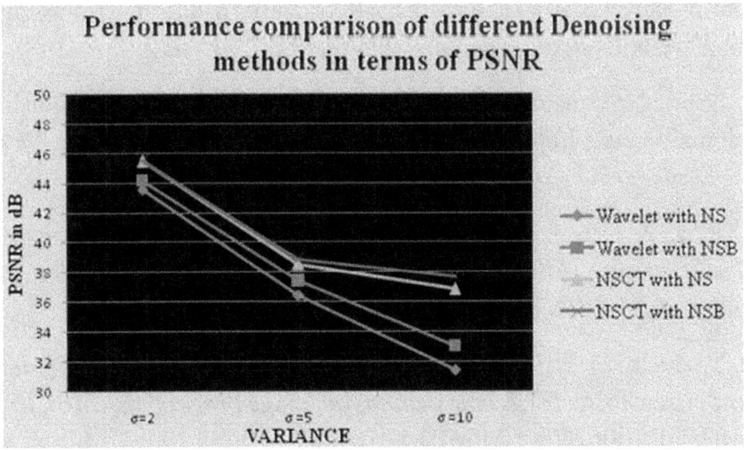

REFERENCES

Chan, W. Y., Law, N. F., & Siu, W. C. (2003). Multiscale Feature Analysis Using Directional Filter Bank. *International Conference on Information, Communications and Signal Processing*, 2, 822-826. 10.1109/ICICS.2003.1292571

Chen, X. W., & Tian, J. W. (2010). Wavelet-contourlet texture image retrieval system. *Computer Engineering and Applications*, *46*, 11–13.

da Cunha, A. L., Zhou, J., & Do, M. N. (2006, October). The Nonsubsampled Contourlet Transform: Theory, Design, and Applications. *IEEE Transactions on Image Processing*, *15*(10), 3089–3101. doi:10.1109/TIP.2006.877507 PMID:17022272

Do, M. N., & Vetterli, M. (2003). The contourlet transform: An efficient directional multiresolution image representation. *IEEE Transactions on Image Processing*, *14*(12), 2091–2106. doi:10.1109/TIP.2005.859376 PMID:16370462

Do, M. N., & Vetterli, M. (2002). Contourlets: A Directional Multiresolution Image Representation. In *International Conference on Image Processing* (Vol. 1). IEEE. 10.1109/ICIP.2002.1038034

Hamdi. (2012). A Comparative Study in Wavelets, Curvelets and Contourlets as Denoising Biomedical Images. *I.J. Image. Graphics and Signal Processing*, *1*, 44–50.

Hiremath, P. S., & Prema, T. (2010). Speckle Reducing Contourlet Transform for Medical Ultrasound Image. *International Journal of Computer and Information Engineering*, *4*, 4.

Jiang, Fang, & Tang. (2010). Texture Image Retrieval by Multi-directional Information Fusion of Wavelet Domain. *Computer Engineering*, 215-217.

Kamran, Nasri, Nezamabadi-Pour, & Saryazdi. (2012). Image denoising in the wavelet domain using Improved Neigh-shrink. *National Conference New Idea In Electrical Engineering (NCNIEE).*

Ma, Y., Xie, J., & Luo, J. (2009). Image Enhancement Based on Nonsubsampled Contourlet Transform. *Fifth International Conference on Information Assurance and Security*. 10.1109/IAS.2009.44

Po, D. D.-Y., & Do, M. N. (2006). Directional multiscale modeling of images using the contourlet transform. *IEEE Transactions on Image Processing*, *15*(6), 1610–1620. doi:10.1109/TIP.2006.873450 PMID:16764285

Riazifar, N., & Yazdi, M. (2009). Effectiveness of Contourlet vs. Wavelet Transform on Medical Image Compression: A Comparative Study. *World Academy of Science, Engineering and Technology*.

Serief, C., Barkat, M., & Bentoutou, Y. (2007). An automatic image registration scheme based on the nonsubsampled contourlet transform. *Proceedings of the 9th International Symposium on Signal Processing and Its Applications*, 1–4. 10.1109/ISSPA.2007.4555446

Tang, L., Zhao, F., & Zhao, Z. G. (2007). The nonsubsampled contourlet transform for image fusion. *International Conference on Wavelet Analysis and Pattern Recognition (ICWAPR '07)*, 305–310.

Tomasi, C., & Manduchi, R. (1998). Bilateral Filtering for Gray and Color Images. *IEEE International Conference on Computer Vision*. 10.1109/ICCV.1998.710815

Wang, H., He, C., & Wei, L. (2010). Locally adaptive bivariate shrinkage algorithm for image denoising based on Nonsubsampled Contourlet Transform. *International Conference on Computer, Mechatronics, Control and Electronic Engineering (CMCE)*, 5.

Wu, Y. Q., & Wu, Y. Y. (2011). Image Retrieval Based on NSCT and Krawtchouk Moments. *Wuhan Daxue Xuebao. Xinxi Kexue Ban*, 691–694.

Yang & Bo. (2013). Image De-Noising Algorithm Using Adaptive Bayes Threshold by subband Based on Nonsubsampled Contourlet Transform. *Third International Conference on Intelligent System Design and Engineering Applications*.

Zhou, Cunha, & Do. (2005). Nonsubsampled contourlet transform: construction and application in enhancement. *IEEE International Conference on Image Processing*, 11-14.

Zhou, D., & Cheng, W. (2008). Image denoising with an optimal threshold and neighbouring window. *Pattern Recognition Letters*, *29*(11), 1694–1697. doi:10.1016/j.patrec.2008.04.014

Section 5
Study on Fundamentals in Image Processing and Its Advancements

Chapter 9
The Fundamentals of Biomedical Image Processing

Kirti Raj Bhatele
Rustamji Institute of Technology, India

Vivek Gupta
Rustamji Institute of Technology, India

Kamlesh Gupta
Rustamji Institute of Technology, India

Prashant Shrivastava
Rustamji Institute of Technology, India

ABSTRACT

This chapter provides a brief introduction to the various fundamentals and concepts related to the basics of the biomedical image processing. Medical imaging processing comprises various techniques and processes that are used to create images of human body for clinical purposes and medical procedures for the purpose of diagnosis or examination of disease. Digital image processing along with its suitable components and computer-simulated algorithms are implemented using computers to perform the image analysis of digital images. The study of normal anatomy and physiology of human body is made as a part of diagnosis process. Though medical imaging of various organs and tissues can be performed for medical examination purposes, the impact of digital images on modern society is tremendous and image processing has become a critical component of science and technology related to the biomedical image processing.

DOI: 10.4018/978-1-5225-5876-7.ch009

INTRODUCTION

As the expanding utilization of direct sophisticated imaging frameworks for therapeutic diagnostics, computerized picture handling turns out to be increasingly essential in social insurance. Notwithstanding initially computerized techniques, for example, Computed Tomography (CT) or Magnetic Resonance Imaging (MRI), at first simple imaging modalities, for example, endoscopy or radiography are these days outfitted with advanced sensors. Computerized pictures are made out of individual pixels (this acronym is shaped from the words "picture" and "component"), to which discrete shine or shading esteems are appointed (Acharya & Ray, 2005). They can be proficiently prepared, unbiased assessed, and made accessible at many places in the meantime by methods for fitting correspondence systems and conventions, for example, Picture Archiving and Communication Systems (PACS) and the Digital Imaging and Communications in Medicine (DICOM) convention, individually. In light of computerized imaging methods, the whole range of advanced picture handling is currently pertinent in solution.

The Image enhancement techniques improve the quality, clarity of biomedical images and human perception as well as machine understanding. Contrast generally refers to the difference in the luminance or grey level values in an image and is an important characteristic that is defined as the ratio of the maximum intensity over an image. Contrast enhancement techniques are also available to improve or adjust proper values of contrast in an adaptive manner.

These techniques are most useful because many medical images when examined on a color display give inadequate information for image interpretation. There is no general theory to improve the fidelity of the image with regard to some ideal form of the image but there exists a wide variety of the image with regard to some ideal form of the image but there exists a wide variety of techniques for improving the image quality. The contrast stretch, density slicing, edge enhancement and spatial filtering are the more commonly used techniques which attempt to provide corrected image against geometric and radiometric distortions. Numerous digital image techniques can be seen in literatures to be most satisfactory than the photographic technique for image enhancement because of the precision and wide variety of digital processes. This chapter also talked about the various factors causing poor quality of image such as problem with data acquisition process, imperfect instrument, and some amount of noise. This poor quality of images cannot be tolerated in medical imaging because it could lead to wrong diagnosis and interpretation. The noise reduction techniques and filters are also discussed in this chapter but since robustness is the biggest challenge in image processing, an efficient filtering method for enhancing the digital images is necessary for the removal of noise.

VARIOUS MODALITIES OF MEDICAL IMAGING

There are number of medical imaging modalities used for different purposes and applications such as ultrasound imaging, mammographic imaging etc. There have been several improvements over the technologies and imaging methods including modern image acquisition systems and sensors with which the medical imaging systems are built. The most commonly used technique for capturing breast X- ray images is Mammography. Although High quality scanners are nowa day's avalaible but improper radiation still poses problems sometimes and hence, the radiation risk is expected to be negligible (Guy, 2005).

Computer aided diagnosis systems used a digital mammographic image as input image to be analysed from a conventional film mammogram and masses, calcifications or other abnormal areas are detected. The Anomalies present may indicate the presence of cancer. The accuracy of breast cancer detection has been enhanced to a significant level with the advent digital mammographic techniques.

Breast Cancer Imaging

Brest Cancer imaging is onc of the most used medical imaging modality for the detection of breast cancer. The image of a female breast organ normally consists of two large semispherical eminences containing mammary glands. These glands are used to secrete milk when stimulated corresponding to the period after giving birth. Each breast image has 15 to 20 sections called lobes. The lobes are organized in a pattern like the petals of a daisy. Lobes consist of even smaller lobules which are terminated by tiny bulb like structures that help in producing milk. These cubes or ducts are further connected to nipples in the dark area at the centre of the breast. The dark area of skin is called areola.

Lobules and ducts are filled in be fats and muscles are not found in breast; However, these lie under breast and are associated with ribs. Blood vessels in bones carry lymph which leads to lymph nodes. These nodes are small bean shaped organs whose clusters are present under the arms and above the collarbones.

When the images are acquired through mammographic image scanning methods, it has been observed that cancerous elements begin in the cells in which building blocks are making tissues. The tissues of breast are connected to the other parts of body and hence, growing cells or tissues affect the other parts also. Normal cells grow, become older and get damaged and finally die; in the meantime, new cells are produced in place of the old dead cells. But sometimes, new cells are not accepted by the body, since the body does not need new cells for the moment and consequently, the cells do not die. This process trigger building up of extra cells which in turn form masses of tissues that are not at all desirable (Kosus, Kosus, & Turhan, 2010).

These tissues masses go on to further construct lump or grow as Anomaly or tumour. The tumors can be classified as an benign tumor i.e., not cancerous or malignant tumour which is cancerous and hence, dangerous. The benign tissues are although extra masses, not harmful to the body, since cancer is not present in them, but malignant tissues are very much harmful. The growth of malignant masses is even more harmful and its removal is required, otherwise it can pose risk to life. Nearby organs and tissues are also damaged if the malignant tissues are not removed and continue to grow. The malignant tissues upon growing enter the blood vessels and other parts of body. The cancer cells may damage other tissues and also cause formation of tumors in the parts other than breast.

If breast cancer is reported in a biopsy, then it is required to know the stage of cancer also. Radiologists need to know the staging so that the patient can be diagnosed accordingly and the best treatment can be provided. Generally, the stages of cancer depend on size of the cancerous regions or tissues and whether these tissues have affected other tissues.

Ultrasound Imaging

Ultrasound has been utilized to picture the human body for over 50 years. Dr. Karl Theo Dussik, an Austrian neurologist, was the first to apply ultrasound as a therapeutic indicative device to picture the brain.Today, ultrasound (US) is a standout among the most broadly utilized imaging advances in pharmaceutical. It is versatile, free of radiation chance, and generally reasonable when contrasted and other imaging modalities, for example, attractive reverberation and registered tomography. Besides, US pictures are tomographic, i.e., offering a "cross-sectional" perspective of anatomical structures. The pictures can be obtained "progressively," accordingly giving immediate visual direction to numerous intervention systems including those for provincial anesthesia and torment administration. In this part, we depict a portion of the basic standards and material science fundamental US innovation that are important to the agony professional Mammographic Imaging(Preim, & Bartz, 2007).

Ultrasound Imaging depends on the utilization of high frequency sound to help in the determination, diagnosis and treatment of patients. Ultrasound frequencies ranges from 2 to around 15 MHz, albeit considerably higher frequencies might be utilized as a part of a few circumstances. The ultrasound bar starts from mechanical motions of various precious stones in a transducer, which is energized by electrical heartbeats (piezoelectric impact). The transducer changes over one kind of vitality into another (electrical <- - > mechanical/sound).

The ultrasound waves (beats of sound) are sent from the transducer, proliferate through various tissues, and after that arrival to the transducer as reflected echoes. The returned echoes are changed over once more into electrical motivations by the transducer gems and are additionally prepared to shape the ultrasound picture exhibited on the screen.

Ultrasound transducers contain a scope of ultrasound frequencies, named data transfer capacity. For example, 2.5-3.5 MHz for general stomach imaging and 5.0-7.5 MHz for shallow imaging. Ultrasound waves are reflected at the surfaces between the tissues of different thickness, the reflection being comparing to the refinement in impedance. In the event that the distinction in thickness is expanded, the extent of reflected sound is expanded, and the extent of transmitted sound is proportionately diminished. On the off chance that the distinction in tissue thickness is altogether different, at that point the sound is totally reflected, bringing about aggregate acoustic shadowing. Acoustic shadowing is accessible behind bones, calculi (stones in kidneys, gallbladder, et cetera.) and air (intestinal gas). Echoes are not conveyed if there is no refinement in a tissue or between tissues.Homogenous liquids like blood, bile, pee, substance of straightforward growths, and pleural emanation are viewed as resound free structures (Beutel, Kundel, Van Metter, 2000).

Magnetic Resonance Imaging

The NMR spectroscopy (Nuclear magnetic resonance) is the establishment based of the Magnetic resonance imaging (MRI), in which by simply spatially encoding the NMR signal coming from nuclei (e.g. protons) present in the object to be imaged through the application of time-varying linear magnetic field gradients, medical images are generated. A very high spatial resolution and the ability to distinguish soft tissues are the main advantages of MRI. However, sometimes insufficient contrast is observed and, thus, the use of contrast agents (CAs) is of great assistance in many applications of MRI. A number of such substances have been developed and research continues in order to find more selective contrast media that will allow a better delineation of diseases, thus helping radiologists to make a more precise diagnosis. We depict underneath the distinctive classes of CAs and give a few illustrations, giving an outline not just of current clinical CAs, CAs experiencing clinical assessment and mixes following new thoughts, yet in addition of some of their applications. Currently available MR CAs can be classified in different ways, according to their various features, such as

1. The presence and nature of their metal centre,
2. Their magnetic properties,
3. Their effect on the image,
4. Their chemical structure and ligands present or
5. Their bio distribution and applications.

The above classification is simplify in order to avoid unnecessary repetition as many of these above mentioned items are related closely. We will start by using together the criteria of the CAs chemical composition (including metal centre and ligands present), the resulting magnetic properties and the corresponding effects on the MRI image.

Breast Thermograph Imaging

The idea of Digital Infrared Imaging depends on the rule that metabolic movement and vascular dissemination in both pre-destructive tissue and the region encompassing a creating bosom malignancy is quite often higher than in ordinary breast tissue. The harmful tumors increment course to their cells by holding open existing veins, opening lethargic vessels, and making new ones (neoangiogenesis) in a consistently expanding requirement for supplements. There is an increase in the regional surface temperatures of the breast because of the above mention process. Digital Infrared Imaging employs ultra-sensitive medical infrared cameras and sophisticated computers to analyze, detect and produce high-resolution images of these temperature variations. These temperature variations may be among the earliest signs of breast cancer and/or a pre-cancerous state of the breast can be early detected because of the Digital Infrared Imaging extreme sensitivity (Kosus, Kosus, & Turhan, 2010).

The current strategies utilize to recognize suspicious indications of bosom tumor depend basically on the mix of both physical examination and mammography. The backbone of early bosom growth recognition has turned into this approach and greater progression is required. Since the outright counteractive action of bosom disease has not turned into a reality starting at yet, endeavors must be coordinated at identifying bosom malignancy at its most punctual stage. The Inclusion of Digital Infrared Imaging (Breast Thermography) to the cutting edge of early bosom malignancy identification brings a lot of uplifting news for ladies.

While mammography, MRI, ultrasound and other basic imaging apparatuses depend basically on finding the physical tumor then again the Digital Infrared Imaging depends on identifying the warmth created by expanded vein flow and metabolic changes related with a tumor's beginning and development By detecting minute variations in normal blood vessel activity, infrared imaging may find thermal signs suggesting a pre-cancerous state of the breast or the presence an early tumor that is not yet large enough to be detected by physical examination, mammography, or other types of structural imaging (Nyirjesy, 1986).

The Mammography methodology must have the capacity to distinguish 80% kinds of diseases and the rest around 20% can't be recognized for different reasons, however some of these malignancies can be effortlessly found by the utilization of Digital Infrared Imaging. Mammography additionally experiences a few negative marks, for example, a few troubles in perusing mammograms can happen extraordinarily in ladies who are on hormone substitution, nursing or have fibrocystic, extensive, thick, or improved bosoms. These bad marks can be effectively overwhelmed with the assistance of Digital Infrared Imaging.

Studies have grandstand that a not typical infrared picture is the absolute most vital marker of high hazard for creating bosom tumor, 10 times more noteworthy than a family history of the infection. In patients with a persevering anomalous thermogram side effect, the examination comes about turn into a marker of higher future disease chance. Contingent on specific components, reevaluations are performed at fitting interims to screen the bosoms. This actually grants woman time to take a pro-active approach by working with her doctor to improve her breast health. By maintaining close monitoring of her breast health with infrared imaging, self breast exams, clinical examinations, mammography, and other tests, a woman has a much better chance of detecting cancer at its earliest stage and preventing invasive tumor growth. Advanced Infrared Imaging is as exceptional as a unique finger impression, every patient has a specific infrared guide of their bosoms. Any change of this infrared guide on serial imaging (pictures assumed control a very long time to years) may constitute an early indication of an irregularity. In any case, if pathology is suspected, this data is utilized to suggest promote examinations and tests.

Positron Emission Tomography

In disease conclusion, neuroimaging and atomic imaging research, the Positron emanation tomography (PET) assumes a critical part particularly in early recognition and analysis. In this imaging modality tracer (a diagnostic drug), which is labelled by positron emitters such as 18F is injected. For example, fludeoxyglucose (FDG), which is synthesized from glucose, is used for cancer imaging. Through the positron annihilation, two 511 keV photons (gamma-rays) are emitted at the same time toward almost opposite directions. By making incident recognition of a couple of photons, the source position can be restricted along the line interfacing the two locators utilized for occurrence discovery. By simply measuring millions of lines enables tomographic image reconstruction and the 3D distribution of positron emitters is imaged However potential focuses stay for which enormous enhancements of PET could be made, including spatial determination, affectability and assembling costs. For instance, the affectability of present PET scanners does not surpass 10%.This means that more than 90% of the gamma-rays emitted from a subject are not utilized for imaging. There is need of more research on next generation PET technologies, which still remains a hot topic worldwide (Kim & Horii, 2000).

Computed Tomography

Computed tomography is popular imaging modalities that generates cross-sectional images and all the local X-ray attenuation properties of the body is represented in each pixel. In 1970, the first experimental set-up of Hounsfield worked with the so-called translation/rotation principle. Through the use of a collimator, a thin beam of X-rays was generated and a single detector element was used to measure the attenuated intensity. By changing this set-up, different positions were measured. After acquiring an entire set of parallel measurements, the set-up was rotated to acquire the next parallel projection. The 1st generation of CT scanners is based on this very principle discussed before. The 2nd generation CT scanners differed only slightly from that initial design in that a small number of measurement values could be obtained simultaneously. The first commercially available scanner a total of 180 projections were obtained in steps of 1° with 160 measurement values each in Hounsfield's. The acquisition of those 28.800 measurement values took five minutes. From that data an image of 80 × 80 pixels was reconstructed. A normal head examination requiring six slices took about half an hour with such a scanner.

Therefore, physicists were aspiring at shortening the examination times. This was achieved with the introduction of the 3rd generation CT scanners: a 1D array of detector elements positioned on an arc covers the entire measurement field and acquires a complete 'fan-beam' projection. This not only avoided the slow translation movements, but also improved the efficiency of using the output of the X-ray tube. As figure 2 shows a modern 3rd generation CT scanner is a machine consisting of a donut-shaped gantry with a big hole. The Head, body, arms or legs have to be in the middle of the scanner to make a cross-sectional image. The patient is moved in and out on a motor-controlled table. The slice thickness is usually 0.5 to several mm and the spatial resolution (in the cross section) is roughly 1 mm at 512 × 512 pixels per slice. Within the ring of the CT scanner an X-ray tube is placed opposite a detector array with up to 1200 detecting elements, which receive the photons that went through the patient. If one measurement has been done this way, the source and detector rotate over a small angle (roughly 1°) and a new measurement is taken. The scanner repeats this procedure until a rotation of 180° has been reached. Then all thousands of measurements for reconstructing one slice have been done. The table on which the patient lies can then move a little further through the ring for measuring a new slice (Preim & Bartz, 2007).

Radiography

The Wilhelm Conrad Roentgen on November 8, 1895 found the utilization of X-Rays. Since the basic starting revelation has progressed rapidly. Radiography fuses both symptomatic radiography and furthermore extra imaging modalities, for example, Magnetic reverberation imaging (MRI), vascular-interventional radiography, PET-CT, PET-MRI, heart interventional radiography, quality administration (QM), bone densitometry, atomic drug (NM), sonography, processed tomography (CT), mammography and radiation treatment. Radiography has become an indispensable diagnostic tool of modern medicine nowadays. Radiography thus helps the physician to diagnose and know the exact conditions in various medical cases such as broken bones can be aligned, ulcers can be detected and many other injuries.

Radiography is an imaging methodology in view of viably utilizing radiation to give pictures of the tissues, inside organs, bones, and vessels that contain the human body. Doctors and Radiologists, who have experienced uncommon preparing in the understanding of analytic pictures, read or analyze of these pictures. Tolerant treatment relies upon the exact and exact generation of radiographic pictures (Preim & Bartz, 2007).

Echocardiogram

Echocardiogram pictures delivered with the assistance of Echocardiography helps in the discovery of cardiomyopathies, for example, hypertrophic cardiomyopathy and widened cardiomyopathy. Stress echocardiography may likewise help in deciding if any chest torment or related side effects are identified with the coronary illness. The Ultrasound images created by the echocardiogram of heart structures and produce accurate assessment of the blood flowing through the heart using pulsed or continuous wave Doppler ultrasound. This can help in the assessment of both normal and abnormal blood flow through the heart (Bryan, 2010).

PROBLEMS WITH MEDICAL IMAGES

Digital images are very important in the field of medical image diagnosis systems. The early identification of malignancy and different inconsistencies in the interior parts of human body can be prior recognized to significant degree and afterward help the radiologist in the exact conclusion of infection. However, there are some hitches or difficulties in the imaging systems and its associated processes that could cause problems in the semi automatic and automatic process of diagnosis and then following a precise clinical decision making. In medicine and biology, pictorial data acts as an important source of information but getting correct pictures or images is a very difficult task, though with the help of modern and sophisticated equipments are available this task is somewhat simple nowadays.

Image quality and processing speed are the major problem areas of medical image processing. If the image size is big enough to contain image properties, then the time for retrieval and other processing make the system time to increase. Poor quality of image poses even bigger challenge, as it could affect the decision making process adversely. Mass screening of medical images helps in the reduction of viewing time. High noise levels, low contrast, poor resolution, etc. are some other factors causing problems in the medical image processing. The usefulness of biomedical images can be achieved using contrast enhancements, sharpness enhancements, image magnification and reduction of distortion (Bankman, 2008).

IMAGE ENHANCEMENT

The poor quality of the image simply increases the possibility of wrong decision making in the medical image diagnosis. Therefore Image Enhancement becomes an imperative method to be applied over all the medical images before their interpretation or diagnosis (Gonzalez & Woods, 2008).

The primary goal of utilizing picture upgrade is to process a picture with the goal that the outcome is more appropriate than the first picture for a particular application, for example, discovery of variation from the norm or bosom tumor location or lung disease identification. The upgrade can enhance the difference or shine of the first picture by growing dynamic range splendor esteems. Once in a while, the picked set of highlights may likewise be enhanced utilizing improvement systems. The impact of upgrade is either the changes of human visual discernment or the improved comprehension from the perspective of processing gadgets. In restorative picture investigation and applications, an investigator needs to separate between the zones at first having a little distinction in the thickness and it winds up productive and less demanding in the wake of applying a reasonable picture improvement strategy. Picture upgrade is predominantly of two sorts which is as per the following:

Spatial Domain Methods

Spatial area strategies specifically work on the comprising picture pixels. These pixel esteems are changed and controlled to accomplish wanted level of upgrade. Spatial space methods like the logarithmic changes, control law changes, histogram leveling, depend on the immediate control of the pixels in the picture. Spatial methods are especially helpful for specifically changing the dim level estimations of individual pixels and consequently the general difference of the whole picture(Jain, 2005). In any case, they as a rule improve the entire picture in a uniform way which by and large delivers bothersome outcomes. It is not possible to selectively enhance edges or other required information effectively. Some of the Spatial Domain Techniques are:

Log Transformation

Log transformation is one of the elementary image enhancement techniques of the spatial domain that can be effectively used for contrast enhancements of dark images. The log change is basically a dim level change which implies that the dim levels of picture pixels are modified. This change maps a limited scope of low dim level esteems in the information picture to a more extensive scope of yield levels (Jayaraman, S., Esakkirajan & Veerakima, 2010). The general form of the log transformation can be mathematically represented as:

$$S= c \log (1+r) \tag{1}$$

where, S is the output grey level, r is the input grey level and c is a constant. It is assumed that $r \geq 0$.

Power Law Transformation Technique

The *n*th power and *n*th root curves can be given by the expression,

$$S = C * r^{\gamma} \tag{2}$$

Where, S is the output grey level, r is the input grey level and c and $^{\gamma}$ are constants. This transformation function is also called as *gamma* correction. For various values of γ different levels of enhancements can be obtained. This technique is quite commonly called as *Gamma Correction*. The difference between the log-transformation function and the power-law functions is that using the power-law function a family of possible transformation curves can be obtained just by varying the value of λ.

Histogram Transforms and Processing

In an image, there may be a number of pixels which have the same intensity values. The number of pixels is plotted against the intensity value which is known as histogram. Histogram is a graph or a kind of bar diagram representing an eight-bit grayscale image, 256 different possible intensities are there and hence, the grayscale value. The histogram of a digital image shows the probability of occurrence of grayscale values of pixels in the range 0 to 255. Intensity values are the measured grayscale statistics in an image or regions in an image. The measurements include minimum intensity values, maximum intensity value and mean intensity value and standard deviation of the intensity values. Histogram Equalizations is another method for contrast enhancement of an image.

Histogram based methods applied to enhance images are mainly used for increasing the dynamic range of gray-scale values in an image. Following are the few limitations of histogram equalizations method:

1. The histogram equalization method may result in in over enhancement and saturation artefacts.
2. The brightness of an image may unnecessarily be changed. (Jayaraman, Esakkirajan, & Veerakima, 2010)

SOURCES OF NOISE AND FILTERS USED FOR NOISE REDUCTION

Medical image processing and its analysis is used in several important applications such as early detection of breast cancer and lung cancer. The nature of picture required in these applications is high, since a minor variety may bring about wrong determination. The picture quality might be corrupted because of essence of clamor that may be included the therapeutic pictures either by the picture securing framework itself or by some different reasons. The abrupt variation in system conditions such as lighting, pose or poor illumination may contribute noise to the signals. This random variation has generally no particular pattern and it causes image quality to reduce. Almost all the images captured contain noise in some form or other. This may be easily seen as grainy, textured or snowy appearance. The presence of noise-like patterns, called speckle noise, is a big challenge in ultrasound images which adversely affect the individual interpretation and diagnosis. Digital cameras can produce some common noise signals, namely, random noise, fixed pattern noise and banding noise (Gonzalez & Woods, 2008).

The main characteristics of random noise are the fluctuations in intensity and colour. These variations may be due to short exposure to illumination and hence, the intensity or colour varies above and below the desired or actual image intensity. Another kind of clamor is the settled example commotion that shows hot pixels having considerably higher force than the power at encompassing irregular commotion vacillations. This kind of clamor is caused because of long exposures and is exacerbated by higher temperatures. Aside from this, there is a banding kind of commotion likewise that is because of the catching gadget and the clamor is included as a result of splendor shadows. This clamor is obvious at high speeds and as shadows.Dark noise is found as the accumulation of the heat generated electrons in the sensor which contribute a snow-like appearance to the image. Photon noise is caused by the difference in the arrival time of light to the sensor. Random noise varies from image to image and is contributed by many influences. The noise signals in medical images can be reduced by using image enhancement techniques or filtering methods. The main objective of this filtering operation is to process an image so that the result becomes more suitable than the original image for a specific application such as cancer detection. Image filters are of two types mainly- spatial domain filters and frequency domain filters. The filters used to remove noise are discussed in this chapter in a little elaborated way along with the results for few cases and their evaluation (Gonzalez, & Woods, 2008).

SPATIAL DOMAIN FILTERS

Spatial domain filters directly operate over pixels of an image, i.e. the intensity values are directly modified in spatial domain. The picture clamor evacuation goes for concealment of commotion that may have debased a picture amid its obtaining or transmission. In spatial space, sifting task is performed utilizing convolution veil connected to the entire picture. This mask is a small subimage of any suitable size and it covers the whole image either by moving the mask from top to bottom or by any other means.

An image consists of gray scale values which may be high frequency components or low frequency components. High frequency components are generally found in the edges and other sharp details are highlighted and the low frequency components are suppressed or attenuated. Similarly, smooth areas or slowly varying areas are the low frequency components and these can be retained by using a suitable low pass filters which attenuates the high frequency components.

An example of the mark used in the spatial domain filtering can be seen in the Figure 4. This mask is represented in the form of matrix consisting of coefficients or elements. Table 1 illustrates a mask of size (3*3) where C1,C2……… C9 are the coefficients of mask.

If the grayscale values or intensities of pixels are assumed as D_1,D_2…..D_9 then the average values can be calculated as

Table 1. An Example of mask used in spatial domain filters

C_1	C_2	C_3
C_4	C_5	C_6
C_7	C_8	C_9

$$D_a = (1/9) * (C_1*D_1+C_2*D_2+C_3*D_3+..........+C_9*D_9) \quad (3)$$

This mask moves to the whole image observing some mechanism and the new pixel values are computed accordingly and finally, a new image is constructed. There are a number of filters for removing the noise present in the medical images in spatial domain such as low pass filter,high pass filter,high boost filter, variance filter, etc. These filters are discussed by here along with the practical results of real-time medical image of our database (Gonzalez, R., & Woods, R., 2008).

Low Pass Filter

Low pass filter; as this name suggests, is used to pass low frequency details and remove high frequency components such as sharp transitions or edges. The filer works using a mask or window a which a new grayscale is calculated as a simple average or arithmetic mean of the cells in the filter window or mask. A smooth image is obtained and hence, the filters are also called smoothing filters. Although sharp transitions (which are not desired) are removed, but the low pass filters may produce some amount of blurring and degrade the useful image information and reduce the contrast as well. A sample of mask for low pass filter is shown in Table 2.

High Pass Filter

High pass filters are used to pass high frequency component in special domain and reject or attenuate low frequency details of an image. The calculation of filter coefficients is done by selecting the value of a centre pixel or cell and subtracting its form it half the average value of surrounding pixels. If there is any variation in the centre cell, than this difference will be accentuated in the output image, while the areas of uniform brightness are changed very little(Gonzalez, R., & Woods, R., 2008). The sharp details such as edges and the high contrast details are retained. A mask of size (3x3) . The enhancement of desired features is improved if the filter window size is increased but the processing time may increase in such condition. A sample mask for high pass filter is illustrated by Table 3.

Table 2. A sample of mask for low pass filter

1	1	1
1	1	1
1	1	1

Table 3. A sample of mask for high pass filter

-1	-1	-1
-1	-8	-1
-1	-1	-1

High Boost Filter

The result of high pass filter may have a background present in the image which is darker than the original image. This difficulty or limitation of high pass filter is overcome by using another filter called high boost filter that can restore the original background and the sharpness of image, as desired, can also be achieved. High boost filter enhance the high frequency content along with the low frequency information of the background also (Jain, A.K., 2005). The filter operation is given below and its sample mask is illustrated by Table 4:

HIGH BOOST FILTER = (A – 1) Original image + high pass filter output

= A[Original image] – low pass filter output (4)

where A is the high boost coefficient. For A=1, it becomes standard high pass filter and for A>1, the high boost image becomes approx equal to the original image multiplied by a constant. The result can also be seen for the other medical images.

Frost Filter

The Frost filter is an adaptive and exponentially weighted averaging filter based on the variation coefficient. This coefficient of variation is the ratio of the local standard deviation to the local mean of the degraded or noisy image. The filter replaces the pixel of consideration with a weighted sum of the values within the moving kernel of suitable file. A set of weight values for each pixel within the filter

Table 4. A sample of mask for High Boost filter

-1	-1	-1
-1	9-A	-1
-1	-1	-1

window surrounding each pixel is calculated assuming the multiplicative stationary noise (Jain, 2005).

Variance Filter

A variance filter is used to highlight the edged in the X-ray and CT SCAN images of the brain. The areas of varying reflectance become brighter than the uniform areas that appear darker. A local homogeneity of the intensity in an image can be measured with the help of results of variance filter. This filter is also referred to as non-linear and non-directional edge detector. Basically, a central pixel value is replaced with the variance of specified set of pixel values surrounding it in a window on the image (Pratt, 2002).

Median Filter

Median filters can be used as a substitute for the low pass filter, since they are not suitable for the reducing the strong spike type noise pattern. Median value of the pixel in the window is computed and then, the centre pixel of the window is replaced with the computed median value. This can be done by sorting all the pixel values from the surrounding neighbourhood and replacing the pixel with the middle pixel value. Figure shows a mask where the pixels are arranged in the ascending order and the median values are calculated. The centre pixel of the mask are replaced by the median value and this procedure is repeated for moving the mask one position after another until the last pixel in the image is processed (Pratt, 2002).

For example, in a given mask shown in Figure 8, arranging the pixels in ascending order gives a sequence -16, 18,25,32,37,40,47,51,54 and the median value 37 is selected. Finally, the centre pixel of the mask are replaced by the median value illustrated by Table 5.

Table 5. A sample of mask

25	16	18
32	40	37
54	47	51

FREQUENCY DOMAIN FILTERS

Frequency domain filtering does not operate directly over the pixel values like spatial domain. Frequency domain filters operate on the Fourier transform of input images to be enhanced. The Fourier transform or filter transfer function is also calculated and multiplied with the Fourier transform of the original image. The inverse transform of product gives an enhanced or filtered image (Gonzalez & Woods, 2008). The frequency domain filters have specific advantages as compared to the spatial domain filters. Some of them are as under:

1. Convolution can be easily calculated in the frequency domain.
2. The periodic pattern of noise can be reduced to a limited set of high spatial frequencies which-makes the filtering easy and effective.
3. Computationally more efficient to implement.
4. Features extraction is easier in the frequency domain which is very much required in the image analyses and understanding.
5. Digitization makes the task of filtering very easy and simple, since Fourier transform is computed as fast Fourier transform(FFT) and discrete Fourier transform(DFT) in the digital domain.
6. Digitization process provides all the benefits of digital versus analog implementation of filtering or similar operations.
7. Enhanced utility of working in the frequency domain to perform certain image measurement and processing. Some operations could be performed with significantly greater computational effort in the spatial domain such as convolution.
8. The use of frequency domain filtering methods can offer benefits in many real time applications in one need not to deal with the mathematics deeply.

Discussion of frequency domain filters includes basics of convolution theorems, smoothing domain filter, sharpening domain filters and homomorphic filtering.

Convolution Theorem

Fourier transform used in the frequency domain filtering helps in converting images from spatial domain into frequency domain or vice-versa if the inverse transform id used. In spatial domain, filter function directly operates over the pixel values and hence, the convolution is required to compute in the time domain which is little complex than that of the frequency domain(Gonzalez & Woods, 2008). Basically, convolution is defined as the integral of one functions at time t and another function at time t-τ.

$$f * g = \int_{-\infty}^{\infty} f(\tau)g(t-\tau)d\tau = \int_{-\infty}^{\infty} g(\tau)f(t-\tau)d\tau \qquad (5)$$

where f and g are the two functions in the time domain and f*g is convolution between the two.

Convolution, directly in the spatial domain, is very difficult to calculate but this is simplified using Fourier transform. This can be done as follows:

$$F(f * g) = F(f) \cdot F(g) = F \cdot G \qquad (6)$$

where F and G are Fourier transform of functions f and g, respectively, dot (.) denotes the element-by-element multiplication and F is Fourier transform operator.

Now, by using the inverse Fourier transform F^{-1} , we can obtain

$$F^{-1}(F \cdot G) = F * g \qquad (7)$$

If an image to be enhanced is represented as f(x, y) and the two-dimensional **filter** function is expressed as h(x, y), then the convolution between the two is computed in digital domain using discrete Fourier transform as follows:

$$f(x,y) * h(x,y) = \frac{1}{MN} \sum_{m=0}^{M-1} \sum_{n=0}^{N-1} f(m,n)h(x-m, y-n) \qquad (8)$$

where MN is the size of two functions f(x, y) and h(x, y).

Frequency domain filters are mainly divided into three different types as listed below:

1. Smoothing domain filters or low pass filters
2. Sharpening domain filters or high pass filters
3. Homomorphic filters

We have discussed here about the smoothing domain filters, sharpening domain filters and homomorphic filters in terms of their suitable transfer function and the response of filters. Colour image enhancement is not separately discussed because it exploits any of the remaining three filters(Gonzalez & Woods, 2008).

Smoothing Domain Filters

Smoothing domain filters are also called as low pass filters, since the pass components of digital images are retained and the high frequency components are eliminated from the images. The filters can result in the blurring of image and hence, the sharp transitions associated with the noise are reduced. Sharp transitions in an image are the high frequency details and they are removed by smoothing domain filters and therefore, referred to as low pass filters. Ideally, a low pass filters would retain all the low frequency components and eliminate all the high frequency components but practical low pass filters can't do this and problems, namely, blurring and ringing are there in the results obtained after applying these filters (Jain, A.K., 2005). The edges, other sharp transitions and similar noise components are the high frequency details which are not required in several applications and are attenuated by the smoothing domain filters. Their types are discussed below in terms of filter transfer function and its response:

Ideal Low Pass Filter (ILPF)

This filter is used to block all the frequency details i.e., the frequencies higher than the cut-off frequency r_0 and the other terms are retained. Filter transfer function may be expressed as follows:

$$H = (u, v) = \begin{cases} 1, & if\ D(u, v) \leq r_0 \\ 0, & if\ D(u, v) > r_0 \end{cases} \tag{9}$$

where r_0 is the cut-off frequency which is a positive quantity and D(u, v) is the distance from point (u, v) to the frequency rectangle in the frequency domain of image. Assuming image size of (M X N), the distance can be measured as

$$D(u, v) = \sqrt{\left(u - \frac{M}{2}\right)^2 + \left(v - \frac{N}{2}\right)^2} \tag{10}$$

Low pass filters are generally radial symmetric, which illustrates filter cross section as a function of distance from the origin, image equivalent of filter and perspective plot or filter response.

Ringing effect is the major drawback of an ideal low pass filter that occur along the edges of the enhanced images. This effect is like one of the characteristics of ILPF. The filter operation involves computation of convolution in the frequency domain and multiple peaks of the ideal low filter in the spatial domain produce ringing effect along the intensity edges in the enhanced images. The results are always seen visualised in the spatial domain even if the filtering is performed in the frequency domain (Jain, 2005).

The cut-off frequency determines the amount of frequency components which are passed by the filter. Smaller the value of cut-off frequency, more is the number of image components eliminated by the filter. With the decreasing value of cut-off frequency, the enhanced image is more blurred and ringing is more severe.

Butterworth Low Pass Filter (BLPF)

Butterworth low pass filter also eliminates the high frequency components whose transfer function of filter order n is given as

$$H(u,v) = \frac{1}{1+\left[\frac{D(u,v)}{D_0}\right]^{2n}} \tag{11}$$

where D_0 corresponds to the cut-off frequency r_0.

Normally, Butterworth low pass filter has no ringing effect foe small filter order and a little ringing effect appears with the increase in filter order, which increases more if the order further increases. (Gonzalez & Woods, 2008).

Sharpening Domain Filters

It is known to everyone that the high frequency components are contributed due to the edges, sharp transitions and other similar noise signals. Image sharpening filters attenuate the low frequency components but the edges or high frequency details are retained. It works in opposition to the low pass filtering and therefore, it attenuates the object and the background which does not have sharp characteristics and enhance the edges (Gonzalez & Woods, 2008). The random noise signals associated with the image are also enhanced by the sharpening domain or high pass filters. A transfer function as the inverse of transfer function of the low pass filter is given as

$$H_{hp}(u,v) = 1 - H_{lp}(u,v) \tag{12}$$

Where $H_{lp}(u,v)$ is the transfer function of low pass filter and $H_{hp}(u,v)$ the transfer function of high pass filter. Generally, ideal high pass filter has the same ringing properties as ILPF.

Homomorphic Filtering

An image as a function can be expressed as the product of illumination and reflectance components as follows:

$$F(x,y) = I(x,y) * R(x,y) \tag{13}$$

The above equation cannot be used directly to operate separately on the frequency components of illumination and reflectance because the Fourier transform of the product of two functions is not separable (Jain, A.K., 2005). Instead the function can be represented as a logarithmic function wherein the product of the Fourier transform can be represented as the sum of the illumination and reflectance components as shown below:

$$\ln(x,y) = \ln(I(x,y)) + \ln(R(x,y)) \tag{14}$$

The Fourier transform of above equation is

$$Z(u,v) = Fi(u,v) + Fr(u,v) \tag{15}$$

The fourier transformed signal is processed by means of a filter function H(u,v) and the resulting function is inverse fourier transformed. Finally, inverse exponential operation yields an enhanced image. This enhancement approach is termed as homomorphic filtering.

CONCLUSION

This chapter begins with the introduction to the various types of medical imaging modalities used for Clinical purposes and medical procedures such as Ultrasound imaging, Mammographic imaging, Radiography, Computed tomography etc. The digital images generated by these modalities are very significant in the medical image diagnosis systems. The detection of cancer and other anomalies in the interior parts of body can be easily detected to considerable extent and help the radiologists in the diagnosis of disease. Table 6 provides a brief comparison among the general Bio-Medical Image modalities discussed in this chapter.

Table 6. Comparison of Bio-Medical Image modalities

S. No.	Medical Image Modality	Description	Merits	Demerits
1	X - Ray	Employ X-rays to display the images of some tumors and other dense matter, bones,	Very Quick, painless and non-invasive. Especially used to diagnose various injuries, including broken bones, some cancers and infections.	Due to the exposure to ionizing radiation (X- rays), there is a Very small increased risk of cancer in future
2	MAGNETIC RESONANCE IMAGING (MRI)	Employ magnetic fields and radio waves to show detailed images of soft tissues, bones, ligaments, organs and cartilage.	Uses no ionizing radiation. It helps to diagnose and guide treatment for a wide range of conditions. It provides similar information to Computed Tomography in some types of investigations.	It is time consuming and noisy procedure. Slight movement can ruin the image which requires retesting. Can make some people feel claustrophobic Sedation or anesthesia may be required for young children or others who can't remain still.
3	COMPUTED TOMOGRAPHY (CT SCANS)	Employs the multiple X-rays to generate the cross-sectional layers that display the detailed images of bones, organs, tissues, and tumors inside the body.	It helps in diagnose and guide the treatment for a wider range of conditions than plain X-ray. It is very Quick and painless.	There is a small risk of cancer in future from the exposure to X- rays. This procedure requires the injection of a contrast medium (dye), which can cause the kidney problems or result in allergic.
4	POSITRON-EMISSION TOMOGRAPHY (PET)	The PET involves inhaling, injecting, swallowing a radioactive 'tracer'. In it, the PET scanner capitalizes the gamma-rays emitted by tracer to show images of bones and organs.	The PET helps in treat, diagnose or predict the outcome for a wide range of conditions. The PET can illustrates the functioning of the different parts of the body and can detect problems much earlier. It is also used to predict how far a cancer has spread and how well treatment is working.	The PET involves exposure to gamma-rays which may cause allergic or injection-site reactions in some people.
5	UL TRASOUND	It employs the use of high-frequency sound waves to generate the motion images of the inside of the body onto a screen, including soft tissues, bones, organs and even an unborn baby.	Usually it is safe, non-invasive and relatively painless. Uses of non-ionizing radiation. Does not usually require injection of a contrast medium (dye). It helps in diagnosis a range of conditions in different parts of the body, such as the abdomen, pelvis, blood vessels, breast, kidneys, muscles, bones and joints. It can be used to monitor the growth of a baby during pregnancy.	Interpretation and Quality of the Medical images highly depends on the skill of the person doing the scan. Other factors can affect image quality, including the presence of air and calcified areas in the body (e.g. bones, plaques and Hardened arteries), and a person's body size. Use of a special probe (e.g. for the esophagus, rectum or vagina) is required in some Ultrasounds. Special preparations may be required before a procedure (e.g. fasting or a full bladder.)

If the quality of images is poor, then the possibility of wrong diagnosis increases hence various image enhancement and noise reducing techniques came into existence and applied over all the medical images prior their interpretation and diagnosis. Primarily Spatial domain and Frequency domain methods are used, former method directly operate over the pixels and later method based on the Fourier transform and convolution theorem in order to enhance the medical images.

REFERENCES

Acharya, T., & Ray, A. K. (2005). *Image processing: Principles and Applications*. Wiley-Inter Science. doi:10.1002/0471745790

Bankman, N. (2008). *Handbook of Medical Image Processing and Analysis* (2nd ed.). New York: Academic Press.

Beolchi, L., & Kuhn, M. H. (1995). *Medical Imaging: Analysis of Multimodality 2D/3D Images*. IOS Press.

Beutel, J., Kundel, H. L., & Van Metter, R. L. (2000). Handbook of Medical Imaging.: Vol. 1. *Physics and Psychophysics*. Bellingham: SPIE Press.

Bryan, R. N. (2010). *Introduction to the Science of Medical Imaging*. Cambridge, UK: Cambridge University Press.

Choras, R. S. (2007). Image feature Extraction techniques and their applications for CBIR and Biometrics system. *International Journal of Biology and Biomedical Engineering*, *1*(1), 231-238.

Dougherty, D. (2009). *Digital Image Processing for Medical Applications*. Cambridge, UK: Cambridge University Press.

Gautherie, M. (1983). Thermobiological Assessment of Benign and Malignant Breast Diseases. *American Journal of Obstetrics and Gynecology*, *8*(8), 861–869. doi:10.1016/0002-9378(83)90236-3 PMID:6650622

Gonzalez, R., & Woods, R. (2008). *Digital image processing* (3rd ed.). Prentice Hall of India.

Gonzalez, R. C., & Woods, R. E. (2002). *Digital Image processing* (2nd ed.). Prentice Hall of India.

Guy, C. (2005). *Introduction to the Principles of Medical Imaging*. London: Imperial College Press. doi:10.1142/p363

Jain, A.K. (2005). *Fundamentals of Digital Image Processing* (4th ed.). Pearson Education.

Jan, J. (2005). *Medical Image Processing, Reconstruction and Restoration: Concepts and Methods*. CRC Press. doi:10.1201/9781420030679

Jayaraman, S., Esakkirajan, S., & Veerakima, T. (2010). Digital Image Processing (3rd ed.). Tata McGraw Hill Education Private Limited.

Kim, Y., & Horii, S. C. (2000). Handbook of Medical Imaging: Vol. 3. *Display and PACS*. Bellingham: SPIE Press.

Kosus, N., Kosus, A., & Turhan, N. (2010). Comparison of standard mammography with digital mammography and digital infrared thermal imaging for breast cancer screening. *Journal of Turk Ger Gynecol Assoc.*, 152–157.

Lehmann, T. M., Wein, B., Dhaman, J., Bredno, J., Vogelsang, F., & Kohnen, M. (2000). Content Based image retrival in medical applications: A novel multistep approach. *Proceedings of the Society for Photo-Instrumentation Engineers*, *3972*, 312–320. doi:10.1117/12.373563

Meyerbaese, A. (2003). *Pattern Recognition in Medical Imaging*. San Diego, CA: Academic Press.

Nyirjesy, M. D. (1986). Clinical Evaluation, Mammography and Thermography in the Diagnosis of Breast Carcinoma. *Thermology*, *1*, 170–173.

Pratt, W. K. (2002). *Digital Iamge Processing*. John Wiley & Sons.

Preim, B., & Bartz, D. (2007). *Visualization in Medicine: Theory, Algorithms, and Applications*. Amsterdam: Morgan Kaufmann.

Chapter 10
A Survey on Female Breast Cancer:
Computer-Aided Diagnosis Using Digital Breast Tomosynthesis

Kalaivani Anbarasan
Saveetha School of Engineering, India

Ramya S.
Saveetha School of Engineering, India

ABSTRACT

The mortality rate of breast cancer can be effectively reduced by early diagnosis. Imaging modalities are used to diagnose through computer for women breast cancer. Digital mammography is the best imaging model for breast cancer screening technique and diagnosis. Digital breast tomosynthesis (DBT), a three-dimensional (3-D) mammography, is an advanced form of breast imaging where multiple images of the breast from different angles are captured and reconstructed (synthesized) into a three-dimensional image set. This chapter discusses the research work carried out on the computer diagnosis of women breast cancer through digital breast tomosynthesis and concludes with further improvement in the computer-aided diagnosis.

INTRODUCTION

Cancer is a deadly disease, which can start in any internal organ; slowly it spreads to the entire body and the patient dies. Each year American Cancer Society publish more number of new cancer cases and deaths caused by it. For the year 2015-2016,

DOI: 10.4018/978-1-5225-5876-7.ch010

they forecast 1,658,370 new cancer cases and 589,430 cancer deaths only in the United States. Therefore, it is expected that the Statistics will be very high for the entire world (Siegel, 2015). Among all types of cancer, breast cancer is the Second leading cause of death in the United States. Current solutions to diagnosing cancer are not adequate due to less promising computer technology and high false negative results.

Breast cancer found in Indian females based on age factor is 25 women's for 1,00,000 women's and the mortality rate is 12 women's for 1,00,000 women's. Statistical Data analysed from latest National Cancer Registries and the report is based on age and mortality factor. The age is adjusted based on the incidence rate of carcinoma of the breast which was found as high as 41 per 100,000 women in Delhi, followed by Chennai (37.9), Bangalore (34.4) and Thiruvananthapuram District (33.7). A statistically significant increase in age adjusted rate over time (1982–2014) in all the places namely Bangalore (annual percentage change: 2.84%), Barshi (1.87%), Bhopal (2.00%), Chennai (2.44%), Delhi (1.44%) and Mumbai (1.42%) was observed. Mortality-to-incidence ratio was found to be as high as 66 in rural registries whereas as low as 8 in urban registries. Young age is found as a major risk factor for breast cancer in Indian women. Breast cancer projection for India during time periods 2020 suggests the number to go as high as 1797900. Better health awareness and availability of breast cancer screening programmes and treatment facilities would cause a favourable and positive clinical picture in the country. The statistics of women breast cancer in India of different age groups are shown in Figure 1.

Breast cancer is two types: non-invasive breast cancer and invasive breast cancer are shown in Figure 2. Non-invasive breast cancer does not invade or spread to other cells. Invasive breast cancer breaks the wall of the tissue and spread all over the breast; it very common type breast cancer (Williams, 2007). The following figure shows healthy milk ducts, non-invasive cancer milk duct, and invasive milk duct.

The chapter introduced the overview of Breast Cancer in Introduction section. The imaging modalities used for Breast Cancer is discussed in section ii such as Ultrasound, Magnetic Resonance Imaging, Digital Mammography and Breast Tomosynthesis. Section iii discuss the most important breast cancer lesions such as micro-calcification, masses, architecture distortion and bilateral symmetry. Nowadays, computer aided diagnosis plays a vital role and their significance and functionalities are discussed in section iv. Researchers carried out a mass volume of work in this field and their highlights are specified in section v. The paper finally concludes with the future direction of breast cancer diagnosis.

Figure 1. Statistics of Breast Cancer in India
Malvia, 2017.

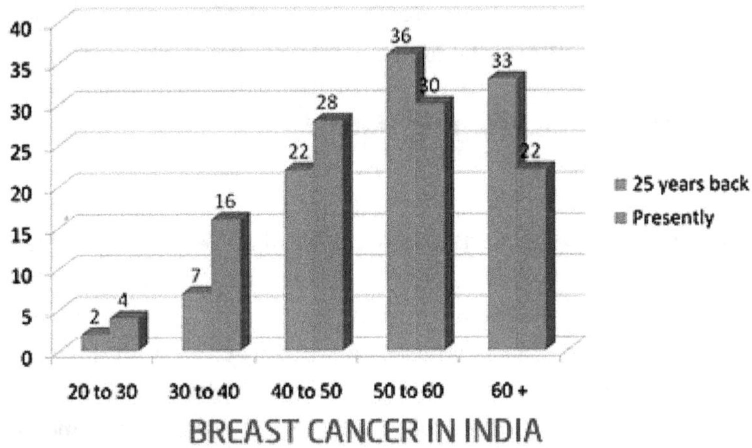

Figure 2. Breast Cancer Types: a. Normal b. Non-invasive milk duct c. invasive milk duct
Williams, 2007.

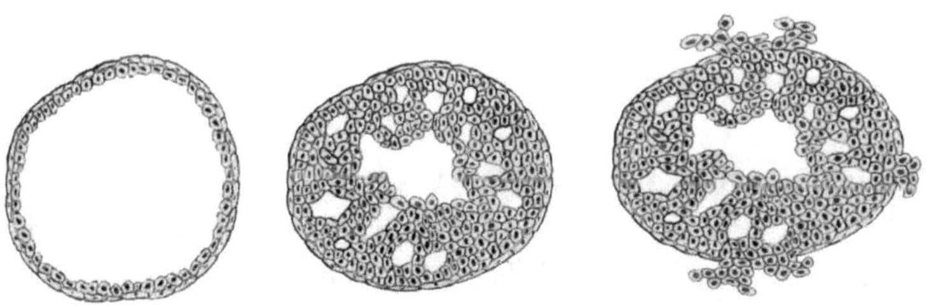

BREAST CANCER DIAGNOSIS IMAGING MODALITIES

Breast cancer diagnosis starts with the screening process. During the screening process, breast anatomical imaging is performed using different imaging modalities. Few common imaging modalities are ultrasound, magnetic resonance imaging, digital mammography and breast tomosynthesis.

Ultrasound

Ultrasound is a beneficial tool to evaluate breast issues and to follow up finding in physical exam or mammography. It is also recommended for breast screening during pregnancy and lactation. Ultrasound is suggested before diagnostic fine needle biopsy and it can be used for biopsy guidance and mass locating. The development of colour Doppler imaging and ultrasound echo-enhancing (contrast agents) provides additional information of anatomical and vascular flow related, which assists the differential diagnosis of breast lesions (Svensson,1997). A sample women breast screening images using ultrasound are shown in Figure 3.

Magnetic Resonance Imaging (MRI)

Since nearly three decades, MRI screening has been employed for detection and diagnosis of breast cancer lesions (Heywang et al., 1989). MRI is suggested for screening women who have a high risk of developing breast cancer, or it can be used to investigate suspicious areas found by the mammogram to help measure the size of the mass. Breast MRI is advised to women with family history of breast cancer and has a high rate of sensitivity (78-98%) and low specificity (43-75%) (Kuhl, 2007). The interpretation process of MRI image is very time-consuming and requires a high level of radiologist experience to detect and differentiate benign and malignant lesions (Meeuwis et al.,2010). In recent studies, computer systems have been developed to facilitate MRI image analysis and improve the diagnosis productivity (Meeuwis et al., 2010; Wang et al., 2009; Williams et al., 2007). A sample women breast cancer screening images using MRI are shown in Figure 4.

Digital Mammography

Full-field digital mammography (FFDM) is a mammography system in which mammographic pictures of the breast are captured. These systems are similar to those found in digital cameras and their efficiency enables better picture with a

Figure 3. Ultrasound images (a) Normal breast (b) Cancer tumour
Svensson, 1997.

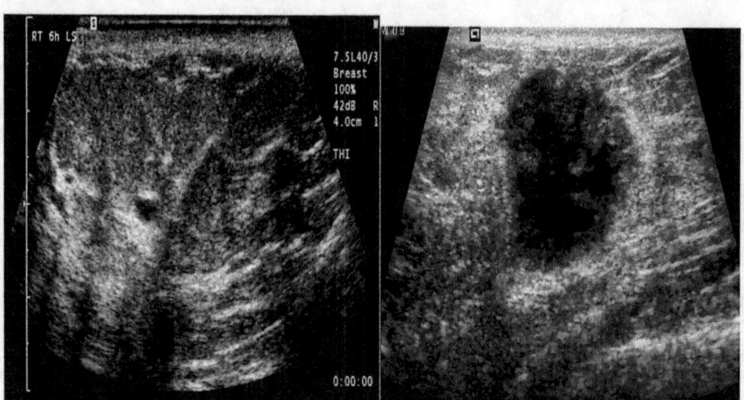

Figure 4. Breast cancer screening using MRI

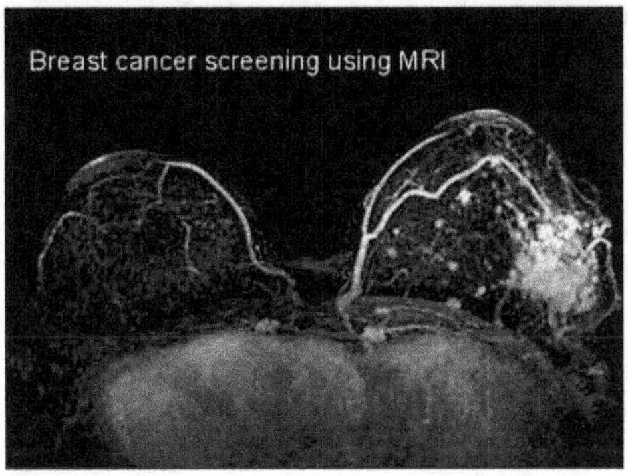

lower radiation dose. The breast images are transferred to a computer for review by the radiologist and for long term storage. A sample women breast cancer screening images using Digital Mammography are shown in Figure 5.

Breast Tomosynthesis

Breast tomosynthesis also called three dimensional (3-D) mammography and digital breast tomosynthesis (DBT) is an advanced form of breast imaging where multiple images of the breast from different angles are captured and reconstructed (synthesized) into a three dimensional image set. In this way 3D breast imaging is similar to computed tomography (CT) imaging in which a series of this slices are assembled together to create a 3D reconstruction of the body. Large population

Figure 5. Digital mammograms. (a) Normal breast and (b) Cancer tumour

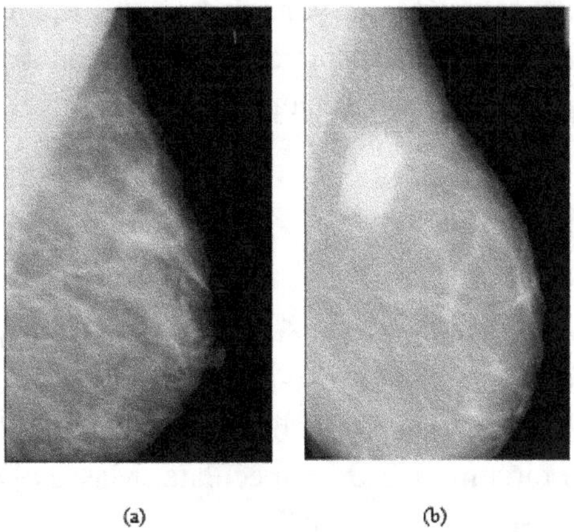

studies have shown that screening with the breast tomosynthesis result in improved breast cancer detection rates and fewer call-backs instances where women are called back from screening for additional testing because of a potentially abnormal finding.

Advantages of Breast Tomosynthesis

- Greater accuracy in pinpointing the size, shape and location of breast abnormalities. Fewer unnecessary biopsies or additional tests.
- Greater likelihood of detecting multiple breast tumours.
- Clearer image of abnormalities within dense breast tissue.

BREAST CANCER LESIONS

Breast cancer lesions are micro calcifications, masses, architectural distortions and bilateral asymmetry.

Micro-Calcifications

Micro calcifications are small calcium deposits of white specks on a mammogram. which are of 0.33 to 0.7mm in size, slightly brighter than surrounding tissues Micro calcifications presence is not a cancer but if they appear in certain patterns and are clustered may be a pre-cancerous cells or early breast cancer. Breast calcifications do not cause symptoms as they are too small to be felt during a routine breast exam. Breast calcifications are first noticed on a mammogram. The calcifications will be determined to be benign, probably benign or suspicious. Benign are harmless, no treatment or further evaluation. Probably Benign have less than 2% risk should be monitored every six months for at least one year. After a year of follow up and assuming no changes are found your doctor will recommend you to have a routine mammogram once a year. Suspicious calcifications identified by the doctor recommends for biopsy. An original mammography images and ground truth are shown in Figure 6.

Masses

Masses are lesions more difficult to detect in monographs than micro calcifications because the features of a mass bear semblance to those of the normal breast parenchyma. In general, mass shape can be round, oval, lobulated or irregular, and margins can be from circumscribed to speculate. Masses Descriptions based on BI-RADS standard are shown in Figure 7.

Figure 6. (a) Original Mammography Image (b) Correspondent ground truth (from MIAS Database)
Dos Santos Teixeira 2012.

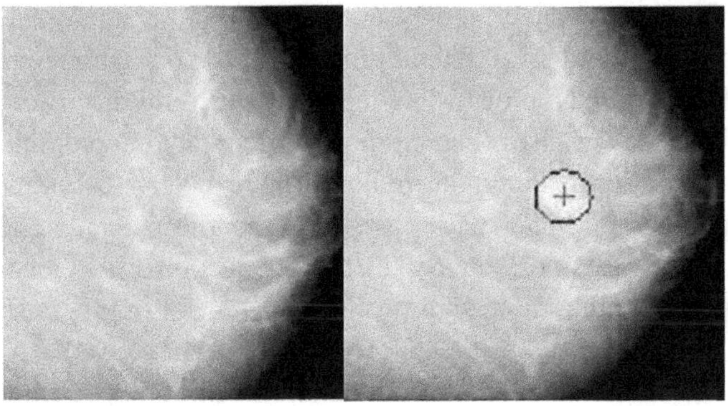

Figure 7. BI-RADS standardized description of masses
Jatoi, 2010.

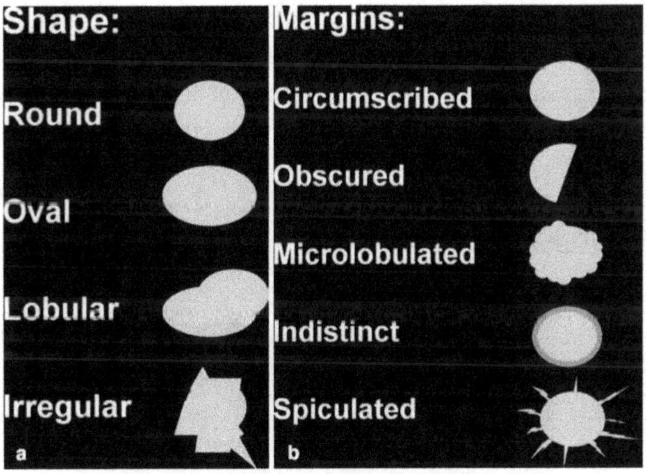

Masses are difficult to distinguish between benignant or malignant due to the differences in the shape and texture features between them. Benign masses are typically smooth and distinct, and their shapes are similar to the round. On the other hand, malignant masses are irregular and their boundaries are usually blurry. A mass with regular shape has a higher probability of being benign whereas a mass with an irregular shape has a high probability of being malignant (Saki, 2010; Sun, 2010; Zhao, 2011).

Architectural Distortions

Architectural distortion is the third most common mammographic appearance of non-palpable breast cancer, representing nearly 6% of abnormalities detected on screening mammography. Although its prevalence on mammography is small compared with calcification or visible mass, architectural distortion is also more difficult to diagnose because it can be subtle and variable in presentation. Indeed, architectural distortion is common finding in retrospective assessments of false-negative mammography and may represent the earliest manifestation of breast cancer. Moreover, some studies suggest that early detection of architectural distortion may be associated with a more significant improvement in prognosis than earlier detection of calcifications. Several automated approaches have been developed to increase the detection rate of architectural distortion, but they remain imperfect. A sample Architectural Distortion are shown in the Figure 8.

Bilateral Asymmetry

Bilateral asymmetry is the difference between corresponding regions in left and right breast which are classified as global asymmetry and focal asymmetry. The former, happens when a greater volume of fibro glandular tissue is present in one breast compared to another in the same region. The latter, corresponds to a circumscribed

Figure 8. Architectural distortion
Bozek, 2009.

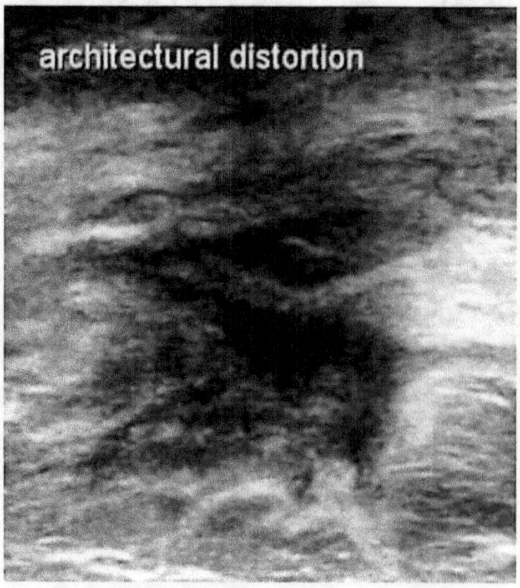

area of asymmetry seen on two views, and usually is an island of healthy fibro glandular tissue that is superimposed with surrounding fatty tissue (Bozek, 2009; Li, 2009). A sample figure of Bilateral Asymmetry are shown in the figure 9.

COMPUTER-AIDED DIAGNOSIS

Recent advances in the resolution of medical imaging modality have revolutionised the diagnostic accuracy. Efficient usage of imaging data to improve the diagnosis is very important. In recent years, computer-aided diagnosis systems (CADs) have developed a new context in radiology to take advantage of the data to be applied to different imaging modality and the diagnosis of different diseases.

The efficiency of radiologists' interpretation can be improved in terms of accuracy and consistency in detection or diagnosis while productivity can be improved by reducing the time required to read the images (Doi, 2009). The outcomes are derived using various techniques in computer vision to present some of the significant parameters such as the location of suspicious lesions and the likelihood of malignancy of the detected lesions.

Figure 9. Bilateral Asymmetry

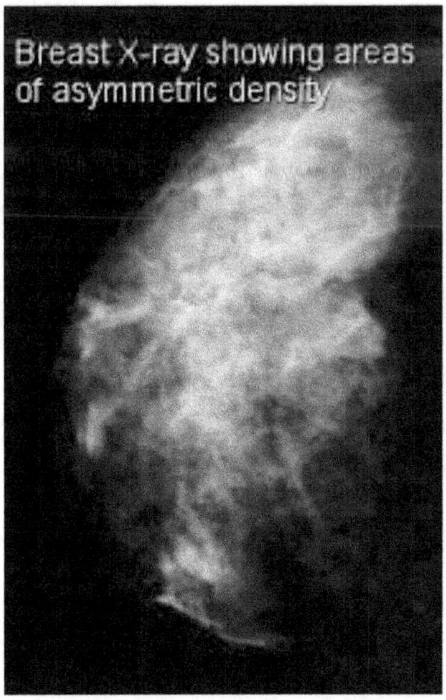

In relation to breast cancer, the main objective of CAD system is to design accurate and reliable approach, to decrease observational oversights and assist in discriminating benign and malignant lesions. In the following, we present some of the recent proposed CAD systems for breast cancer detection or diagnosis on various modalities such as mammography, ultrasound, MRI, and biopsy histopathological images.

Medical image processing requires prior knowledge on the content and nature of image to select appropriate methods to implement the CAD system. In order to achieve a high level of efficiency for automated diagnosis, it is significant to employ efficacious image processing approaches in the main steps of CADs system. The block diagram for Computer Diagnosis System is shown in Figure 10.

Diagnosis

The main stages of a Computer Aided Diagnosis System are as follows:

1. **Image Pre-Processing:** This step is essential for some modality such as ultrasound for the purpose of enhancing the image and reducing the noise with minimum distortion of image features. Pre-processing stage is performed to remove noise and defect caused in image acquisition procedure, image resizing, and enhance the image intensity. Some of the CAD systems do not have a pre-processing stage.
2. **Image Segmentation:** Image segmentation is a vital step towards efficient development of CAD systems. The main purpose of segmentation is the separation of the region of interest (ROI) commensurate with the desired properties (Nie, 2009). Recently, imaging modalities such as magnetic resonance

Figure 10. Computer aided diagnosis system

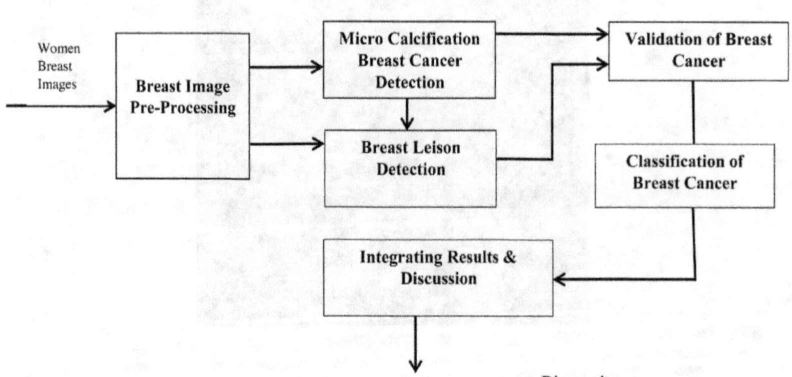

imaging (MRI), computed tomography (CT), 3D ultrasound, and many more modalities are capable of producing images in the form of 3D. Therefore, 3D segmentation methods are desirable for more accurate segmentation in volumetric imagery.

3. **Feature Extraction and Selection:** In this step, different features are extracted according to the characteristics of lesions from the image. These features are used to distinguish benign or malignant lesions. Features are characteristics of the whole image or region of interests. The proper selection of features has an important influence on (1) memory size, (2) accuracy of classification, (3) computational cost of classification and (4) robustness. Feature descriptors and metrics widely depend on the specific application.
4. **Classification:** Classification is the last stage in CAD systems that differentiates and labels of the abnormality. Classification methods play an important role in the diagnosis and educational purposes in medicine. Generally, in the implementation of classifier in clinical image processing, supervised classification or unsupervised classification techniques are used.
5. **Performance Evaluation:** Evaluating the true performance of the classifier is the last stage in CAD system. True positive (Jinsamol et al., 2015) value indicates the number of correctly predicted abnormality and true negative (TN) value shows the number of correctly predicted as a normal instance. The number of incorrect prediction of abnormality is shown by false negative (FN) and the number of incorrect prediction of normal objects is presented with false positive (FP) value. The main evaluation metrics that are used to assess performance of CAD systems include true positive fraction, false positive fraction, sensitivity, specificity, accuracy, receiver operating characteristics (Doi, 2014; James et al., 2001), and area under receiver operating characteristics (AUROC) (Gonçalves et al., 2014).

RELATED SURVEY

Researchers contributed for the breast cancer lesions masses, micro-calcification, architectural distortion and combination of the lesions detection at the larger extent.

Masses

Computer-aided detection of masses (Chan, 2007) approaches are evaluated in this study. In the first approach, mass candidate identification and feature analysis are performed in the reconstructed three-dimensional (3D) DBT volume. In the second approach, pre-screening of mass candidate and feature analysis are first performed on the individual two-dimensional (2D) projection view (PV) images. In the third approach, the mass likelihood scores estimated by the 3D and 2D approaches, described above, at the corresponding 3D location are combined and evaluated using FROC analysis. The average FP rates achieved by combining the 3D and 2D information were 1.23 and 2.04 per breast with 80% and 90% sensitivities. The combined system is a promising approach to improving automated mass detection on DBTs (Chan, 2007). ROC curves for classification of breast masses are shown in Figure 11.

A novel mass detection approach (Kim, 2014) using slice conspicuity in the 3D reconstructed digital breast volumes used to overcome the limited resolution towards depth direction. Experimental results demonstrate that the proposed approach outperforms the conventional 3D approach by achieving a high sensitivity with a small number of false positives (Kim, 2014).

A computer-aided detection (CAD) system (Samala, 2016) is developed to identify masses in digital breast tomosynthesis (DBT) volume by using a deep convolutional neural network (DCNN) from mammograms. The difference between the performances for the two systems was statistically significant ($p\text{-value} < 0.05$) (Samala, 2016).

An improved mass detection is proposed with combined feature representations from projection views with reconstructed volume in the DBT. Experimental results demonstrate that the proposed mass detection can achieve high sensitivity with a small number of false positives. In addition, the experimental results demonstrate

Figure 11. ROC curves for classification of breast masses

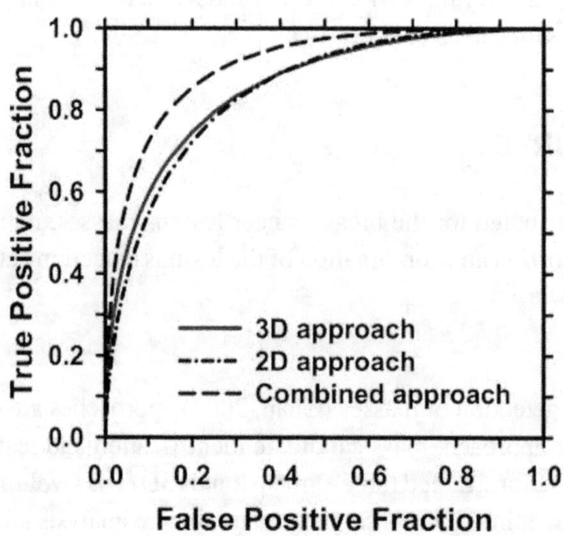

that the selected feature representations for classifying masses complementarily come from both projection views and reconstructed volume.

Micro Calcifications

A computer-aided detection (CAD) algorithm (Jeong, 2016) is proposed a for micro calcification (MC) clusters using reconstructed digital breast tomosynthesis (DBT) images. The algorithm consists of pre-screening, MC detection, clustering, and false-positive (FP) reduction steps. In this paper, a simple and efficient FP reduction scheme coupled with a detection algorithm for MCCs in a reconstructed DBT volume using 3D objectness and SNR enhanced images is suggested. A datasets of two view DBTs of 69 breasts with or without MCCs are viewed and sensitivity of 83.3% was achieved at 2.47 FPs per DBT volume (Jeong, 2016)

A CADe system was designed to detect micro calcification clusters in the reconstructed volume. The system consisted of pre-screening, clustering, and false-positive reduction stages. In the pre-screening stage, the conspicuity of micro calcification-like objects was increased by an enhancement-modulated 3D calcification response function (Sahiner, 2012).

Architectural Distortion

The Contourlet Transform based method (Anand, 2013) is used to detect the location of the architectural distortion in mammograms. The dominant angle is detected in this Contourlet decomposition which comprises of Laplacian Pyramidal Filter bank and Steerable Gaussian Filter. The textural features will not show any deviation in the distorted area. Here the methods proposed will assist the Radiologist to identify the unidentified potential sites of distortion. Therefore the main aim of this work becomes the reduction of the region of interests. In this project 39 cases were testes in which 19 are Architectural Distorted image from the MIAS database and 17 Normal images. The proposed algorithm detected 1502 regions of interest (ROIs) with 247 True Positives and 1255 False Positives. In this paper 26 textural features were considered and result is obtained as 0.77 with an artificial neural network.

Masses and Microcalcification

A DBT CAD system can detects large percentage 89% of breast cancers by detecting masses and micro calcification clusters, with an acceptable false-positive rate of 2.7%. Further studies with larger datasets acquired with equipment from multiple vendors are needed to replicate the findings and to study the interaction of radiologists and

CAD systems. Women Breast images captures through Digital Breast Tomosynthesis are shown in Figure 12.

Masses and Architectural Distortion

Towards this aim, this paper focuses on the detection of masses and architectural distortions in DBT images. A complete detection scheme is proposed, consisting of two parts, called channels, each dedicated to one type of lesions, which are then merged in a final decision step, thus handling correctly the potential overlap between the two types of lesions. The first detection channel exploits the dense kernel nature of masses and the intrinsic imprecision of their attributes in a fuzzy approach. The experimental results on 101 breasts, including 53 lesions, demonstrate the usefulness of the proposed approach, which leads to a high sensitivity with a reduced number of false positives, and compares favourably to existing (Palma, 2014) . The procedure for detection of Masses and Architectural Distortion are shown in Figure 13.

Masses, Micro Calcification, Architectural Distortion, and Bilateral Asymmetry

The proposed method (Shanthi, 2014) is based on multiscale surrounding region dependence method, Gabor filters, multi fractal analysis, directional and morphological analysis. The extracted features are input to self-adaptive resource allocation network (SRAN) classifier for classification. The approach is extensively demonstrated using the two benchmark data sets Mammographic Image Analysis Society (MIAS) and Digital Database for Screening Mammography (DDSM) and the results have been proved to be progressive. The region of Interest identified in different signs of breast abnormalities are shown in Figure 14.

Figure 12. Digital Breast Tomosynthesis images

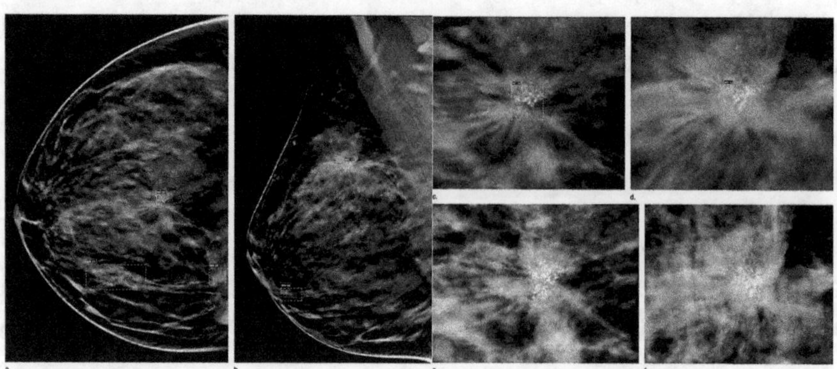

Figure 13. Detection of masses and architectural distortion

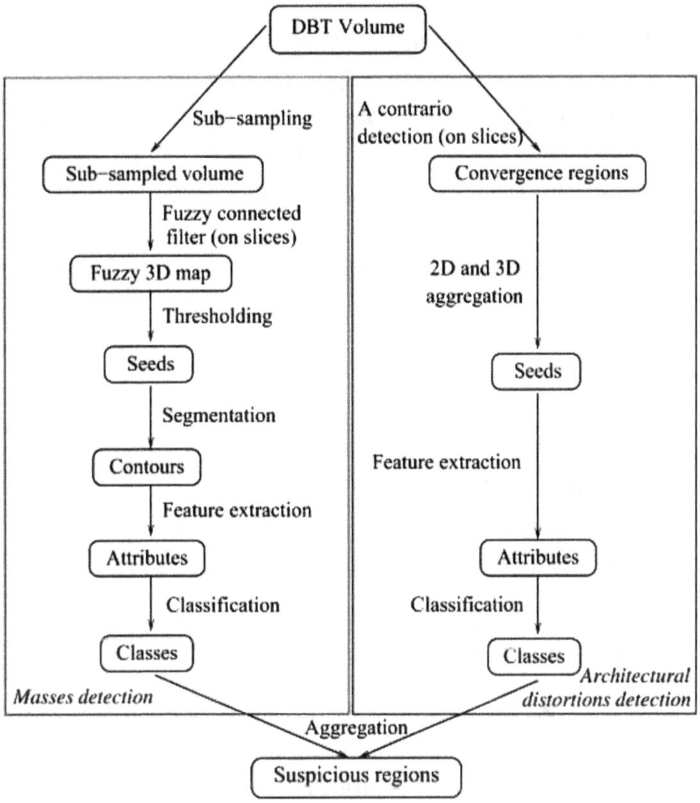

Figure 14. ROI of different signs of abnormalities: (a) Microcalcification, (b) Masses and (c) Architectural distortion

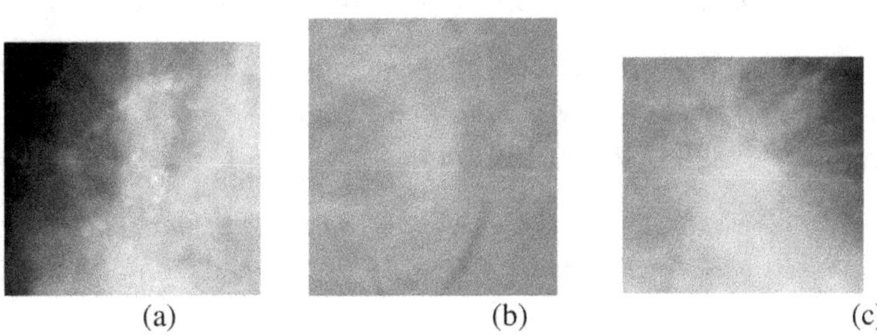

CONCLUSION

Breast cancer disease is the common malignancy of women and cause many deaths. The early detection is the best solution in order to avoid mastectomy, reduce the probability to return, and decrease the rate of mortality. CAD system has intended to support the doctor and other technicians in detecting of mammary lesions, a second opinion. Though diagnosis is done through digital breast tomosynthesis, but still there is a problem in the improvement of the accuracy using diagnosis system. It reduces the additional evaluation and improvement in screening parameters in all fatty breasts.

REFERENCES

Anand, S., & Rathna, R. A. V. (2013). Architectural Distortion Detection in Mammogram using Contourlet Transform and Texture Features. *International Journal of Computers and Applications*, *74*(5).

Bozek, J., & Dumic, E. (2009). Bilateral asymmetry detection in digital mammography using B-spline interpolation. In Systems, Signals and Image (pp. 1-4). IEEE.

Chan, H. P., Wei, J., Zhang, Y., Helvie, M. A., Moore, R. H., Sahiner, B., & Kopans, D. B. (2008). Computer-aided detection of masses in digital tomosynthesis mammography: Comparison of three approaches. *Medical Physics*, *35*(9), 4087–4095. doi:10.1118/1.2968098 PMID:18841861

Doi, K. (2009). *Computer-aided diagnosis in medical imaging: achievements and challenges*. Paper presented at the World Congress on Medical Physics and Biomedical Engineering, Munich, Germany. 10.1007/978-3-642-03904-1_26

Doi, K. (2014). Current status and future potential of computer-aided diagnosis in medical imaging. *The British Journal of Radiology*, *78*(suppl_1), S3–S19. doi:10.1259/bjr/82933343 PMID:15917443

Dos Santos Teixeira, R. F. (2012). *Computer analysis of mammography images to aid diagnosis*. MSc in Biomedical Engineering, Faculdade de Engenharia da Universidade do Porto, 35.

Gonçalves, V. M., Delamaro, M. E., & Nuns, F. L. S. (2014). A systematic review on the evaluation and characteristics of computer-aided diagnosis systems. *Revista Brasileira de Engenharia Biomédica*, *30*(4), 355–383. doi:10.1590/1517-3151.0517

Heywang, S. H., Wolf, A., Pruss, E., Hilbertz, T., Eiermann, W., & Permanetter, W. (1989). MR imaging of the breast with Gd-DTPA: Use and limitations. *Radiology, 171*(1), 95–103. doi:10.1148/radiology.171.1.2648479 PMID:2648479

James, D., Clymer, B. D., & Schmalbrock, P. (2001). Texture detection of simulated microcalcification susceptibility effects in magnetic resonance imaging of breasts. *Journal of Magnetic Resonance Imaging, 13*(6), 876–881. doi:10.1002/jmri.1125 PMID:11382947

Jatoi, I., & Kaufmann, M. (2010). Management of breast diseases. Springer. doi:10.1007/978-3-540-69743-5

Jeong, J. W., Chae, S. H., Chae, E. Y., Kim, H. H., Choi, Y. W., & Lee, S. (2016). Three-Dimensional Computer-Aided Detection of Microcalcification Clusters in Digital Breast Tomosynthesis. *BioMed Research International, 2016*, 1–8. doi:10.1155/2016/8651573 PMID:27274993

Jinsamol, K., Shiji, T., & Thomas, V. (2015). CAD system for breast ultrasound images using multi-scale blob detection and active contour segmentation algorithm. *International Conference on Information Science (ICIS' 14).*

Kim, D. H., Kim, S. T., & Ro, Y. M. (2015). Improving mass detection using combined feature representations from projection views and reconstructed volume of DBT and boosting based classification with feature selection. *Physics in Medicine and Biology, 60*(22), 8809–8832. doi:10.1088/0031-9155/60/22/8809 PMID:26529080

Kim, S. T., Kim, D. H., & Ro, Y. M. (2014). Breast mass detection using slice conspicuity in 3D reconstructed digital breast volumes. *Physics in Medicine and Biology, 59*(17), 5003–5023. doi:10.1088/0031-9155/59/17/5003 PMID:25119017

Kuhl, C. K. (2007). Current status of breast MR imaging, Pt. 2:Clinical applications. *Radiology, 244*, 672–691. doi:10.1148/radiol.2443051661 PMID:17709824

Malvia, S., Bagadi, S. A., Dubey, U. S., & Saxena, S. (2017). Epidemiology of breast cancer in Indian women. *Asia Pacific Journal of Clinical Oncology, 13*(4), 289–295. doi:10.1111/ajco.12661 PMID:28181405

Meeuwis, C., van de Ven, S. M., Stapper, G., Fernandez Gallardo, A. M., van den Bosch, M. A. A. J., Mali, W. P. T. M., & Veldhuis, W. B. (2010). Computer-aided detection (CAD) for breast MRI:evaluation of efficacy at 3.0 T. *European Radiology, 20*(3), 522–528. doi:10.100700330-009-1573-5 PMID:19727750

Nie, K. (2009). *Development of breast MRI computer-aided diagnosis system* (Thesis). Irvine, CA: University of California.

Palma, G., Bloch, I., & Muller, S. (2014). Detection of masses and architectural distortions in digital breast tomosynthesis images using fuzzy and a contrario approaches. *Pattern Recognition*, *47*(7), 2467–2480. doi:10.1016/j.patcog.2014.01.009

Sahiner, B., Chan, H. P., Hadjiiski, L. M., Helvie, M. A., Wei, J., Zhou, C., & Lu, Y. (2012). Computer-aided detection of clustered microcalcifications in digital breast tomosynthesis: A 3D approach. *Medical Physics*, *39*(1), 28–39. doi:10.1118/1.3662072 PMID:22225272

Saki, F., & Tahmasbi, A. (2010). *A novel opposition-based classifier for mass diagnosis in mammography images*. ICBME.

Samala, R. K., Chan, H. P., Hadjiiski, L., Helvie, M. A., Wei, J., & Cha, K. (2016). Mass detection in digital breast tomosynthesis: Deep convolutional neural network with transfer learning from mammography. *Medical Physics*, *43*(12), 6654–6666. doi:10.1118/1.4967345 PMID:27908154

Shanthi, S., & Muralibhaskaran, V. (2014). Automatic Detection and Classification of Microcalcification, Mass, Architectural Distortion and Bilateral Asymmetry in Digital Mammogram. *World Academy of Science, Engineering and Technology, International Journal of Medical, Health, Biomedical, Bioengineering and Pharmaceutical Engineering*, *8*(11), 822–827.

Siegel, R. L., Miller, K. D., & Jemal, A. (2015). Cancer statistics, 2015. *CA: A Cancer Journal for Clinicians*, *65*(1), 5–29. doi:10.3322/caac.21254 PMID:25559415

Svensson, W. (1997). A review of the current status of breast ultrasound. *European Journal of Ultrasound*, *6*(2), 77–101. doi:10.1016/S0929-8266(97)10009-X

Wang, L. C., DeMartini, W. B., Partridge, S. C., Peacock, S., & Lehman, C. D. (2009). MRI-detected suspicious breast lesions: Predictive values of kinetic features measured by computer-aided evaluation. *AJR. American Journal of Roentgenology*, *193*(3), 826–831. doi:10.2214/AJR.08.1335 PMID:19696298

Zhao, H., Xu, W., Li, L., & Zhang, J. (2011). Classification of Breast Masses Based on Multi-View Information Fusion Using Multi-Agent Method. In *2011 5th International Conference on Bioinformatics and Biomedical Engineering* (pp. 1-4). IEEE.

Section 6

Medical Image Registration and Retrieval for Improved Clinical Diagnosis

Chapter 11
A Comparative Study of Medical Image Retrieval Using Distance, Transform, Texture, and Shape

A. Swarnambiga
Indian Institute of Technology Madras, India

Vasuki S.
Vellammal College of Engineering and Technology, India

ABSTRACT

Content-based medical image retrieval (CBMIR) is the application of computer vision techniques to the problem of medical image search in large databases. Three main techniques are applied to check the applicability. The first technique implemented is distance metrics-based retrieval. The second technique implemented is transform-based retrieval. The transform which has lesser performance is combined with higher performance, to check the applicability of the results. The third technique implemented is content-based medical image retrieval. Texture and shape-based retrieval techniques are also applied. Shape-based retrieval is processed using canny edge with the Otsu method. The multifeature-based technique is also applied and analyzed. The best retrieval rate is achieved by multifeature-based retrieval with 100/50%. Based on more relevant retrieved images all the three, brain, liver, and knee, images are found to be retrieved more with 100/50%.

DOI: 10.4018/978-1-5225-5876-7.ch011

INTRODUCTION

The various techniques of retrieval such as Distance metrics based retrieval, Transform based retrieval and Content based retrieval are introduced and applied in this article. It is often difficult to assess their performance since it usually depends on the chosen test images. But this has been handled well and justified by the retrieved results with the Observers' classification. CAD systems are distinguished into two main types and the research is especially focused on computer aided diagnosis (Gletsos, 2003). CAD (Computer Aided Diagnosis) provides automated interpretation of imaging examinations as a second opinion to radiologists (Depeursinge, 2011) .

RELATED WORK

Although image retrieval have been frequently proposed for use in medical image management, only a few systems have been developed specifically for medical images Manjunath (1996); Shyu (1999); Smelders (2000); Shao Hong (2005); Dimitrovski (2015) and Van kitanovski (2017). Techniques applied for huge image based databases for exact clinical diagnosis with medical justification in this research is provided. A brief survey is given in Table 1.

MATERIALS AND METHODS

Computer-aided diagnosis helps in supporting clinical decision making (Shao Hong 2005). One clinical decision-making technique is case-based reasoning, which searches for previous, already-solved problems similar to the current one and tries to apply those solutions to the current problem (Ceyhun Burak, 2011; Worring & Smeulders, 2000).

For the satisfaction with the search results, have provided Observers' classification to the retrieval system, which contains a mechanism to learn the radiologists and physician information needs. The schema of the medical image retrieval system is shown in Figure 1.

An overview of the retrieval framework implemented with the identification of state-of-the art modules and methods for input data, feature extraction and query image processing is discussed in the Figure 2. Three approaches are implemented and followed for medical image retrieval. The first approach includes distance based medical image retrieval. The second approach includes transform based retrieval. The third approach is implemented using CBMIR. At the end of the chapter, presented best methods used to retrieve medical images. An analysis of the most

Table 1. Brief summary of the image feature descriptors used in medical domain

S. No.	Year	Author	Title of the Paper	Comments
1	1999	Comaniciu D	Image guided decision support system for pathology	(a) Representation by color. (b)Using histogram.
2	2003	Gletsos M	A computer aided diagnostic system to characterize CT focal liver lesions: design and optimization of a neural network classifier	(a) Representation by gray scale. (b) Moments based.
3	1999	Shyu C R	ASSERT: A physician in the loop content based image retrieval system for HRCT image databases.	(a) Representation by gray scale (b) Texture Co-occurrence
4	2002	Kwak D.M	Content-based ultrasound image retrieval using a coarse to fine approach	(a) Representation by gray scale (b) Wavelet based
5	2005	Cauvin JM	Computer-assisted diagnosis system in digestive endoscopy	(a) Anatomic location, shape and color are the descriptors used (b) Block based
6	2007	Rahman M	A framework for medical image retrieval using machine learning and statistical similarity matching techniques with relevance feedback.	(a) Using edge histograms (b)By contours/curves
7	2000	Wang J Z	Pathfinder: multiresolution region –based searching for pathology images using IRM.	(a) By region and parts (b) By wavelet based region descriptors
8	2005	Pokrajac D	Applying spatial distribution analysis techniques to classification of 3-D medical images.	(a) By region and parts (b)Spatial distribution of ROI.
9	2007	Toews M	A statistical parts-based model of anatomical variability.	(a) By region and parts (b) By statistical anatomical parts model
10	2005	Qian X N	Optimal embedding for shape indexing in medical image databases.	(a) By point sets (b) By shape spaces

representative techniques for specific medical imaging is yet to be effective (Rui & Huang, 1999; Liu, 2001). This role cannot be denied at this stage corresponding to exploratory research for clinical diagnosis, extending for medical image registration based retrieval.

A short summary of the database system is discussed here. The database is created with 10 sets of databases. Each database set includes Brain images, Chest, Liver, Knee and Spine images comprising of 100 images with each 5 sets with a total of 500 images. This medical image system design is constructed by considering the two layer system, the database with front end and back end relies on design concept. Back end system embodies higher end programs than that of the front end system. The front end design is correlative text and image information, which

Figure 1. Conceptual framework for content based medical image retrieval system

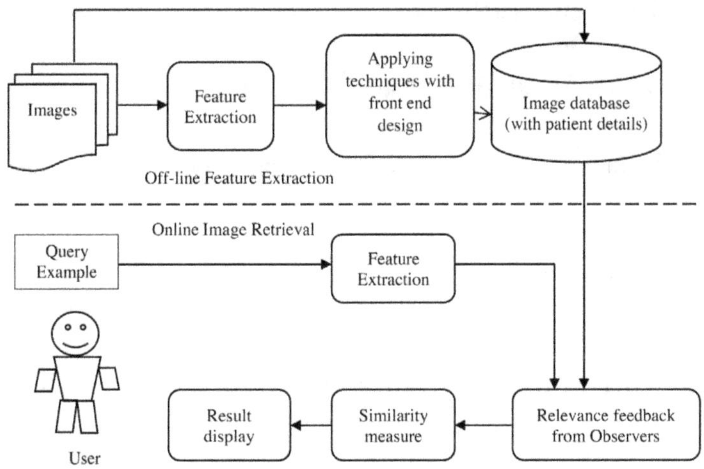

Figure 2. Schema of retrieval system

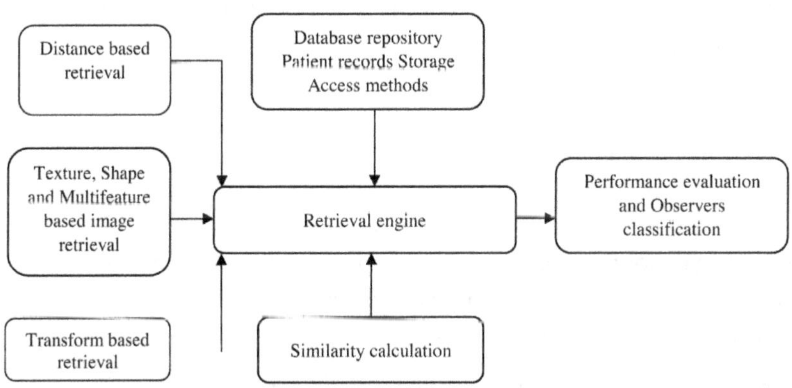

connects with the back end design in registration, retrieval and registration based retrieval for improving retrieval precision and recall. The back end design includes the techniques used for feature extraction and retrieval Schema for effective retrieval. The system is the most simple and the basis, but it is indispensable, and can obtain image file directly, including: (1) Medical treatment device, for example, MR and CT; (2) Organ examined or images examined; (3) Patient Primary details. This design increases the retrieval scope and picks up retrieval speed. This layer offers assistant description information. The images used to form the database are Brain, Chest, Liver, Knee and Spine images and their specific criteria considered for justifying the results are given below. Throughout this experiment for retrieval the same set of database is used. The web reference database and personally collected images are used as images in the database.

Distance Based Medical Image Retrieval

1. The Euclidean distance measure (d_E) is defined in Equation (1)

$$d_E\left(X,Y\right) = \sqrt{\sum_{i=1}^{n}(x_i - y_i)^2} \quad (1)$$

x_i and y_i are the database image and Query image. The minimum distance value signifies an exact match with the query.

2. The Manhattan measure (d_M) computes the similarity scores between two images and they are widely used in similarity calculation for medical images. Here x_i and y_i are the images of the database image and query image and is defined in Equation (2).

$$d_M\left(X,Y\right) = \sum_{i=1}^{n}\left|x_i - y_i\right| \quad (2)$$

3. The Mahalanobis distance metric is appropriate when each dimension of the image feature vector is dependent of each other and has different importance in medical imaging. Here F_i and F_j are the images of the database image and query image and is defined in Equation (3) and (4).

$$D\left(i,j\right) = \sqrt{\left(F_i - F_j\right)^T c^{-1}\left(F_i - F_j\right)} \quad (3)$$

where C is the covariance matrix of the feature vector. In this case, only the variance of each feature component c_i is used. Mahalanobis metric is represented as $D\left(i,j\right)$.

$$D\left(i,j\right) = \sum_{i=1}^{N}\frac{\left(F_i - F_j^2\right)}{c_i} \quad (4)$$

4. The numerator signifies the difference and the denominator normalizes the difference in Canberra distance metric (δ_C). It assigns a greater weighting to large relative differences between corresponding components. Here x_{r_i} and x_{s_i} are the images of the database image and query image and is defined in Equation (5).

$$\delta_C = \sum_{i=1}^{n} \frac{\left|x_{ri} - x_{si}\right|}{\left|x_{ri}\right| + \left|x_{si}\right|} \tag{5}$$

5. The Bray-Curtis measure (δ_{BS}) usage on medical images found to be lesser. The numerator signifies the difference and the denominator normalizes the difference. It also assigns a greater weighting to large relative differences between corresponding components. Here x_{r_i} and x_{s_i} are the images of the database image and query image and is defined in Equation (6).

$$\delta_{BS} = \frac{\sum_{1=1}^{n} \left|x_{ri} - x_{si}\right|}{\sum_{i=1}^{n} x_{ri} + x_{si}} \tag{6}$$

6. The Squared Chord distance measure $\left(d_{sc}\right)$ is highly useful for image database applications. Distance values never exceed one and it is equal to one if any one of the attributes is zero. Here x_i and y_i are the images of the database image and query image and is defined in Equation (7).

$$d_{sc}\left(X,Y\right) = \sum_{i=1}^{n} \sqrt[2]{x_i} - \sqrt{y_i} \tag{7}$$

7. Within the distance metrics the Chi-Squared distance (d_{ch}) have been used with thelesser implementation in medical image retrieval. Here x_i and y_i are the images of the database image and query image and is defined in Equation (8).

$$d_{ch}\left(X,Y\right) = \sum_{i=1}^{n} \frac{\left(x_i - y_i\right)^2}{x_i + y_i} \tag{8}$$

Transform Based Medical Image Retrieval

Due to limitation in space, I have not discussed in detail the transform based derivations, In this experimentation have used DFT, DCT, DWT, CWT, RCWF and Curvelet transforms. They are used as fundamental level without any change in their parameters.

Texture Feature Extraction Using GLCM

The third technique implemented is content based medical image retrieval. GLCM, LBP and GLCM with LBP are used for texture based retrieval. GLCM creates a matrix with the direction and distances between pixels, and then extracts meaningful statistics from the matrix as texture features. GLCM texture features commonly used are shown in the following: GLCM is composed of the probability value, it is defined by $P(i,j \mid d,\theta)$ which expresses the probability of the couple pixels at θ direction and d interval. When θ and d is determined, $P(i,j \mid d,\theta)$ showed by $P_{i,j}$. Distinctly GLCM is a symmetry matrix; its level is determined by the image gray-level. Elements in the matrix are computed by the Equation (9).

$$P\left(i,j \mid d,\theta\right) = \frac{P(i,j \mid d,\theta)}{\sum_i \sum_j P(i,j \mid d,\theta)} \tag{9}$$

GLCM expresses the texture feature according the correlation of the couple pixels gray-level at different positions. It describes the texture feature in quantified manner. Energy is a grayscale image texture measure of homogeneity changing, reflecting the distribution of image grayscale uniformity of weight and texture and is given in Equation (10). P(x,y) is the gray level value at coordinate (x,y).

$$\text{Energy } E = \sum_x \sum_y p\left(x,y\right)^2 \tag{10}$$

LBP Based Feature Extraction

Two-dimensional surface textures can be described by two complementary measures. They are gray scale contrast and local spatial patterns. The LBP value for the center pixel $\left(a,b\right)$ of the image $f\left(a,b\right)$ is calculated using the Equation (11),

$$LBP\left(a,b\right)=\sum_{i=0}^{n}U\left(f\left(a,b\right)-f\left(a_i,b_i\right)\right)2^i \tag{11}$$

where $U\left(x\right)$ is the thresholding function which is defined in the Equation (12).

$$U\left(x\right)=\begin{cases}1\,if\;x\geq 0\\ 0\,if\;x<0\end{cases}\left(\right)$$

Shape Based Retrieval

Shape based retrieval is processed using canny edge with the Otsu method. The features extracted from each technique are combined and used in the retrieval process. The Canny edge detection algorithm is given in steps (1) –(3) as follows:

1. Compute the gradient of the resultant smooth image. Store the edge magnitude and edge orientation separately in two arrays, $M\left(x,y\right)$ and $\alpha\left(x,y\right)$, respectively.
2. Examining every edge point orientation is a computationally intensive task.
3. Apply hysteresis thresholding. In hysteresis thresholding only a large amount of change in the gradient magnitude matters in edge detection and small changes does not affect the quality of edge detection. Now this is combined with Otsu method.

The Otsu method has the important property that is based entirely on computations performed on the histogram of an image. It selects a global threshold value by maximizing the separability of clusters in gray levels.

Multi Feature Extraction

Texture and shape are the most important visual features and have already described them separately. In texture feature extraction techniques, have introduced two different extraction methods they are gray GLCM and LBP. For shape feature extraction techniques, have introduced Canny edge with the Otsu method.

The image has varied dramatic ups and downs in gray-level, showing a very strong texture characteristic. Using only the simple features of image information alone cannot get comprehensive description of image content. The features are extracted from the query image and database image and are effectively computed using texture based retrieval techniques and shape based retrieval techniques, leading to multifeature extraction. Those features are normalized and then the features of query image and the database image are effectively calculated using Euclidean similarity measure.

EXPERIMENTATION AND PERFORMANCE MEASURES

The performance of the medical image retrieval system techniques is analyzed by the following measures.

1. The level of retrieval accuracy which is achieved by a system is important to establish its performance illustrated by (Muller et al., 2004). In CBMIR, precision-recall is the most widely used measurement methods to evaluate the retrieval accuracy. Precision P is defined as the ratio of the number of retrieved relevant images r to the total number of retrieved images n . Precision measures the accuracy of the retrieval and it is given in below Equation (13).

$$P = \frac{Number\ of\ relevant\ images\ retrieved}{Total\ number\ of\ images\ retrieved} = \frac{r}{n} \tag{13}$$

The recall is defined by (Muller et al. 2004) and is denoted as R). Recall measures the robustness of the retrieval and is given in Equation (14).

$$R = \frac{Number\ of\ relevant\ images\ retrieved}{Total\ number\ of\ relevant\ images\ in\ Database} = \frac{r}{m} \tag{14}$$

Generally, the precision value falls with increases in the recall values. A retrieval system can be called 'ideal' if both the precision and recall values remain high. However, in reality, no such image retrieval systems have yet been found. Precision-recall pair is a good standard of performance evaluation.

2. The error rate is also reintroduced by (Muller et al., 2000) which is common in medical image processing. It is in fact a single precision value, so it is important to know where the value is measured and is given in Equation (15)

$$Error\ rate = \frac{Number\ of\ irrelevant\ images\ retrieved}{Total\ number\ of\ images\ retrieved} \tag{15}$$

3. The retrieval efficiency is defined in Equation (4) by (Muller et al., 2004). If the number of images retrieved is lower than or equal to the number of relevant images, this value is the precision; otherwise it is the recall of a query. This definition can be misleading since it mixes two standard measures.

$$Retrieval\,efficiencey = \begin{cases} \dfrac{Number\,of\,relevant\,images\,retrieved}{Total\,number\,of\,images\,retrieved} & if\ No.retrieved > No.relevant \\ \dfrac{Number\,of\,relevant\,images\,retrieved}{Total\,number\,of\,relevant\,images} & Otherwise \end{cases} \tag{16}$$

4. The average precision AP for a single query q is the mean over the precision scores after each retrieved relevant item and is defined in Equation (17) and (18). N_R is the total number of relevant images for the query. APR is the average of all precision values. ARR is the average of all recall values from the experimentation.

$$APR(q) = \frac{1}{N_R}\sum_{n=1}^{N_R}(P_q) \tag{17}$$

$$ARR(q) = \frac{1}{N_R}\sum_{n=1}^{N_R}(R_n), \tag{18}$$

5. The classification error rate CER is defined by Desealers (2003). To classify a query image correctly, the first retrieved image should be relevant. Otherwise the query is misclassified and it is defined in Equation (19).

$$CER = \frac{1}{|Q|}\sum_{q\in Q}\begin{cases} 0 & if\ the\ most\ similar\ image\ is\ {}^{relevant}/_{from}\ the\ correct\ modality \\ 1 & Otherwise \end{cases} \tag{19}$$

6. Muller et al. (2000) has classified the retrieved images based on the factor "relevant" and "irrelevant". Relevance judgment with Observers' classification is a vital part of performance evaluation. For example, suppose the retrieved image exactly belongs to the query image then score is 1. If the retrieved image does not fall any of the above criteria and exactly different then the score is 0.

This is also known as Observers' classification. The same set of Observers' are used, which is similarly followed in registration.

The visual similarity is defined as similarity found in a query and from all the retrieved images and is shown in Table 2 and 3. If maximally both are similar then it is (1-best or higher similarity), if maximally they are found to be dissimilar then it is (0-worst or lesser similarity) (Muller, 2000, 2004).

The relevant images are defined as, the retrieved first image is relevant to query image then it is 1 if it differs then it is 0. The similarity difference is defined as if the query image is of one modality and the retrieved image is extremely of another modality then it is found to be dissimilar and given as zero and if they are extremely similar modality then it is given as 1. If there are minimal number of irrelevant images to the query image and then the criteria is 1, if they extremely counts more from the query image then it is 0. Lesser redundant image can be checked with the images whether it is repeated or also checked with file name in the case reports for finding more relevant images without any repetition. If it is so then it is given as 1 and if the repetition of relevant image is found then it is 0. Now the overall criteria ranging is done. If the maximal number of 1 then the score are 5. If the minimal number of 1 found from the average then the classification from the criteria is 0. If there is extremely lesser number of 1 then the classification from the criteria is 0. Average of Observers' parameters scores ranges between (0-5) for Brain, Liver and for Knee from Observers' criteria classification.

7. Muller et al. (2004) defined, as many of the presented systems uses classifications of images, accuracy is very often used to evaluate the system. This is defined in Equation (20).

$$Accuracy = \frac{Number\ of\ images\ classified\ correctly}{Total\ number\ of\ images\ classified} \tag{20}$$

Table 2. Criteria for measurement of performance evaluation using Observers' classification for CBMIR

Score	Criteria
1.0	The retrieved image belongs to the class of the query image.
0	The retrieved image does not belong to any related images.

Table 3. Result image rating: Observers' scores for individual images from distance metrics

Observer Parameters	Brain	Liver	Knee
Visual similarity	(0/1)	(0/1)	(0/1)
Relevant images	(0/1)	(0/1)	(0/1)
Similarity difference	(0/1)	(0/1)	(0/1)
Minimal irrelevant images	(0/1)	(0/1)	(0/1)
Lesser redundant image	(0/1)	(0/1)	(0/1)
Average score for each type of image	(0-5)	(0-5)	(0-5)

Figure 3. Retrieved images related to Liver image using distance metrics

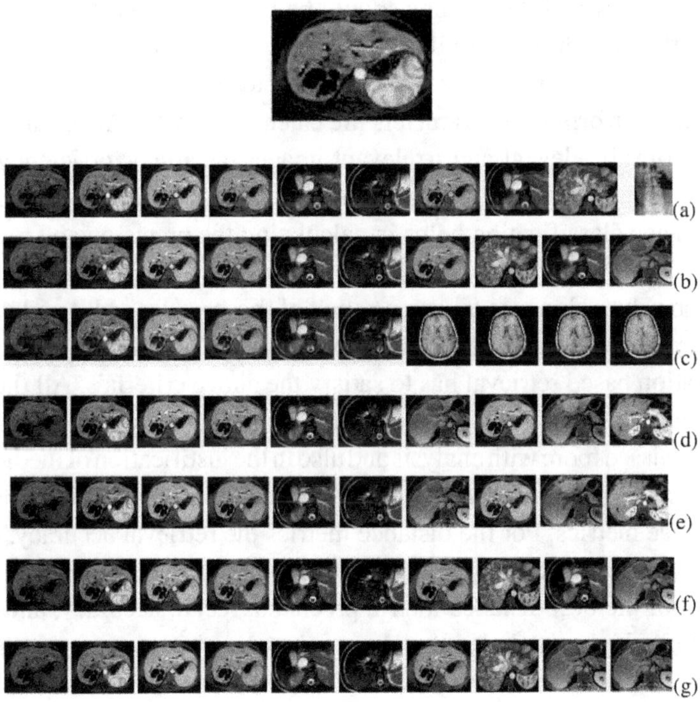

Accurate medical image retrieval plays an important role in clinical diagnosis because an error in this process will be propagated further. Visual evaluation of retrieval results is very often used for the assessment of the retrieval process. Unfortunately different people can evaluate differently. Sometimes, the retrieval is indirectly evaluated and it relies upon the results of further processing. (P/R) denotes Precision/Recall values, (R/IR) denotes retrieved Relevant and Irrelevant images, T denotes Time taken for retrieval and is denoted in seconds, A denotes Accuracy and E denotes Efficiency values and they are denoted in percentage, ER denotes Error Rate and CER denoted Classification by Error Rate. APR denotes the Average Precision Rate and ARR denote the Average Retrieval Rate and is represented in percentage.

The precision and recall values should be higher and they are depicted in percentage. The half the precision values is the recall value logically. The relevant image and irrelevant image are noticed separately for effective evaluation. The relevant image should be more than the irrelevant image. For a single retrieval the number of retrieval system window size is 10 for distance metrics, texture based, shape and multifeature based retrieval and 12 for transform. Efficiency

In the classification of error rate, 0 means perfect retrieval if 1 means it is not an effective retrieval. The next criterion is time taken for retrieval and it should be lesser. The APR and ARR value should be higher for best retrieval of images. APR and ARR on column wise denotes the values for images. APR and ARR on row wise denotes the values for various retrieval techniques from retrieved images. The following performance parameters are calculated. APR, ARR values, the time taken for retrieval, relevant and irrelevant images, accuracy, efficiency error rate and classification by the error rate are experimented and analyzed. The relevant and irrelevant image classification helps in calculating the precision and recall values. The value of accuracy and efficiency are found equal to the precision value. Hence the precision values alone are taken on behalf of those values. APR and ARR values are considered in the overall performance calculation. The best technique in retrieval and registration based retrieval has to satisfy the above criteria's. All these criteria are measured from the experimentation. The precision and recall values are the main criteria's discussed more with analysis and also in the justification of medical images. Other criteria's are taken as reference. Time taken for retrieval is found to be same for all distance metrics. For the distance metrics the retrieval accuracy, efficiency, error rate and classification by error rate also found to be more similar with lesser variations. For the best distance metric precision, recall, accuracy, and efficiency are found to be higher and also they have a lesser error rate and classification by error rate. It is observed that the precision and recall values of Brain images for all distance metrics found to be similar and higher. Hence all metrics perform well in the retrieval of Brain images. The best performance in relevant image retrieval for Liver images is given by Canberra and Bray-Curtis metrics and is shown in Figure 3.

However, better performance is given by Euclidean, Manhattan, Squared Chord and Chi-Squared metrics respectively. The poor performance is given by Mahalanobis metric. For Knee images the precision and recall values for all distance metrics found to be same with lesser variations and hence all the distance metrics performs well for them. But the poor performance is given by Mahalanobis metric. Table 4 shows the performance evaluation of the retrieved Brain, Liver and Knee images using distance metrics.

Table 5 shows the overall precision and recall calculation from the performance evaluation using distance metrics for Brain, Liver and Knee images. All the distance metrics are applied, experimented and analyzed for all images. This overall evaluation criterion falls into two categories. The first category is evaluating, analyzing the overall precision and recall calculation for all distance metrics and the second category is evaluating, analyzing the overall precision and recall calculation for all the images. The overall best performance is given by the Manhattan, Canberra, Bray-Curtis, Squared Chord and Chi-Squared distance metrics with (100/50)% based on (APR/ARR). The next best performance is given by Euclidean and Mahalanobis metric. Based on retrieval of more relevant images Brain and Knee are retrieved more than Liver images. The justification of the results in medical terms is given below.

When the metrics applied to the medical images, they calculate the difference between the pixel intensity rather than feature extraction. The metric like Manhattan calculate the normalized pixel difference, Canberra metric calculates the normalized intensity difference, Euclidean calculates their squared intensity difference, Squared Chord and Chi-Squared calculate the squared intensity of database images and query images. This directly gives the pixel difference. But, for Manhalanobis, image feature vector is dependent of each other and has different importance in medical imaging. Hence the overall best performance is given by the Manhattan, Canberra, Bray-Curtis, Squared Chord and Chi-Squared distance metrics.

Now it is important to justify the retrieved results based on the images. The orientations of the Brain have more tissue matters and cranial properties. The intensity distribution is also evenly distributed for both Brain and Knee images. No other organs or structures are found whose intensity might vary. These are the reasons for the best obtained results for Brain and Knee images respectively. Since the Liver images have more internally distributed structures and their pixel distribution varies drastically for each and every slice. Hence the Brain and Knee images are found to have more relevant images retrieved with (94/47) % of (APR/ARR). Only the next most relevant retrieved images are found for Liver images. The rating is given by observers from the experimentation results. They have given higher sore (5) for Knee images confirming our results from the evaluation measures. Table 6 shows the Observers' classification from retrieved images applied to all images. Average of Observer parameters score ranges between (0-5) is 4 for Brain and Liver and 5 for Knee from observers' criteria classification, Knee images found to be retrieved more in Distance based retrieval than Brain and Liver images.

Table 7 shows the performance evaluation of the retrieved Brain, Liver and Knee images using transform techniques. The time taken for retrieval is found to be more similar with lesser variations in seconds for all transform based techniques. The best

Table 4. Performance evaluation from retrieved Brain, Liver and Knee images using various distance metrics

Distance Metrics	(P/R)	(R/IR)	T	A	E	ER	CER
Retrieval Results for Brain Images							
Euclidean	100/50	10/0	0.5	100	100	0	0
Manhattan	100/50	10/0	0.5	100	100	0	0
Mahalanobis	60/40	6/4	0.5	60	60	40	0
Canberra	100/50	10/0	0.5	100	100	0	0
Bray-Curtis	100/50	10/0	0.5	100	100	0	0
Squared Chord	100/50	10/0	0.5	100	100	0	0
Chi-Squared	100/50	10/0	0.5	100	100	0	0
Retrieval Results for Liver Images							
Euclidean	90/45	9/1	0.5	90	90	10	0
Manhattan	100/50	10/0	0.5	100	100	0	0
Mahalanobis	60/30	6/4	0.5	60	60	40	0
Canberra	100/50	10/0	0.5	100	100	0	0
Bray-Curtis	100/50	10/0	0.5	100	100	0	0
Squared Chord	100/50	10/0	0.5	100	100	0	0
Chi-Squared	100/50	10/0	0.5	100	100	0	0
Retrieval Results for Knee Images							
Euclidean	100/50	10/0	0.5	100	100	0	0
Manhattan	100/50	10/0	0.5	100	100	0	0
Mahalanobis	60/30	6/4	0.5	60	60	40	0
Canberra	100/50	10/0	0.5	100	100	0	0
Bray-Curtis	100/50	10/0	0.5	100	100	0	0
Squared Chord	100/50	10/0	0.5	100	100	0	0
Chi-Squared	100/50	10/0	0.5	100	100	0	0

retrieval using transform techniques have precision, recall, accuracy, and efficiency values found to be higher and also they have a lesser classification by error rate. Overall CWT and DFT have higher precision and recall with lesser time taken for retrieval. DCT+CWT also have next higher precision and recall with greater time taken for retrieval.

Table 8 shows the overall precision and recall calculation from the performance evaluation using transform based retrieval techniques for Brain, Liver and Knee images. T1 denotes DFT, T2 denotes DCT, T3 denotes DWT, T4 denotes RCWF, T5

Table 5. Overall performance evaluation using (Precision /Recall) calculation from retrieved images by various distance metrics

Images	EU	MAN	MAH	CA	BR	SQ	CHI	APR	ARR
(Precision/Recall) Values									
Brain	100/50	100/50	60/30	100/50	100/50	100/50	100/50	94	47
Liver	90/45	100/50	60/30	100/50	100/50	100/50	100/50	93	46
Knee	100/50	100/50	60/30	100/50	100/50	100/50	100/50	94	47
APR	97	100	60	100	100	100	100	-	-
ARR	48	50	30	50	50	50	50	-	-

Table 6. Result image rating: Observers' scores for individual images from distance metrics

Observer Parameters	Brain	Liver	Knee
Visual similarity	1	1	1
Relevant images	1	1	1
Similarity difference	0	0	1
Minimal irrelevant images	1	1	1
Lesser redundant image	1	1	1
Average score for each type of image	4	4	5

denotes CWT, T6 denotes Curvelet, T7 denotes DCT+CWT, T8 denotes DCT+DWT, and T9 denotes Curvelet +DWT. As already the properties of medical images are discussed in the previous section now, let us straightly see for transforms related with the images. CWT retains information in six different directions with good directional selectivity observed to be performing better. Though RCWF also retains information than CWT, it does not suit for retrieval. DWT has good textural characteristics, but it performs next to above said transform because of its lack in orientation. Since the DFT collects the pattern information from the frequency components of the images it does not work well. DCT preserves global features rather than local features it lacks in retrieval. Curvelet preserves and retain information or images based only on edges and curves. From the overall analysis based on (APR/ARR) with (47/28) % CWT found to retrieve more relevant images and the next best performance is given by DFT, DCT+CWT, DCT, DWT, RCWF, Curvelet, DCT+DWT, Curvelet +DWT respectively. Now justification is based on images. Knee image is found to be retrieved more. This is because of lesser internal details than Liver and Brain images. The orientation also differs only in a lesser way. More internal organs are

Table 7. Performance evaluations from retrieved Brain, Liver and Knee images using various transform techniques

Transform	(P/R)	(R/IR)	T	A	E	ER	CER
Retrieval Results for Brain Images							
DFT	50/30	6/6	0.2	50	50	50	0
DCT	17/10	2/10	0.5	17	17	83	0
DWT	50/30	6/10	0.2	50	50	83	0
RCWF	25/15	3/9	0.6	25	25	75	0
CWT	50/30	6/6	0.3	50	50	50	0
CURVELET	25/15	3/9	0.6	25	25	75	0
DCT+CWT	42/25	5/7	0.6	42	42	58	0
DCT+DWT	17/10	2/10	0.6	17	17	83	0
CURVELET+DWT	17/10	2/10	0.6	17	17	83	0
Retrieval Results for Liver Images							
DFT	42/25	5/7	0.2	42	42	58	0
DCT	50/30	6/6	0.5	50	50	50	0
DWT	42/25	5/7	0.2	42	42	58	0
RCWF	33/20	4/8	0.6	33	33	67	0
CWT	50/30	6/6	0.3	50	50	50	0
CURVELET	33/20	4/8	0.6	33	33	67	0
DCT+CWT	50/30	6/6	0.6	50	50	50	0
DCT+DWT	8/5	1/11	0.6	8	8	92	0
CURVELET+DWT	8/5	1/11	0.6	8	8	92	0
Retrieval Results for Knee Images							
DFT	42/25	5/7	0.2	42	42	58	0
DCT	42/25	5/7	0.5	42	42	58	0
DWT	17/10	2/10	0.2	17	17	83	0
RCWF	17/10	2/10	0.6	17	17	83	0
CWT	42/25	5/7	0.3	42	42	58	0
CURVELET	17/10	2/10	0.6	17	17	83	0
DCT+CWT	42/25	5/7	0.6	42	42	58	0
DCT+DWT	42/25	5/7	0.6	42	42	58	0
CURVELET+DWT	42/25	5/7	0.6	42	42	58	0

present in Liver and its intensity varies drastically. But the intensity variations are gradual in Brain images. Based on more relevant retrieved images, Knee images with (43/26) % are retrieved more than Liver and Brain images respectively.

Higher the score (5) means more number of relevant images are retrieved. Table 8 shows the Observers' classification from retrieved images applied to all images.

Table 8. Overall Performance evaluations by (Precision /Recall) calculation from retrieved images by various transform techniques

Images	T1	T2	T3	T4	T5	T6	T7	T8	T9	APR	ARR
(Precision/Recall) Values											
Brain	50/30	17/10	50/30	25/15	50/30	25/15	42/25	17/10	17/10	33	19
Liver	42/25	50/30	42/5	33/20	50/30	33/20	50/30	8/5	8/5	35	21
Knee	42/25	42/25	17/10	17/10	42/25	17/10	42/25	42/25	42/25	43	26
APR	45	36	36	25	47	25	45	22	22	-	-
ARR	27	22	15	15	28	15	27	13	13	-	-

Table 9. Result image rating: Observers' scores for individual images from transform techniques

Observer Parameters	Brain	Liver	Knee
Visual similarity	1	1	1
Relevant images	1	1	1
Similarity difference	0	0	0
Minimal irrelevant images	0	0	1
Lesser redundant image	1	1	1
Average score for each type of image	3	3	4

Average of Observers' parameters score ranges from (0-5) is 4 for Knee and 3 for Brain and Liver from Observers' criteria classification from Table 8 and 9, the classification criteria as described already in previous section. The observers' also confirms that, the Knee image is found to be retrieved more in transform based retrieval than Brain and Liver images.

Table 10 shows the performance evaluation of the retrieved Brain, Liver and Knee image using texture based techniques. Higher the precision means, the accuracy and efficiency will be increased. Also, error rate and classification by error rate also are observed to be more similar with lesser variations for the above all texture based retrieval technique. The best performance in relevant image retrieval for Brain images is given by GLCM and GLCM+LBP. Only the next best performance is given by LBP. For the best texture technique the precision, recall, accuracy, and efficiency found to be higher and they also have a lesser error rate and classification by error rate. The time taken for retrieval is found to be more similar for all texture based techniques.

Table 10. Performance evaluations from retrieved Brain, Liver and Knee images using texture based extraction techniques

Techniques	(P/R)	(R/IR)	T	A	E	ER	CER
Retrieval Results for Brain Images							
GLCM	100/50	10/0	2	100	100	0	0
LBP	80/40	8/2	2	80	80	20	0
GLCM+LBP	100/50	10/0	2	100	100	0	0
Retrieval Results for Liver Images							
GLCM	100/50	10/0	2	100	100	0	0
LBP	30/15	3/7	2	100	100	70	0
GLCM+LBP	100/50	10/0	2	100	100	0	0
Retrieval Results for Knee Images							
GLCM	100/50	10/0	2	100	100	0	0
LBP	100/50	10/0	2	100	100	0	0
GLCM+LBP	100/50	10/0	2	100	100	0	0

Table 11 shows the overall precision and recall calculation from the performance evaluation using texture based retrieval techniques for Brain, Liver and Knee images. GLCM performs well in texture based retrieval; it calculates statistics based on distance and direction between pixels. LBP is based on the orientation of pattern distribution has lesser retrieval rate. But, when GLCM is combined with LBP, they perform well because of its combined advantage. Based on the (APR/ARR) GLCM and GLCM+LBP with (100/50)% found to perform well in retrieval of Brain, Liver and Knee images. Based on more relevant retrieved images, Knee images are found to be retrieved more with (100/50) %.

The textural property of gray scale contrast is more in Knee images than Brain and Liver images. The supporting proof for this is provided in Histogram plot in later section. Moreover this technique is able to differentiate the different textures within the image. Hence the bony structures and the tissues are exactly identified. The Knee images with (100/50) % found to be retrieved more than Brain and Liver images.

Table 12 shows the Observers' classification from retrieval technique applied to all images. Average of Observers' parameters score ranges from (0-5) is 4 for Brain and Liver and 5 for Knee from Observers' criteria classification from Table 10 and 11 as already described in previous sections. Brain and Liver images found to be retrieved lesser in texture based retrieval than Knee images. The observers' also confirms that, the Knee image is found to be retrieved more in texture based

Table 11. Overall Performance evaluation by (precision /recall) calculation from retrieved images using texture based extraction techniques

Images	GLCM	LBP	GLCM+LBP	APR	ARR
(Precision/Recall) Values					
Brain	100/50	80/40	100/50	93	47
Liver	100/50	30/45	100/50	77	38
Knee	100/50	100/50	100/50	100	50
APR	100	70	100	-	-
ARR	50	35	50	-	-

Table 12. Result image rating: Observers' scores for individual images from texture based retrieval techniques

Observer Parameters	Brain	Liver	Knee
Visual similarity	1	1	1
Relevant images	1	1	1
Similarity difference	1	1	1
Minimal irrelevant images	0	0	1
Lesser redundant image	1	1	1
Average score for each type of image	4	4	5

retrieval than Brain and Liver images, which are similar. Higher the score (5) means more number of relevant images are retrieved.

Table 13 shows the performance evaluation by retrieval using shape based retrieval techniques. Canny edge with Otsu method is used for shape based medical image retrieval. The time taken for retrieval is found to be more similar for all images. Retrieval accuracy, efficiency is found to be higher for Liver images. Error rate and classification by error rate also found to be more similar with lesser variations for the above shape based retrieval techniques. Liver images are observed to have more relevant images; hence the precision values will be higher.

Table 14 shows the overall precision and recall calculation from the performance evaluation using shape based retrieval techniques for Brain, Liver and Knee images. From the retrieval techniques used, shape is found to have a very lesser retrieval rate. From the suggestions taken from other researchers, for shape based medical image retrieval have combined two shape based techniques. Because the features used in shape based retrieval search for exact size and shape which is not possible in medical images because of their difference in orientation. This makes the retrieval

Table 13. Performance evaluation from retrieved Brain, Liver and Knee images using shape based extraction technique

Images	(P/R)	(R/IR)	T	A	E	ER	CER
Brain	70/35	7/3	3	70	70	30	0
Liver	100/50	10/0	3	100	100	0	0
Knee	20/10	2/8	3	20	20	80	0

Table 14. Overall Performance evaluation by (precision /recall) calculation from retrieved images using shape based extraction technique

Images	(Precision/Recall) Values	APR	ARR
Brain	70/35	70	35
Liver	100/50	100	50
Knee	20/10	20	10
APR	63	-	-
ARR	32	-	-

difficult and retrieves only the lesser image which is most similar image for the given query alone. This is an added advantage but, only lesser images are retrieved. More relevant retrieved images are found for Liver than Brain and Knee images respectively. Canny edge preserves edge details and Otsu on selected global threshold value by maximizing the separability of clusters in gray levels. The (APR/ARR) of shape is observed to be (63/32) % which is lesser than other retrieval techniques.

Higher the score (5) means more number of relevant images are retrieved. The observers' also confirms that, the Liver image is found to be retrieved more in shape based retrieval than Brain and Knee images. Table 15 shows the Observers' classification from retrieved results applied to all images. Average of Observer parameters score ranges from (0-5) is 4 for Brain, 3 for Knee and 5 for Liver from Observers' criteria classification from Tables 2 and 3.

More texture characteristics are present in medical images, it is better to go for combined feature extraction. From the simulated results it is found that no irrelevant images are retrieved for multifeature extraction. The multi feature based technique is implemented and analyzed for all the imaging modalities. The best and similar retrieval results are found from Figures 3.25, 3.26 and 3.27 for GLCM+Canny edge with Otsu method based multifeature extraction for all three images.

Table 16 shows the overall precision and recall calculation from the performance evaluation using multi feature based retrieval techniques for Brain, Liver and Knee

Table 15. Result image rating: Observers' scores for individual images from shape based retrieval techniques

Observer Parameters	Brain	Liver	Knee
Visual similarity	1	1	1
Relevant images	1	1	0
Similarity difference	1	1	1
Minimal irrelevant images	0	1	0
Lesser redundant image	1	1	1
Average score for each type of image	4	5	3

Table 16. Performance evaluation from retrieved Brain, Liver and Knee images using multifeature based extraction technique

Images	(P/R)	(R/IR)	T	A	E	ER	CER
Brain	100/50	10/0	3	100	100	0	0
Liver	100/50	10/0	3	100	100	0	0
Knee	100/50	10/0	3	100	100	0	0

images. Accuracy and efficiency are found to be same and is equivalent to precision values. Time taken for retrieval using distance metrics is found to be equal for Brain, Liver and Knee images. CER and ER is found to be 0 for all images. Brain, Liver and Knee images found to retrieve more relevant images. Higher the relevancy means, efficiency will be higher.

The reason for more relevant retrieved images for Brain images is because of the extraction of textural and shape features, and they supports well for Brain images. Also when both the properties are combined they plays an immense role in the images, where both textural and shape features are extracted for all the three images. The same is approved from the Observers' criteria. The (APR/ARR) of Multifeature is (100/50) % and is shown in Table 16. The reason is since GLCM preserves the textural properties of images which plays the major role in retrieval of images and Canny edge preserving edge details and Otsu on selected global threshold value by maximizing the separability of clusters in gray levels, all the three images found to be retrieved more with (100/50)% of (APR/ARR). The textural and shape are the two major properties while dealing with images and hence when combined produces best results.

Table 17. Overall Performance evaluation by (precision /recall) calculation from retrieved images using multifeature based extraction technique

Images	(Precision/Recall) Values	APR	ARR
Brain	100/50	100	50
Knee	100/50	100	50
Liver	100/50	100	50
APR	100/50	100	50
ARR	100/50	100	50

The above rating is given by observers' from the retrieved images. Since the score is high (5) for all the three organs, Table 18 shows the Observers' classification from retrieved techniques applied to all images. Average of Observers' parameters score ranges from (0-5) is 5 for Brain, Liver and Knee from Observers' criteria classification from Tables 2 and 3. Brain, Liver and Knee images found to be retrieved more in multifeature based retrieval.

SUMMARY AND DISCUSSION

This section presents the summary of the above described techniques and their results.

Figure 4 shows overall best analyzed results from medical image retrieval systems using distance, transform and CBMIR. The values of precision are taken. Figure 5 shows overall best analyzed results from medical image retrieval systems using distance, transform and CBMIR. The values of recall are taken. From the precision and recall analysis chart it is evident that distance, texture and multifeature performs better than texture and shape based techniques. Figure 6 shows overall more relevant retrieved images from medical image retrieval systems using distance, transform and CBMIR. It is evident that for distance and multifeature based retrieval system; all the three imaging organs have been retrieved more than texture, shape and transform techniques.

To avoid controversies in visual observable variation between experts and also to support observers results, Histogram is provided. Due to enormous experimentation and to reduce complexity, the Histogram in Figure 7,8,9,10,11,12,13,14 and 15 are used to display only the best results obtained. The histogram is taken only as a supporting visual observance for confirming the similarity matching. Also the Histogram distribution shows the similarity match between Query image and retrieved images.

Table 18. Result image rating: Observers' scores for individual images from multifeature based retrieval technique

Observer Parameters	Brain	Liver	Knee
Visual similarity	1	1	1
Relevant images	1	1	1
Similarity difference	1	1	1
Minimal irrelevant images	1	1	1
Lesser redundant image	1	1	1
Average score for each type of image	5	5	5

Figure 4. Overall best analyzed results (Precision) from medical image retrieval system using distance, transform and CBMIR

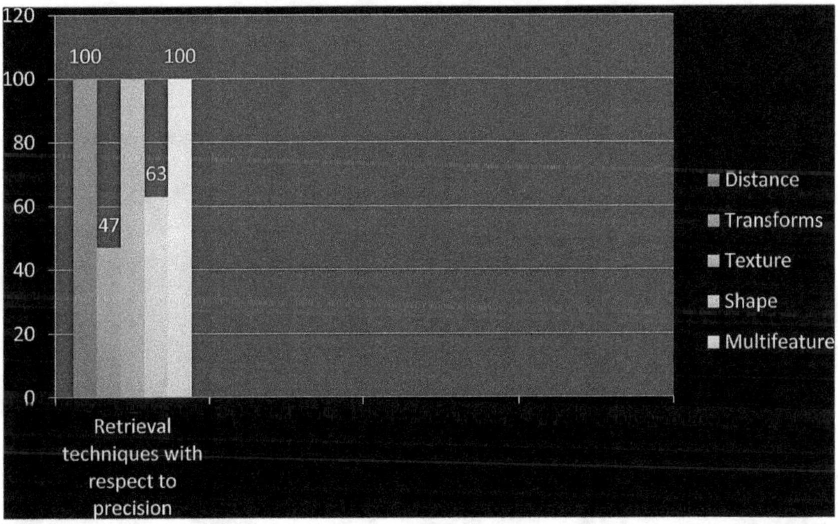

Histogram plot for Distance metrics based retrieval for Brain images shows the more similarity to the query image. Histogram plot for Distance metrics based retrieval for Knee images also has the higher similarity when compared to the given query image. Histogram plot for Transform based retrieval for Knee images have lesser similar plot, with more dissimilar plot when compared with the query image plot. For Texture based retrieval for Knee images confirms the relevancy between the query image and retrieved images. More contrast is found for Knee images than the Liver images. This is also observed from the plot using the visual observance. Histogram plot for Texture based retrieval for Liver images confirms that the plot has lesser intensity variation when compared with the query image. Histogram for

Figure 5. Overall best analyzed results (Recall) from medical image retrieval system using distance, transform and CBMIR

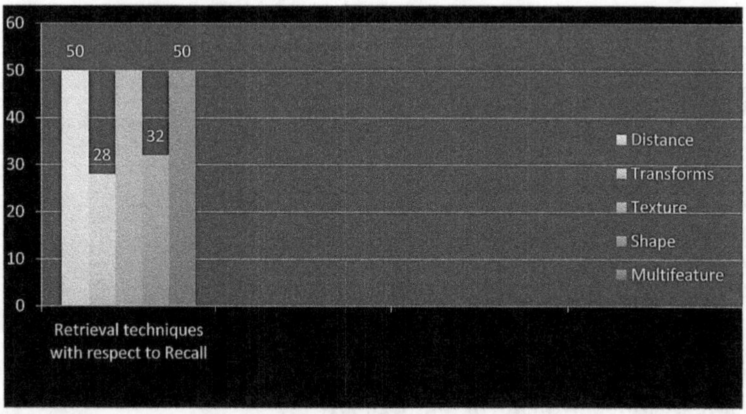

Figure 6. Overall more relevant retrieved image from medical image retrieval system using distance, transform and CBMIR

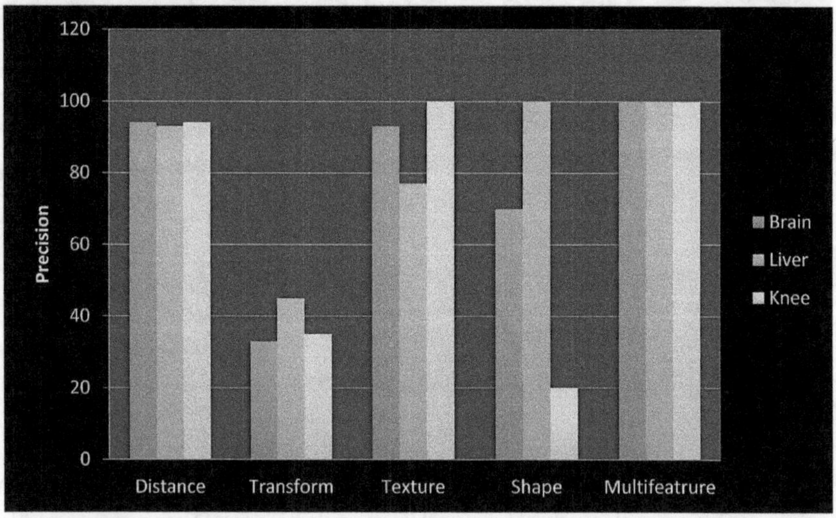

shape based retrieval confirms that, the plot is found to be less similar from the query image. For multifeature based retrieval, the plot is found to be more similar compared to the query image.

Table 19 shows the overall best performed techniques and modalities for medical image retrieval using distance metrics, transform, texture, shape and multi feature based retrieval techniques applied to medical images.

Figure 7. Histogram plot for Distance metrics based retrieval for Brain images.

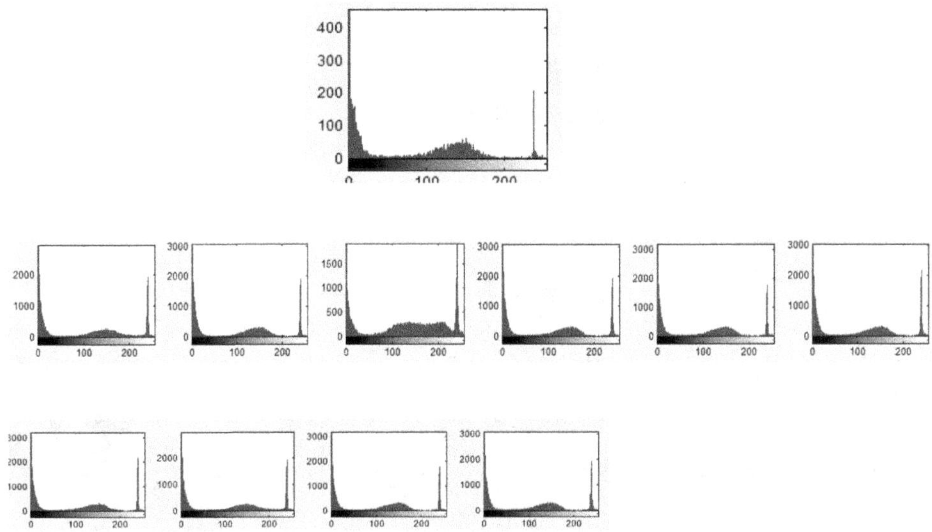

Figure 8. Histogram plot for Distance metrics based retrieval for Knee images

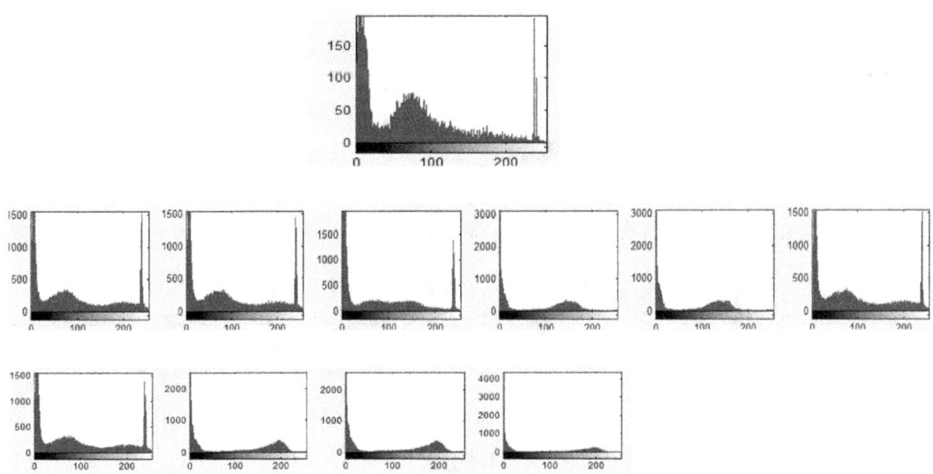

The modification towards development of new knowledge is focused on registration based retrieval for computer assisted clinical diagnosis. Hence while introducing an entirely new knowledge; several proven conventional techniques are implemented. The ultimate aim for performing all these retrieval technique

Figure 9. Histogram plot for Transform based retrieval for Knee images

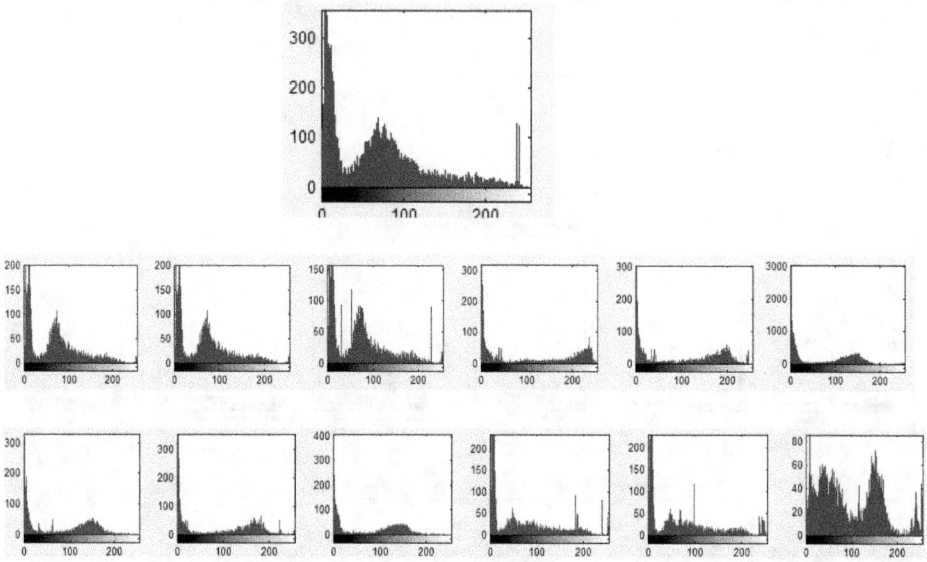

Figure 10. Histogram plot for texture based retrieval for Knee images

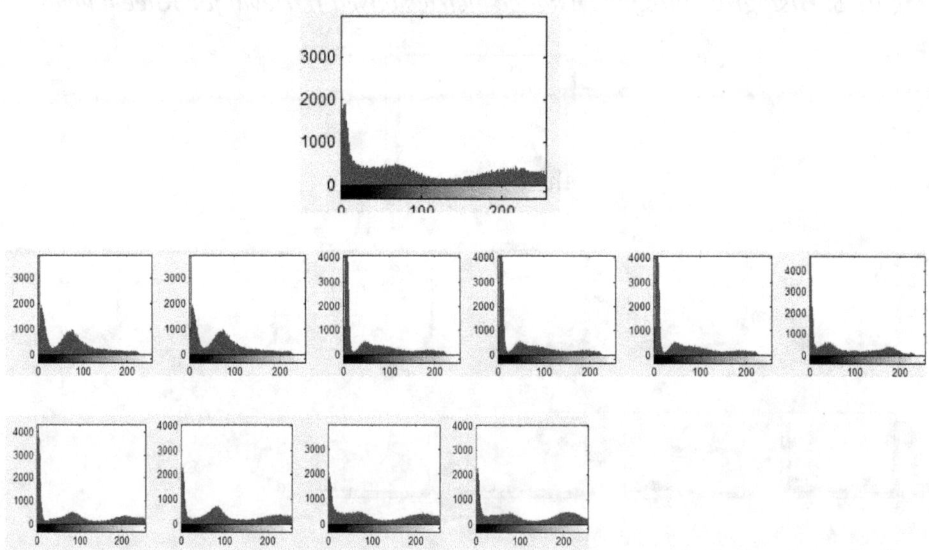

Figure 11. Histogram plot for texture based retrieval for Liver images

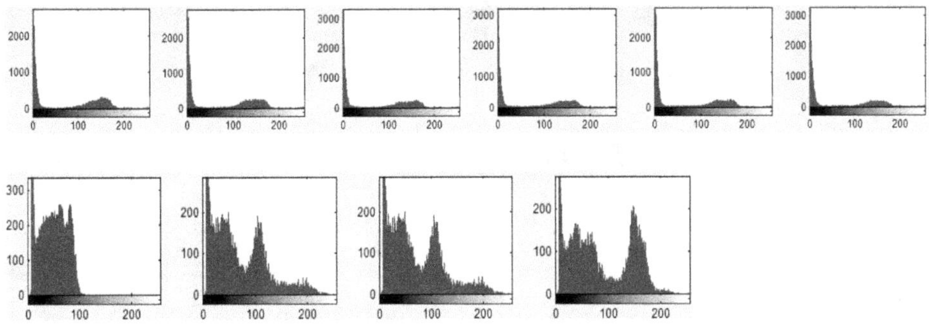

Figure 12. Histogram plot for shape based retrieval for Liver images

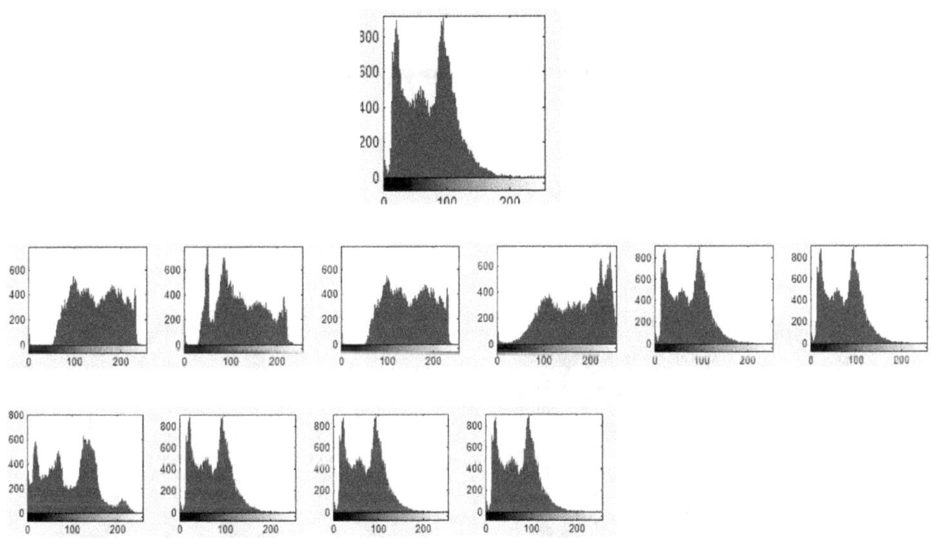

is to improve the retrieval rate. So far in experimentation, the database is created by using only one or two modality for a particular organ. But, here have created database with three various modalities with Five different anatomical objects. Hence proven conventional methods which suits for all organs have been proposed. This is an interesting observation which is not provided so far found in a single system (Ceyhun Burak, 2011)

The combinations of several conventional measures have been tried to improve the retrieval rate. It is found that the several combinations of Transform failed to perform well. The lesser performed transform pulled down the results of higher performed transform. Hence it is observed that combinations of transform do not

Figure 13. Histogram plot for multifeature based retrieval for Brain images

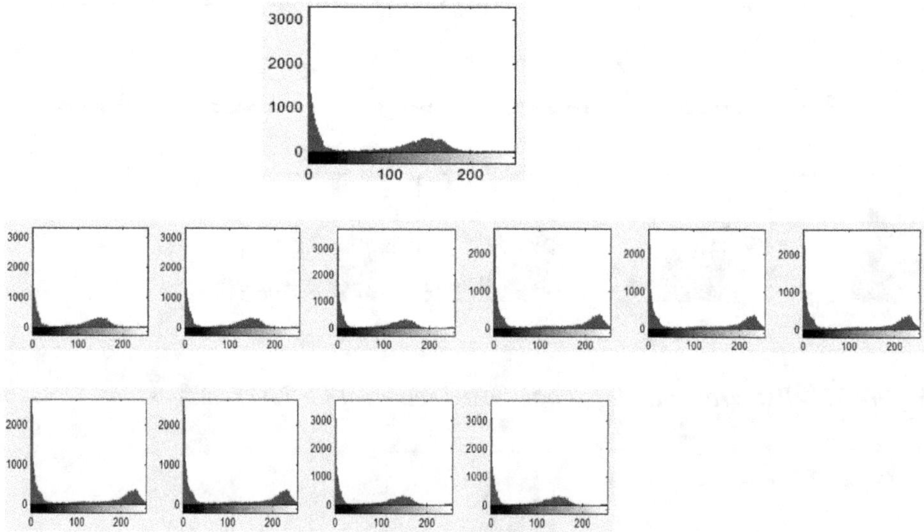

Figure 14. Histogram plot for multifeature based retrieval for liver images

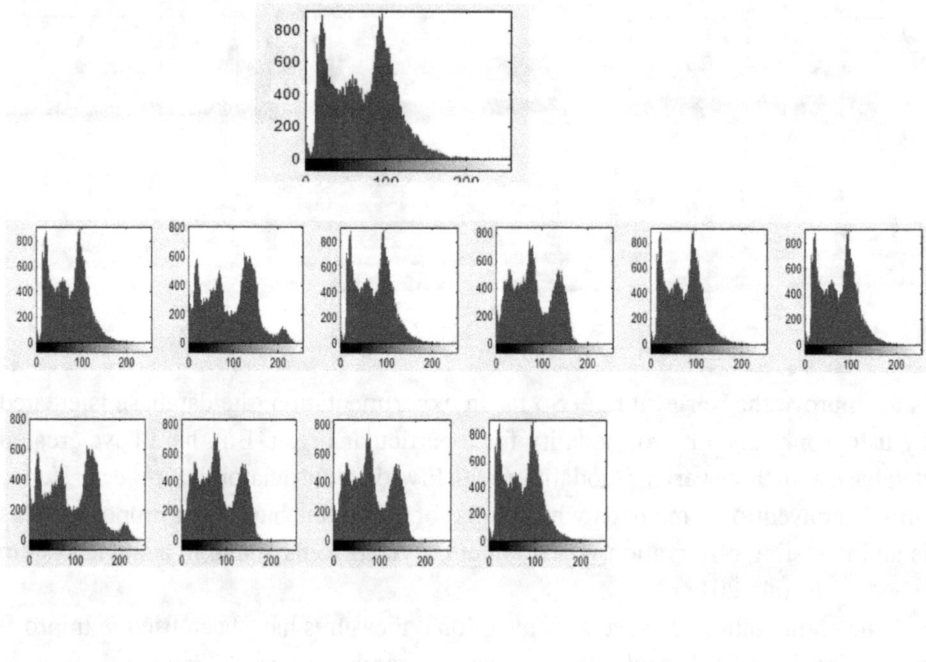

Figure 15. Histogram plot for multifeature based retrieval for knee images

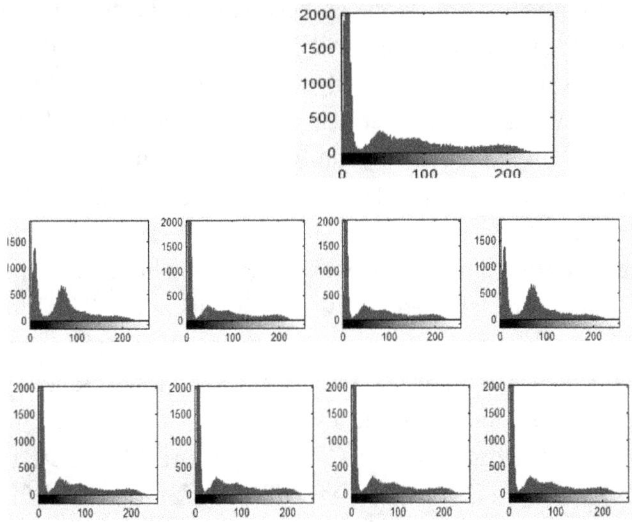

Table 19. Best performed techniques and images from medical image retrieval using distance metrics, transform, texture, shape and multi feature based retrieval techniques

S.No	Types	Methods	Images
1	Distance	Manhattan, Canberra, Bray-Curtis, Squared Chord and Chi-Squared (100/50)	Brain (100/50) Knee (100/50)
2	Transform	CWT (47/38)	Knee (43/26)
3	Texture	GLCM, GLCM+LBP (100/50)	Knee (100/50)
4	Shape	Canny edge with Otsu method (63/32)	Liver (100/50)
5	Multi feature	GLCM+Canny edge with Otsu method(100/50)	Brain (100/50) Liver(100/50) Knee (100/50)

provide best retrieval results. Though there is no new knowledge in the techniques implemented, but the way experiment is approached, carried, analyzed, examined, discussed, justified both qualitatively and quantitatively is the variation shown in this research. The new knowledge provided from the experimentation is the selecting the best technique which suits for particular organ can be easily observed and this one particular system can effectively serves for five anatomical objects on effective clinical diagnosis.

A similarity metric is used to compute similarity between pixels of two images. Hence, calculating the squared intensity differences between pixels directly on medical images produces best retrieval rate. Especially for medical images there will be gradual changes in the texture and drastic change in the inner shape regions. Using distance based retrieval Manhattan, Canberra, Bray-Curtis, Squared Chord and Chi-Squared distance metrics outperform Euclidean, Mahalanobis metrics. Brain images are found to be retrieved more the retrieval than Liver and Knee images. The comparative analysis is exactly based on average precision rate and average recall rate.

Scale values determine the degree to which the wavelet is stretched. Low scale values compress the wavelet and correlate better with high frequencies. The low scale CWT coefficients represent the fine-scale features in the input signal vector. High scale values stretch the wavelet and correlate better with the low frequency content of the image. Hence CWT produces best retrieval rate than other transform. Using transform based retrieval for medical images, CWT outperforms DFT, DCT, DWT, RCWF, CWT, Curvelet, DCT+CWT, DCT+DWT and Curvelet +DWT. Based on retrieval of more relevant retrieved images, Knee images outperforms Brain and Liver images.

CWT retains information in six different directions with good directional selectivity which has better performance is combined with lower performed DCT. It preserves global features rather than local features and hence it lacks in retrieval. But, when both combined lesser retrieval is obtained. Feature extraction with its ability to localize the structures DWT is combined with DCT, since it preserves global features, whereas feature extraction will be effective only on the whole image, this pull down the image. Curvelet achieve a complete coverage of the spectral domain and it captures more orientation information and localizing the structures with better resolution using feature extraction is achieved by DWT. But, when orientation is combined with Feature extraction, the directional changes and scale changes pulled down the results. The combination of transform which has lesser performance is combined with higher performance to check the applicability of the results. Certain transform technique does not perform well in the retrieval system. But, certain transform techniques do perform well due to their inherent features. It is already proved that DCT and Curvelet found to have lesser retrieval rate. CWT and DWT found to have higher retrieval rate. So, the combination of DCT+CWT, DCT+DWT and Curvelet+ DWT has been implemented.

Based on texture based image retrieval GLCM and GLCM+LBP outperforms LBP. Co-occurrence matrix captures numerical features of a texture using spatial relations of similar gray tones. Hence gray level co-occurrence matrix when combined with local binary pattern produces best retrieval rate. The distribution of texture pattern is gradual in Knee images than liver on applying the matrix, this gray level distribution helps in the retrieval. Hence, Knee images are found to be retrieved more from the retrieval. On shape based image retrieval using Canny edge with Otsu based image retrieval, (APR/ARR) is found to be (63/32) %. Liver images found to be retrieved more than Brain and Knee images. Since the variation change is more inside the medical image rather than the contour region, the minimum retrieval rate is achieved. For multifeature based image retrieval using GLCM as texture based retrieval and Canny edge with Otsu for shape based retrieval, the (APR/ARR) is found to be (100/50)%. The advantage of this technique is that, they describe an image at varying levels of detail and avoid the need to segment the image into regions of interest before shape descriptors can be computed. Hence all the three Brain, Liver and Knee images found to be retrieved more from the retrieval.

CONCLUSION

The information obtained by the radiologists and the users also feels that the framework, suits well depending upon their requirement needed for effective clinical diagnosis. From the above criteria it is observed that retrieval rate given by Observers' classification also scored well similar to the metrics analysis. The best retrieval rate is achieved by multifeature based retrieval with (100/50) %. Based on more relevant retrieved images all the three Brain, Liver and Knee images are found to be retrieved more with (100/50)%.

REFERENCES

Burak, Rubin, Napel, Beaulieu, Greenspan, & Acer. (2011). Content-based image retrieval in radiology: current status and future directions. *Journal of Digital Imaging, 24*(2), 208-222.

Cauvin, J. M., Le Guillou, C., Solaiman, B., Robaszkiewicz, M., Le Beux, P., & Roux, C. (2003). Computer-assisted diagnosis system in digestive endoscopy. *IEEE Transactions on Information Technology in Biomedicine, 7*(4), 256–262. doi:10.1109/TITB.2003.823293 PMID:15000352

Comaniciu, D., Meer, P., & Foran, D. J. (1999). Image-guided decision support system for pathology. *Machine Vision and Applications, 11*(4), 213–224. doi:10.1007001380050104

Depeursinge, A., Fischer, B., Müller, H., & Deserno, T. M. (2011). Prototypes for content-based image retrieval in clinical practice. *Journal of Open Medical Informatics*, *5*(1), 58–72. doi:10.2174/1874431101105010058 PMID:21892374

Deselaers, T. (2003). *Features for image retrieval* (Master thesis). University of Rhine-Westphalia Alsiche Technical University of Aachen.

Diagnostic and Interventional Radiology. (n.d.). Retrieved from www.dirjournal.org

Dimitrovski, I., Kocev, D., Kitanovski, I., Loskovska, S., & Džeroski, S. (2015). Improved medical image modality classification using a combination of visual and textual features. *Computerized Medical Imaging and Graphics*, *39*, 14–26. doi:10.1016/j.compmedimag.2014.06.005 PMID:24997992

Gletsos, M., Mougiakakou, S. G., Matsopoulos, G. K., Nikita, K. S., Nikita, A. S., & Kelekis, D. (2003). A computer-aided diagnostic system to characterize CT focal liver lesions: Design and optimization of a neural network classifier. *IEEE Transactions on Information Technology in Biomedicine*, *7*(3), 153–162. doi:10.1109/TITB.2003.813793 PMID:14518728

Harry's Chest Atlas. (n.d.). *Medical image database*. Retrieved on April 15, 2013 from http://www.Chestatlas.com

Hong, S., Cui, W.-C., & Li, T. (2005). Medical image description in content-based image retrieval. *Proceedings of the IEEE Engineering in Medicine and Biology 27th Annual Conference*, 6336-6339.

Kwak, D. M. (2003). „Content-based ultrasound image retrieval using a coarse to fine approach. *Annals of the New York Academy of Sciences*, 212–224. PMID:12594091

Manjunath, B. S., & Ma, W. Y. (1996). Texture features for browsing and retrieval of image data. *IEEE Transactions on Pattern Analysis and Machine Intelligence*, *8*(8), 837–842. doi:10.1109/34.531803

Muller, H., Michoux, N., Bandon, D., & Geissbuhler, A. (2004). A review of content-based image retrieval applications-clinical benefits and future directions. *International Journal of Medical Informatics*, *73*(1), 1–23. doi:10.1016/j.ijmedinf.2003.11.024 PMID:15036075

Muller, H., Muller, W., Squire, D. M., Marchand, S., Maillet, & Pun, T. (2000). Strategies for positive and negative relevance feedback in image retrieval. In *Proceedings of the 15th International Conference on Pattern Recognition (ICPR2000)*. IEEE. 10.1109/ICPR.2000.905650

Pokrajac, D., Megalooikonomou, V., Lazarevic, A., Kontos, D., & Obradovic, Z. (2005). Applying spatial distribution analysis techniques to classification of 3D medical images. *Artificial Intelligence in Medicine*, *33*(3), 261–280. doi:10.1016/j.artmed.2004.07.001 PMID:15811790

Qian, X. N., & Tagare, H. D. (2005). *Optimal embedding for shape indexing in medical image databases*. Medical Image Computing and Computer Assisted. doi:10.1007/11566489_47

RadiologyInfo.org. (2013). *Medical image database*. Retrieved on April 5, 2013 from www.radiologyinfo.org

Rahman, M., Bhattacharya, P., & Desai, B. C. (2007). A framework for medical image retrieval using machine learning and statistical content-based image retrieval in radiology similarity matching techniques with relevance feedback. *IEEE Transactions on Information Technology in Biomedicine*, *11*(1), 58–69. doi:10.1109/TITB.2006.884364 PMID:17249404

Rui, Y., Huang, T. S., & Chang, S. F. (1999). Image retrieval: Current techniques, promising directions, and open issues. *Journal of Visual Communication and Image Representation*, *10*(1), 39–62. doi:10.1006/jvci.1999.0413

Shyu, C. R., Brodley, C. E., Kak, A. C., Kosaka, A., Aisen, A. M., & Broderick, L. S. (1999). ASSERT: A physician-in-the-loop content-based image retrieval system for HRCT image databases. *Computer Vision and Image Understanding*, *75*(2), 111–132. doi:10.1006/cviu.1999.0768

Shyu, C. R., Kak, A., Brodley, C., & Broderick, L. S. (1999). Testing for human perceptual categories in a physician-in-the-loop CBIR system for medical imagery. *Proceedings of the IEEE Workshop on Content-based Access of Image and Video Libraries (CBAIVL)*, 102-108. 10.1109/IVL.1999.781132

Smeulders, A. W. M., Worring, M., Santini, S., Gupta, A., & Jain, R. (2000). Content-based image retrieval at the end of the early years. *IEEE Transactions on Pattern Analysis and Machine Intelligence*, *22*(12), 1349–1380. doi:10.1109/34.895972

Toews, M., & Arbel, T. (2007). A statistical parts-based model of anatomical variability. *IEEE Transactions on Medical Imaging*, *26*(4), 497–508. doi:10.1109/TMI.2007.892510 PMID:17427737

Van Kitanovski, I. D., Madjarov, G., & Loskovska, S. (2017, January). Multimodal medical image retrieval system. *Multimedia Tools and Applications*, *76*(2), 2955–2978. doi:10.100711042-016-3261-1

Wang, J. Z. (2000). Pathfinder: Multiresolution region based searching of pathology images using IRM. *Proceedings of the AMIA Symposium*, 883-887.

Warwick. (2013). Retrieved in 2013 from www.warwick.ac.uk

Worring, M., Smeulders, W. M., & Santini, S. (2000). Interaction in content-based image retrieval: an evaluation of the state of the art. In R. Laurini (Ed.), *Proceedings of the Fourth International Conference On Visual Information Systems (VISUAL)*. Springer-Verlag. 10.1007/3-540-40053-2_3

ADDITIONAL READING

Ayyachamy, S., & Mannivannan, V. (2013). Medical Image Retrieval Using Transform. *Applied Medical Informatics*, *32*(2), 54–66.

Chapter 12
Medical Image Registration in Clinical Diagnosis: An Introduction

A. Swarnambiga
Indian Institute of Technology Madras, India

Vasuki S.
Vellammal College of Engineering and Technology, India

ABSTRACT

The term medical image covers a wide variety of types of images (modality), especially in medical image registration with very different perspective. In this chapter, spatial technique is approached and analyzed for providing effective clinical diagnosis. The effective conventional methods are chosen for this registration. Researchers have developed and focused this research using proven conventional methods in the respective fields of registration Affine, Demons, and Affine with B-spline. From the overall analysis, it is clear that Affine with B-Spline performs better in registration of medical images than Affine and Demons.

INTRODUCTION

A critical stage in visualizing the process is the alignment or registration of the images. This includes transformation, scaling and skews as well as the rigid body parameters in matrix form by preserving all the parallel lines. Rigid body registration is widely used in medical applications where the structures of interest (region of interest) are either bone or are enclosed in bone as noted in works by Yang (1999); Hill (2001);

DOI: 10.4018/978-1-5225-5876-7.ch012

Zitova (2003); Yang et al. (2007) and Viergever et al. (2016). Furthermore, this article focuses discussion on medical image registration on attempting to provide a clinical justification for diagnosis by observers' classification.

RELATED WORK

This Section aims to provide a survey of recent literature concerning medical image registration. Van Den Elsen et al. (1994) describes the intensity re-mapping for MR–CT registration. High intensities are re-mapped to low intensities using MR–CT registration by transforming the CT image intensities. This creates a virtual image from the CT images that has an intensity distribution more like an MR image (in which bone is dark). By using cross correlation the MR image and the virtual MR image created from CT are then registered.

Maes (1997) proposed a new approach to the problem of multimodality medical image registration using Mutual Information (MI) or relative entropy. The accuracy of the MI criterion is validated for rigid body registration of Computed Tomography, Magnetic Resonance Imaging, Positron Emission Tomography images by comparing with the stereotactic registration solution. Their results demonstrate that considering sub voxel accuracy with respect to the stereotactic reference, the solution can be achieved automatically. Maintz et al.'s (1998) survey is taken as a reference for various medical image registration techniques. The various registration techniques used for specific modality are summarized and is given in Table 1.

MATERIALS AND METHODS

The registered images helps in clinical diagnosis by guiding the physicians and radiologists independently without disturbing the patient. An added advantage of this registration techniques is, they can be effectively used by the radiologists, for the detail they expect to achieve without disturbing the patient and without subjecting the patient to take scan for several times. Thus this registration system helps in effective clinical diagnosis.

Registration System Module

In this section, details on the methodology used, which is essentially based on the widely known general image registration framework is provided. However have evaluated three algorithms from the perspective of the transformation used: such as Affine (AFF), Demons (DEM), and Affine with B-Spline (BSP) is given in Figure

Table 1. Brief summary of the image registration techniques used in medical domain

Registration of Object	Applications	Techniques Used
Registration of head images	Monomodal application: CT	By registration of crest lines (external lines of principle)
		3D morphing of CT skulls
		Local elastic 3D intra subject CTA registration
	Monomodal application: Rigid & affine MR registration	By alignment of principal axes and the center of gravity
		"Head-Hat" surface matching technique
		Rigid registration based on segmented curves, using segmentation, K-means clustering on two dimensions
	Monomodal application: Curved MR registration	By slices elastic deformation of segmented curves is performed
		Curved registration by MR images
	Monomodal application:PET	By affine registration
		By using graphical tools e.g., rendering, cup-plane edges an fully interactive method
		Chamfer matching
		Full image content based achieved by optimizing the cross correlation values in image areas near edges
	Monomodal application: SPECT	A 3D rigid registration on full image content using sum of squared intensity differences
	Monomodal application: Portal Images.	By global affine and global rigid transformation by optimizing the cross-correlation
	Monomodal application: DSA	Using generalized cross - correlation for finding a local curved transformation
		Local curved registration by minimizing the intensity variance
	Other Monomodal application	By using affine registration by locally matching and by checking the cross-correlation values
		By manually segmented contours by minimizing displacement of manually registered contours
	Multimodal applications: CT-MR	By computing transformation and user identified landmarks
		Using invasive fiducial markers
	Multimodal application:CT-PET	Using the images principal axes and centre of gravity
		Using the Head-Hat method.
	Multimodal application: CT-SPECT	By rigid chamber matching on automatically extracted surfaces
	Multimodal application: PET-MR	Rigid transformation by identified anatomical landmarks
		Using fiducial markers
		By using user identified anatomical landmarks and external markers
		Rigid surface based methods
	Multimodal application:SPECT-MR	By using anatomical landmarks
		Elastic registration by minimizing the local squared intensity differences
	Multi-application: US or MR	By using calibrated coordinate systems
		By using used identified anatomical landmarks
	Multi-application: X-ray	Silhouette method to register MR to X-ray images

continued on following page

Table 1. Continued

Registration of Object	Applications	Techniques Used
	Modality to model registration	Using elastic registration
		By using morphological watershed and closing algorithm
	Patient to modality registration	By skin markers
		By anatomical landmarks or fiducially
Registration of thoracic images	Registration of global thoracic images	By 3D rigid registration on monomodalities like PET or SPECT images of thorax by minimization of SA
		Monomodal affine portal using local translation only registration and global affine transformation
		Rigid registration of an portal to X-ray simulator using moment matching
	Registration of cardiac images	By using 3D monomodal scintigraphic images
		2D curved automatic registration on series of X-ray angiographic images
		2D rigid method based on geometrical landmarks
		A 3D automatic voxel property/full image content based
	Registration of breast images	By using full image content.
		Automatic 3D curved registration
Registration of Abdominal images	Renal images	By 2D automatic registration of DSA images of the kidney by minimizing DSC criterion
		By 2D automatic Affine transformation
	Hepatic images	By 3D rigid automatic registration by minimizing the SAD or SSC criterion
Registration of pelvic images		By 2D rigid automatic registration of DSA images by optimizing the DSC criterion.
		2D Affine automatic transformation by chamber matching
Registration of limb images		By performing X-ray to CT registration
		By using invasive fiducials markers
		Using surface registration on manually collected, automatically segmented surfaces of calcareous
		By applying invasive fiducial and surface based method images and then compared
		By applying geometrical landmark, an automatic registration is performed.
Registration of spinal images		By 3D rigid automatic registration on full image content by optimizing the cross correlation
		By performing patient to modulating in a semi-automated way
		3D curved registration

1. Although other algorithm combinations have been tested, and here the ones which significantly improves results compared to the individual methods is presented. The basic components of this registration framework are two input images, one output image, a measure, an optimizer, a transformer and an interpolator. The basic input data of the registration process are two images: one is defined as the moving image $m\left(X\right)$ and the other is the fixed image $f\left(X\right)$, and $\left(X\right)$ represents a position in a n-dimensional space. After the each iteration, matching degree between moving

image and fixed image will be measured. When the differences between moving image and fixed image are quite big and maybe matching degree could not reach the threshold forever, and then set the maximum iteration number to avoid this instance. A geometrical transformation is applied to one of the two images to bring two images into spatial alignment.

Similarity Metric for Registered Images

The measure of similarity between images or regions is a vital component in image registration along with the selection of the transformation function. In the latter section presented the two metrics used in this work, Sum of Squared Differences (SSD) and Mutual Information (MI).

Mutual Information

Registration is assumed to correspond to maximize aaaffine 2.2) by Pluim (2000) and is given in Equation (1)

$$I\left(A,B\right)=H\left(B\right)-H(B\mid A) \tag{1}$$

$H\left(B\right)$: Shannon entropy of image B,

Figure 1. General image registration framework

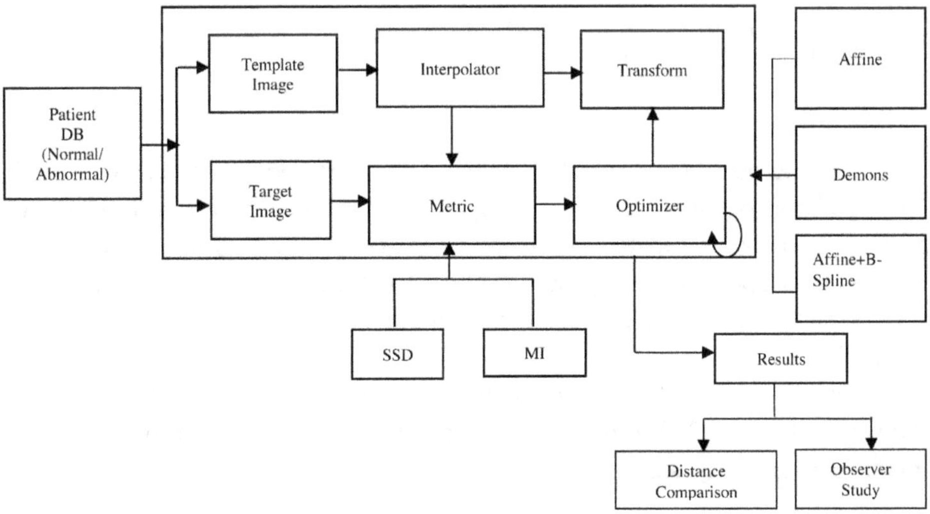

$H(B \mid A)$: Conditional entropy.

The chance of gray value b in image B given that the corresponding pixel in A which has gray value a is $p(b \mid a)$. Mutual information is the amount by which the uncertainty about B decreases when A is given: the amount of information A contains about B. The second form of definition is most closely related to joint entropy and is given in Equation (2)

$$I(A,B) = H(A) + H(B) - H(A,B) \tag{2}$$

$H(A,B)$: Maximizing mutual information and is related to minimizing joint entropy.

$H(A)$ and $H(B)$: Marginal entropy would have lower values when the overlapping part of the image contains only background and high values when it contains anatomical structure.

Sum of Squared Distance

The SSD metric computes the squared differences between intensity values of corresponding pixels. This is a simple, widely used metric that assumes a linear relationship between intensities in the images to be compared and its optimal value is 0 (when images are found to be identical). A and B stand for the images and i iterates over the I pixels in the images, and Equation (3) shows how to compute this metric.

$$SSD(A,B) = \frac{1}{I}\sum_{i=1}^{N}(A_i - B_i)^2 \tag{3}$$

Linear interpolator is used in this framework. When a point on the moving image is mapped from one space to another by a transform, it will in general be in a non-grid position as shown in Figure 2. In general, the grid positions of the moving image will not be mapped onto grid positions of the fixed image. Therefore, interpolation is required to evaluate the image intensity at the mapped position by Pluim (2000) and by Klein (2008).

Gradient descent optimization method is a fast and yet a successful method by Pluim (2000) Klein (2008) and hence it is implemented in this framework of medical image registration system.

Figure 2. Point on the moving image is mapped into the fixed image space after some spatial transformation

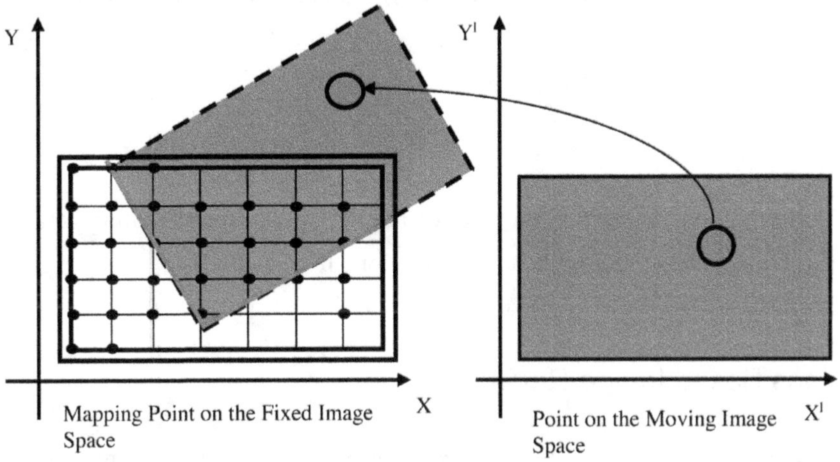

Control Point Selection

Automatic selection of control points is, in most cases, a two-stage process. The first step consists of the identification of significant points or structures in the images. Image matching is the second step, the mutual correspondence between the extracted structures is found and can be implemented either by using correlation-like or symbolic methods.

Affine Based Image Registration

Affine registration model assumes that the above transformation φ is linear and is given in Equation (4).

$$\varphi(X) = \varphi_a(X) = \begin{bmatrix} \varphi_{a_1}(X) \\ \varphi_{a_2}(X) \end{bmatrix} = \begin{bmatrix} a_1 & a_2 \\ a_3 & a_4 \end{bmatrix} \begin{bmatrix} x_1 \\ x_2 \end{bmatrix} + \begin{bmatrix} a_3 \\ a_6 \end{bmatrix} = AX + b \tag{4}$$

where $A = \begin{bmatrix} a_1 & a_2 \\ a_3 & a_4 \end{bmatrix}$ and $B = \begin{bmatrix} a_3 \\ a_6 \end{bmatrix}$ are the Affine transformation matrix and the translation vector respectively, for all $X \in \Omega$. The inverse transform is simply $X = A^{-1}(\varphi_a - b)$ if A is invertible. A can be decomposed into a product of rotation.

a scaling, a shear in $x_1 - \left(and\ /\ or\ x_2 -\right)$ direction or a combination of these simple transformations and is given in Equation (5), Arsigny et al. (2005).

$$A = \begin{bmatrix} a_1 & a_3 \\ a_2 & a_4 \end{bmatrix} = \begin{bmatrix} \cos\theta & -\sin\theta \\ \sin\theta & \cos\theta \end{bmatrix} \begin{bmatrix} s_{x1} & 0 \\ 0 & s_{x2} \end{bmatrix} \begin{bmatrix} 1 & S_{x1} \\ 0 & 1 \end{bmatrix} \quad (5)$$

Rotation scaling shear θ is the rotation angle, s_{x1}, s_{x2} are the scaling parameters, and S_{x1} is the shear factor in $x_1 -$ direction. It is clear that both a rigid-body transformation with $s_{x1} = s_{x1} = 1$ and $s_{x1} = 0$.

Demons Based Image Registration

Contours in the reference image are treated as Semi Permeable Membranes (SMs) and the floating image diffuse into or out of the SMs by the actions of "Demons" situated in the SMs for non-rigid registration and is given in Equation (6) Thirion (1998),

$$\vec{v} = \frac{\left(f - r\right) \times \vec{\nabla} r}{\vec{\nabla} r^2 + \frac{\left(f - r\right)^2}{k^2}} \quad (6)$$

∇r of reference image- Internal force of "Demons" force.
K is a normalization factor

For fixed point P, r is the grayscale of reference image R, and f is for floating image F and the diffusing model of Demons is given in Figure 3.

Figure 3. Diffusing model

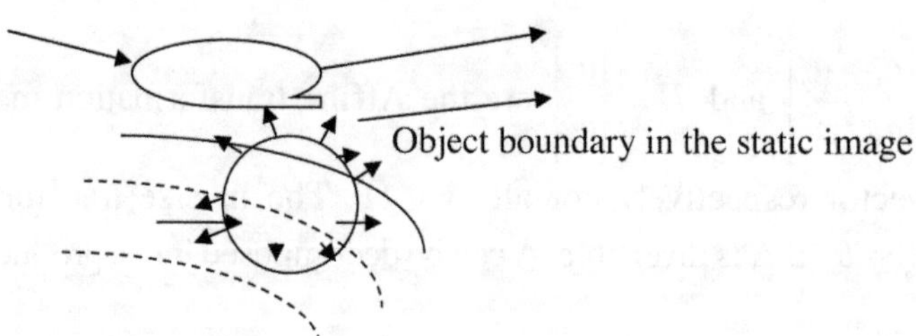

B-Spline Based Image Registration

Affine transformation provide fast image registration. B-Spline bases are used frequently for non-rigid image registration because, locally supported basis function expansions, provides convenient computationality, compact support, fast interpolation schemes, and hierarchical structure for multi-resolution Xie et al. (2004). Though, the deformations with high degrees of freedom can lead to unrealistic transformation results such as folding in the absence of appropriate constraints. The displacements fields u(x,y) and v(x,y) are two dimensional Splines controlled by a smaller number of displacements estimates $\underset{u_i}{\rightarrow}$ and $\underset{v_i}{\rightarrow}$ which lies on a coarse Spline control grid. The value of the displacement of pixel I and is given in Equation (7),

$$u\left(x_i, y_i\right) = \sum_j \underset{u_j}{\rightarrow} B_j\left(x_i, y_i\right) \tag{7}$$

where the $b_j\left(x, y\right)$ are called the basis functions. They are only non-zero over a small interval $W_{ij} = B_j\left(x_i, y_i\right)$ weights to emphasize that the $\left(u_i, v_i\right)$ are known linear combinations of the (u_j, v_j).

Affine With B-Spline Registration

It is proposed a method using a two stage model which do rely on the deformable model demon. Instead, firstly, will estimate an Affine transformation to establish good initial alignment. Subsequently, B-Spline is also used to model the local deformation.

Simulation Results

For the medical image registration, the assessment of registration accuracy is very important. Though the accuracy will vary between techniques and images, but for all considerations it is desirable to know both the expected accuracy (by observers' classification) and also the registration accuracy achieved on each individual set of images.

EXPERIMENTATION AND RESULTS

The most promising approach for ensuring acceptable accuracy is a visual assessment of the registered images before they are used for the desired clinical or research application. The performance measures used are discussed below.

Database

The database is formed from personally collected medical images from clinics and health care centers and benchmarked web image databases especially for particular modalities. Before going for experimental analysis characteristics of medical image are once again discussed briefly which helps in justifying the results.

- The Brain MRI database is composed of 20 T1 and T2 weighted Brain images of 5 different sets.
- The Liver MRI database consists of T2 weighted images. The database is composed of 20 T2 weighted images of 5 different sets.
- The database of Knee MRI is composed of 20 sagittal Knee images of 5 different sets.

MRI allows for a more sensitive evaluation of soft tissue and bone marrow edema and offer more reliable fat suppression. Axial plane of imaging is preferred for a compartmental approach for evaluation and in assessing the neurovascular structures, muscle and facial layers. The coronal plane provides a general overview of the region of interest. Sagittal plane aids in better depicting the cranial caudal extent of muscle and myotendinous junction involvement. Here MR images found in the database includes a combination of TIW and T2W sequences. T1W sequences provide an excellent depiction of anatomic details, bone marrow signal alteration fat, identification of sub-acute blood products and presence of enhanced tissues. T2 W sequences identified tissues with increased water content that can be seen in the setting of a broad range of pathology. Acquisition of T2 W sequences is performed depicts more often cranial caudal properties and also for pathology.

Quantitative Analysis

The following measures are considered in measuring the registered images from its performance parameters which is illustrated by Diez (2011). Evaluating the results of registration methods in MRI images is not an easy task. Hence have initially computed similarity metrics before and after registration to obtain an indication of how the images are similar. A lesser similarity metric is expected after image registration and the method with the lesser similarity metric value is expected to be the most accurate.

However, metric does not always tell the full story as sometimes images that are "closer" in terms of metric functions are perceived to be more different by human observers' like physicians and radiologists. In order to analyze the correlation between similarity metric and visually correct registration, have reviewed the methods using an observers' study where registration results are evaluated by 3 observers' with a different degree of expertise in both medical image analysis and radiology: One expert radiologist, one orthopedic surgeon and bone specialists and one anesthetic with over Twenty Seven years of experience (1), Fifteen years (1) and Thirty Seven years (1) of experience in all medical image analysis. Both subjective and quantitative evaluations are discussed, classified and justified with respect to the contents of the medical image. These are analyzed and discussed with radiologists and physicians to come to a conclusion on registration of medical images. In most of the computer-aided intervention techniques, medical images are crucial for treatment planning and guidance during the surgery. However, images acquired in different stages of diagnosis and treatments are affected by the position of the patient, deformation of soft tissue and the orientation of the imaging device. Therefore, computer aided interventions often involve a registration step in which coordinates systems of two images (of the same or different modalities, intra or inter registration) are matched. Without any constraint, images are chosen for medical image registration depending on the user's selection ensuring the applicability of this developed system.

Figure 4 shows the registration of Brain images using Affine, Demons and Affine with B-Spline registration. The Brain image shown contains the following. This T1 weighted MR image of the Brain shows eyeballs with optic nerve, medulla, vermis, and temporal lobes with hippocampal regions.

There is a clear view identified from the above figure that after performing Affine registration, the images found to have been translated and rotated which will vary according to the control point selection. This selection of control points will vary according to the physicians and radiologists view in finding more detail from images required for clinical diagnosis. For Demons based registration the image found to be registered without translation or rotation. Care should be taken in selecting the control points since, the details found in the original image and registered images should not vary more. So choosing the control point is a main criterion, though it depends on the user's interest. In spite of Demons deforms the image; but due to the care taken in choosing the control points this has been overcome. It is already found that Affine used to change the image view without affecting the details found in the image. It is experimented by combining the Affine with B-Spline which found to enhance the registration of images. This has been proved from the registered images by using similarity criteria as a quantitative measure and by using observers' criteria.

Figure 4. Registration of medical images for Brain image using monomodal registration. (a) represents the reference image. (b) represents the test image to be registered. (c) represents the registered images using Affine, Demons and Affine with B-Spline registration.

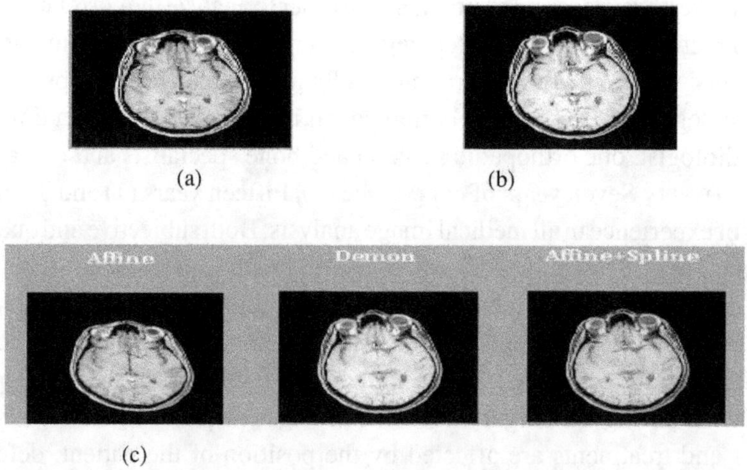

Figure 5. Registration of medical images for Liver image using monomodal registration. (a) represents the reference image. (b) represents the test image to be registered. (c) represents the registered images using Affine, Demons and Affine with B-Spline registration.

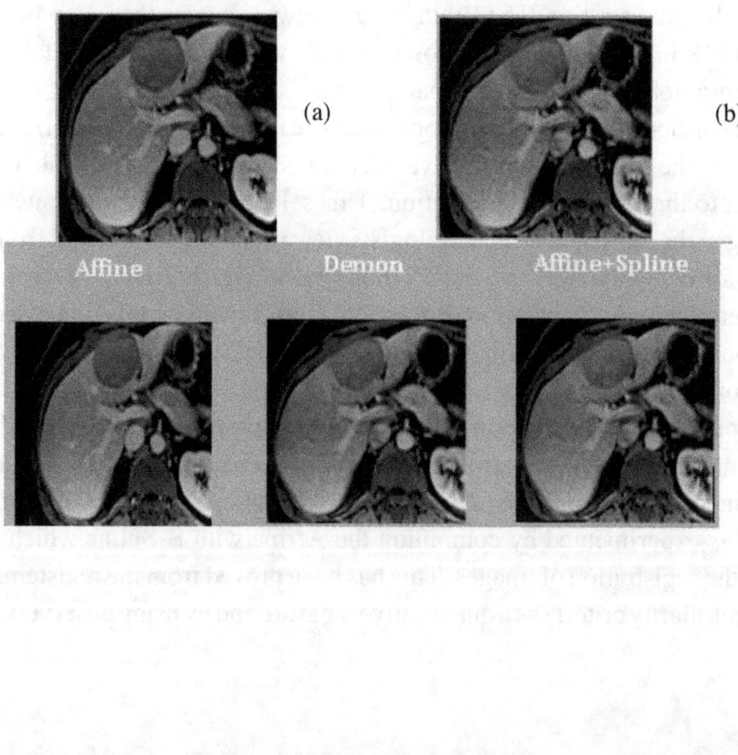

The observers' criterion is based on visual observance. The details are provided in the previous sections.

Figure 6 shows the MR image of the Liver. This T2 weighted slice shows Liver, spleen, aorta, vena cava, stomach, kidneys and thoracic vertebra. Lesser variations in the intensity of images are found for Affine with B-Spline and Demons registered image than Affine. More pathology is found in the Liver images.

Figure 6 shows the MR image of the Knee. It depicts the femur, tibia, fibula, intracondylar notch and menisci with one meniscal tear. Affine with B-Spline registered images found to have lesser changes in the registered image than with the original image. For Demons lesser change in the image is found due to free form deformations. But for Demon

Intensity variations from one patient's to another patient's image detail with possible differences are widely found in MR settings. This limits the use of intensity information in comparing different MR images. This is the reason for performing medical image registration to register the target slice in the MR images and can

Figure 6. Registration of medical images for Knee image using monomodal registration. (a) represents the reference image. (b) represents the test image to be registered. (c) represents the registered images using Affine, Demons and Affine with B-Spline registration.

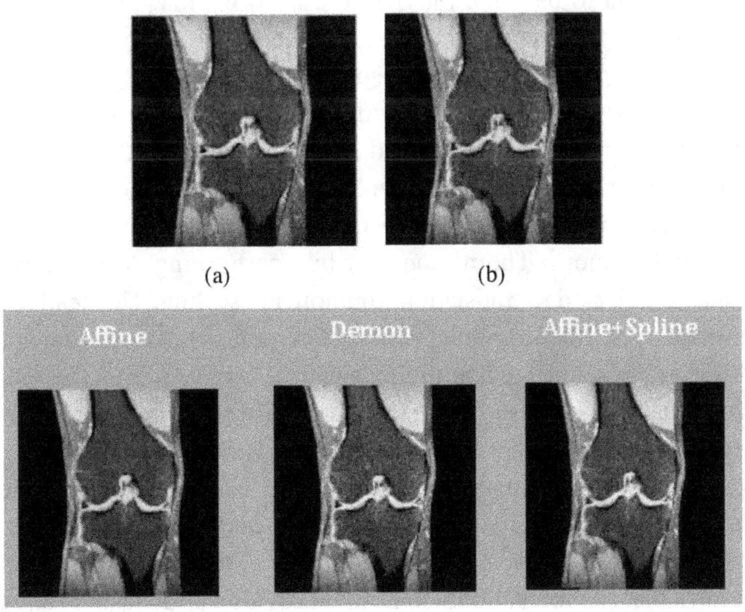

(c)

be effectively used by the radiologists to enhance the clinical diagnosis without disturbing the patient. This is made possible by using this front end design.

Higher similarity between relevant and irrelevant segments in MR images, example such as Brain tissue vs. non-Brain structures in the same slice and relevant slice vs. neighboring slices in the same, makes registration more challenging. Similarly for other images are also compared. In order to have the objective evaluation of the registration system and techniques, experiments have been carried out using medical images. In this section registered images are analyzed using various performance measures. Based on the above analysis results are concluded and justified for clinical assessment and diagnosis. For effective performance measure and registration the condition to be satisfied is, SSD and MI should be found lesser after registration than before registration. The distance before registration will be higher between the images but after applying registration due to the effective change and applying various transformations in the image orientation, SSD and MI metrics i.e. Similarity metrics found to be lesser.

Table 2 shows the measured performance parameter using Affine, Demons and Affine with B-Spline registration applied to the Brain, Liver, and Knee images. The value of SSD and MI before registration is higher while after registration for Affine with B-Spline found to be lesser confirming the best performance for Brain image. It is found that both the similarity metrics SSD and MI found to be lesser for Affine with B-Spline medical image registration than Affine and Demons registration for Brain images. For Liver image the similarity metrics before registration and after registration is found to be same for Affine transformation. The best registration for Liver images is given by Affine with B-Spline registration. The next better is given by Demons registration. For the registration of Knee images the Affine with B-Spline found to be performing better with lesser similarity metrics. The next best performance is given by the Demons and Affine registration respectively.

The above said parameters are shown in Table 2. From the overall analysis it is clear that Affine with B-Spline performs well in registration of medical images than Affine and Demons. The reason is, while performing Affine transform the entire image is subjected to translation, rotation and scaling. This lead to a change in the orientation and hence while selecting control points more care should be given. This led to misaimed registration which is also proved from the SSD metrics and MI metrics, which measures the similarity difference between the registered images and image before registration. B-Spline. Hence this also leads to lesser disorientation of details present in the image. This can be easily identified by the observers' group and qualitatively by metrics SSD and MI. Here comes the reason for the better performance of Affine with B-Spline, the reason is very clear, it is already known that a combination will always provide a good result. Here Affine is chosen because, though it gives orientation changes but, when it is combined with

Table 2. Measured performance parameters using Affine, Demons and Affine with B-Spline based registration for Brain, Liver and Knee images

Performance Parameters Based on Registration	Before Registration (Test Image / Reference Image)	Registration		
		Affine Based Registration	Demons Based Registration	Affine With B-Spline Based Registration
Registration of Brain Image Modality				
SSD	123.1011	135.7515	151.4718	98.5715
MI	1.7181	1.4301	0.6598	1.6902
Registration of Liver Image Modality				
SSD	240.5798	240.299	247.8	124.0495
MI	0.82015	0.9172	0.3434	0.2872
Registration of Knee Image Modality				
SSD	248.57	230.85	187.61	186.06
MI	0.8658	1.5462	0.2052	0.2019

B-Spline which uses basis function with their intimate property of smoothness and multi resolution strategy can able to overcome it. This is the reason for Affine with B-Spline to perform well in monomodal registration of medical images.

Table 3 shows the observers' classification from registered images using Affine, Demons and Affine with B-Spline registration applied to all images. Average of observers' parameters for registration of images score ranges from (0-1) is maximally 1 from observers' classification for Brain, Liver and Knee images. The visual similarity is defined as similarity found in query and all registered image. If maximally both are similar then it is 1 if minimally they are found to be dissimilar then it is 0. Based on the above criteria the visual similarity after performing registration of medical images, does not vary a lot. The information obtained by the radiologists and the users also suits well depending upon their requirement needed for effective clinical

Table 3. Performance parameters from observers' classification using Affine, Demons, Affine with B-Spline based registration for Brain, Liver & Knee images

Observers' Parameters for Images	Observers' Score
Visual similarity of Brain image	1
Visual similarity of Liver image	1
Visual similarity of Knee image	1
Average score of observers' parameters rate	3

diagnosis and hence rated as 1. From the above criteria it is found that registration based on observers' classification also scored well similar to the metrics analysis.

CONCLUSION

The simulated results show the registered images and analysis based on clinical view of the images. A similarity metric is used to compute pixel based / patch based similarity between pixels/patches. In geometry, an affine transformation is a function between affine spaces which preserves points, straight lines and planes. Also, the sets of parallel lines remain parallel after an affine transformation. An affine transformation does not necessarily preserve angles between lines or distances between points, though it does preserve ratios of distances between points lying on a straight line. Hence the variation changes produced by (translation, rotation and shear) pull back its results. In the case of deformable registration, they generally have a regular grid super-imposed over the image and the grid is deformed by solving an optimization problem which is formulated such that the similarity metric and the smoothness penalty imposed over the transformation is minimized (Sotiras, 2013). In deformable registration, once there are deformations over the grid, the final transformation at the pixel level is computed effectively by B-Spline transformation of the grid at the pixel level so that the transformation is smooth and continuous. For each dimension, a 2D array is created which stores B-Splines basis function evaluations for each sample with the weight associated with each control point. Because of local control, many of these weights will be zero indicating that a sample is not affected by a particular control point. This proves the advantage of B-Spline. Hence the B-Spline registration when combined with Affine found to be performed well. It is already found from various experiments by researchers (Diez, 2011; Maintz, 1998; Hill, 2001) that Affine found to have lesser registration results, so have combined lesser performed transformation (Affine) with higher performed transformation (B-Spline) for achieving better results. The advantage of this combination is, the performance of Affine registration is improved by combining with B-Spline by having the added advantage of both transformation functions. The advantage varies on the user's selection of control points in the images. It is also found that Affine with B-Spline equally perform to Demons. Since Contours serves here as a semipermeable membrane, this drives pixels in floating image to move by judging the motion direction of every pixel, and the "Demons" force of every pixel drives floating image to register with reference images, achieving the purpose of non-rigid registration without much deviating from the control points. Since it is a free form Deformation, Demons found to have better results. From the experimental results it is justified that, there is a need for registration in clinical diagnosis. The above justification is proved both by quantitatively and qualitatively. Inter and intra-patient misalignments of the images, because of which anatomical structures are observed at different spatial positions, orientations and scales in the images, can be overcome using medical image registration, which is computationally simple and inexpensive.

The above simulated results show the registered images and analysis based on clinical view of the images. Thus simulated results justifies the need for registration in clinical diagnosis are justified. The advantage varies on the user's selection of control points in the images. The above justification is purely justified by both quantitatively and qualitatively. Inter and intra-patient misalignments of the images, because of which anatomical structures are observed at different spatial positions, orientations and scales in the images, can be overcome using medical image registration. Hence by adopting the registration can solve this problem, which is computationally simple and inexpensive.

REFERENCES

Antonie Maintz & Viergerer. (1998). A survey of medical image registration. *Medical Image Analysis, 2*(1), 1-36.

Arsigny, V., Pennec, X., & Ayache, N. (2005). Polyrigid and PolyAffine Transformations: A novel geometrical tool to deal with non-rigid deformations application to the registration of histological slices. *Medical Image Analysis*, *9*(6), 507–523. doi:10.1016/j.media.2005.04.001 PMID:15948656

Dıez, Y., Martı, R., Oliver, A., & Llado, X. (2010). Comparison of registration methods using mamographic images. *Proceedings of the IEEE international conference image process*, 4421–4424. 10.1109/ICIP.2010.5653325

Hill, Batchelor, Holden, & Hawkes. (2001). Medical image registration. *Physics and Medical Biology, 46*, R1-R45.

Klein, S., Staring, M., & Pluim, J. P. W. (2007). Evaluation of optimization methods for non-rigid medical image registration using mutual information and B-Splines. *IEEE Transactions on Image Processing*, *16*(12), 2879–2890. doi:10.1109/TIP.2007.909412 PMID:18092588

Maes, F., Collignon, A., Vandermeulen, D., Marchal, G., & Suetens, P. (1997). Multimodality image registration by maximization of mutual information. *IEEE Transactions on Medical Imaging*, *16*(2), 187–198. doi:10.1109/42.563664 PMID:9101328

Max, A. (2016). A survey of medical image registration-under review, Medical Image Analysis. *Medical Image Analysis*, *33*, 140–144. PMID:27427472

Pluim, J. P. W., Maintz, J. B. A., & Viergever, M. A. (2000). Interpolation artefacts in mutual information-based image registration. *Computer Vision and Image Understanding*, *77*(2), 211–232. doi:10.1006/cviu.1999.0816

Sotiras, Davatzikos, & Paragios. (2013). Deformable Medical Image Registration: A Survey. IEEE Transactions on Medical Imaging, 32(7), 1153-1190.

Thirion, J. P. (1998). Image matching as a diffusion process: An analogy with Maxwell's demons. *Medical Image Analysis*, *2*(3), 243–260. doi:10.1016/S1361-8415(98)80022-4 PMID:9873902

van den Elsen, P. A., Maintz, J. B. A., Pol, E.-J. D., & Viergever, M. A. (1995). Automatic registration of CT and MR brain images using correlation of geometrical features. *IEEE Transactions on Medical Imaging*, *14*(2), 384–396. doi:10.1109/42.387719 PMID:18215841

Xie, Z., & Farin, G. E. (2004). Image registration using hierarchical B-Splines. *IEEE Transactions on Visualization and Computer Graphics*, *10*(1), 85–94. doi:10.1109/TVCG.2004.1260760 PMID:15382700

Yang, A., Meng, L., Luo, J., & Lin, C. (2007). A rapid registration framework for medical images. *Proceedings of fourth international conference on images and graphics*, 731–736. 10.1109/ICIG.2007.78

Yang, Z., & Cohen, F. S. (1999). Image registration and object recognition using affine invariants and convex hills. *IEEE Transactions on Image Processing*, *8*(7), 934–946. doi:10.1109/83.772236 PMID:18267506

Zitova, B., & Flusser, J. (2003). Image registration methods: A survey. *Image and Vision Computing, Elsevier*, *21*(11), 977–1000. doi:10.1016/S0262-8856(03)00137-9

ADDITIONAL READING

Ayyachamy, S., & Manivannan, V. S. (2013). Medical image registration based retrieval using distance metrics. *International Journal of Imaging Systems and Technology*, *23*(4), 360–371. doi:10.1002/ima.22068

Ayyachamy, S., & Mannivannan, V. (2013). Medical Image Registration Based Retrieval. *Applied Medical Informatics*, *32*(1), 8–20.

Ayyachamy, S., & Mannivannan, V. (2013). Medical Image Retrieval Using Transform. *Applied Medical Informatics*, *32*(2), 54–66.

Ayyachamy, S., & Mannivannan, V. (2013). Content Based Medical Image Retrieval for Histopathological, CT and MRI Images. *Applied Medical Informatics*, *33*(3), 33–45.

Compilation of References

AARP. (n.d.). *Health Tools*. Retrieved from https://www.aarp.org/health/health_tools.html

Acharya & Ray. (2005). *Image processing: Principles and Applications*. Wiley-Inter Science.

Acharya, U. R., Faust, O., Kadri, N. A., Suri, J. S., & Yu, W. (2013). Automated identification of normal and diabetes heart rate signals using nonlinear measures. *Computers in Biology and Medicine*, *43*(10), 1523–1529. doi:10.1016/j.compbiomed.2013.05.024 PMID:24034744

Adnan Tufail, F. R. C. O. (2017). Automated Diabetic Retinopathy Image Assessment Software: Diagnostic Accuracy and Cost-Effectiveness Compared with Human Graders. *American Academy of Ophthalmology*, *124*(3), 343–351. doi:10.1016/j.ophtha.2016.11.014 PMID:28024825

Aeffner, F., Martin, N. T., Peljto, M., Black, J. C., Major, J. K., Jangani, M., ... Young, G. D. (2016). Quantitative assessment of pancreatic cancer precursor lesions in IHC-stained tissue with a tissue image analysis platform. *Laboratory Investigation*, *96*(12), 1327–1336. doi:10.1038/labinvest.2016.111 PMID:27775692

Agar, N., Malcolm, J. G., Mohan, V., Yang, H. W., Johnson, M., Tannenbaum, A., ... Black, P. M. (2010). Imaging of meningioma progression by matrix-assisted laser desorption ionization time-of-flight mass spectrometry. *Analytical Chemistry*, *82*(7), 2621–2625. doi:10.1021/ac100113w PMID:20196536

Ahirwar, A. (2013). Study of Techniques used for Medical Image Segmentation and Computation of Statistical Test for Region Classification of Brain MRI. *I.J. Information Technology and Computer Science*, *5*(5), 44–53. doi:10.5815/ijitcs.2013.05.06

Ahmed, E. (2010). Fast Localization of the Optic Disc Using Projection of Image Features. *IEEE Transactions on Image Processing*, *19*(12), 3285–3289. doi:10.1109/TIP.2010.2052280 PMID:20550999

Ahmed, S. N., Osama, A. H., & Ahmed, H. K. (in press). A decision support system for Acute Leukaemia classification based on digital microscopic images. *Alexandria Engineering Journal*.

Ait-Belkacem, R., Berenguer, C., Villard, C., Ouafik, L., Figarella-Branger, D., Beck, A., ... Lafitte, D. (2014). Monitoring therapeutic monoclonal antibodies in brain tumor. *mAbs*, *6*(6), 1385–1393. doi:10.4161/mabs.34405 PMID:25484065

Amstalden van Hove, E. R., Blackwell, T. R., Klinkert, I., Eijkel, G. B., Heeren, R. M., & Glunde, K. (2010). Multimodal mass spectrometric imaging of small molecules reveals distinct spatio-molecular signatures in differentially metastatic breast tumor models. *Cancer Research*, *70*(22), 9012–9021. doi:10.1158/0008-5472.CAN-10-0360 PMID:21045154

Anand, S., & Rathna, R. A. V. (2013). Architectural Distortion Detection in Mammogram using Contourlet Transform and Texture Features. *International Journal of Computers and Applications*, *74*(5).

Anderson, C. M., Zhang, B., Miller, M., Butko, E., Wu, X., Laver, T., ... Ma, X.-J. (2016). Fully Automated RNAscope In Situ Hybridization Assays for Formalin-Fixed Paraffin-Embedded Cells and Tissues. *Journal of Cellular Biochemistry*, *117*(10), 2201–2208. doi:10.1002/jcb.25606 PMID:27191821

Andrés, G.-F., Ángel, F.-S., Oscar, C.-N., & Cornelio, Y. M. (2017). A machine learning approach to medical image classification: Detecting age-related macular degeneration in fundus images. *Computers & Electrical Engineering*, 1–12.

Angelo, M., Bendall, S. C., Finck, R., Hale, M. B., Hitzman, C., Borowsky, A. D., ... Nolan, G. P. (2014). Multiplexed ion beam imaging (MIBI) of human breast tumors. *Nature Medicine*, *20*(4), 436–442. doi:10.1038/nm.3488 PMID:24584119

Antal, B., & Hajdu, A. (2010). An Ensemble-Based System for Microaneurysm Detection and Diabetic Retinopathy Grading. *IEEE Transactions on Biomedical Engineering*, *59*(6), 1720–1726. doi:10.1109/TBME.2012.2193126 PMID:22481810

Antonie Maintz & Viergerer. (1998). A survey of medical image registration. *Medical Image Analysis, 2*(1), 1-36.

Aquino, A., Gegúndez-Arias, M. E., & Marín, D. (2010). Detecting the Optic Disc Boundary in Digital Fundus Images Using Morphological, Edge Detection, and Feature Extraction Techniques. *IEEE Transactions on Medical Imaging*, *29*(11), 1860–1869. doi:10.1109/TMI.2010.2053042 PMID:20562037

Arsigny, V., Pennec, X., & Ayache, N. (2005). Polyrigid and PolyAffine Transformations: A novel geometrical tool to deal with non-rigid deformations application to the registration of histological slices. *Medical Image Analysis*, *9*(6), 507–523. doi:10.1016/j.media.2005.04.001 PMID:15948656

Associated Osteonecrosis of the Wrist and Knee in Three Pediatric Patients with Recurrent CNS Tumors. (2013). *Journal of Clinical Oncology*, *31*(2).

Axt, J., Murphy, A. J., Seeley, E. H., Martin, C. A., Taylor, C., & Lovvorn, H. N. III. (2011). Race disparities in Wilms tumor incidence and biology. *The Journal of Surgical Research*, *170*(1), 112–119. doi:10.1016/j.jss.2011.03.011 PMID:21529835

Bae, S., Paris, S., & Durand, F. (2006). Two-scale tone management for photographic look. *ACM Transactions on Graphics*, *25*(3), 637. doi:10.1145/1141911.1141935

Balluff, B., Rauser, S., Meding, S., Elsner, M., Schone, C., Feuchtinger, A., ... Walch, A. (2011). MALDI imaging identifies prognostic seven-protein signature of novel tissue markers in intestinal-type gastric cancer. *American Journal of Pathology*, *179*(6), 2720–2729. doi:10.1016/j.ajpath.2011.08.032 PMID:22015459

Bankman, N. (2008). *Handbook of Medical Image Processing and Analysis* (2nd ed.). New York: Academic Press.

Battish, N. (2017). *Analysis of Pre-processing Methods using MRI Images*. Academic Press.

Beolchi, L., & Kuhn, M. H. (1995). *Medical Imaging: Analysis of Multimodality 2D/3D Images*. IOS Press.

Bernal, J., Sánchez, J., & Vilarino, F. (2012). Towards automatic polyp detection with a polyp appearance model. *Pattern Recognition*, *45*(9), 3166–3182. doi:10.1016/j.patcog.2012.03.002

Beutel, J., Kundel, H. L., & Van Metter, R. L. (2000). Handbook of Medical Imaging.: Vol. 1. *Physics and Psychophysics*. Bellingham: SPIE Press.

Bevilacqua, V. (2013). Three-dimensional virtual colonoscopy for automatic polyps detection by artificial neural network approach: New tests on an enlarged cohort of polyps. *Neurocomputing*, *116*, 62–75. doi:10.1016/j.neucom.2012.03.026

Bhonsle, D., Chandra, V., & Sinha, G. R. (2012). Medical Image Denoising Using Bilateral Filter. *I.J. Image, Graphics and Signal Processing, 6*, 36-43. 10.5815/ijigsp.2012.06.06

Bianga, J., Bouslimani, A., Bec, N., Quenet, F., Mounicou, S., Szpunar, J., ... Larroque, C. (2014). Complementarity of MALDI and LA ICP mass spectrometry for platinum anticancer imaging in human tumor. *Metallomics*, *6*(8), 1382–1386. doi:10.1039/C4MT00131A PMID:24984817

Bogoni, L. (n.d.). CAD for Colonography: A tool to address a growing need. *British Journal of Radiology*.

Bohsali, K. I., Wirth, M. A., Rockwood, C. A., Material, S., & Surgery, J. (2010). *Complications of Total Shoulder Arthroplasty*. Academic Press. 10.2106/JBJS.F.00125

Boileau, P., Watkinson, D. J., Hatzidakis, A. M., & Balg, F. (2005). Grammont reverse prosthesis: Design, rationale, and biomechanics. *Journal of Shoulder and Elbow Surgery*, *14*(1S), 147–161. doi:10.1016/j.jse.2004.10.006 PMID:15726075

Boileau, P., Watkinson, D., Hatzidakis, A. M., & Hovorka, I. (2006). Neer Award 2005: The Grammont reverse shoulder prosthesis: Results in cuff tear arthritis, fracture sequelae, and revision arthroplasty. *Journal of Shoulder and Elbow Surgery*, *15*(5), 527–540. doi:10.1016/j.jse.2006.01.003 PMID:16979046

Bolun, C., Ling, C., & Yixin, C. (2013). Efficient ant colony optimization for image feature selection. *Signal Processing*, *93*(6), 1566–1576. doi:10.1016/j.sigpro.2012.10.022

Bond, J. H. (2000). Polyp guideline: Diagnosis, treatment, and surveillance for patients with colorectal polyps. *The American Journal of Gastroenterology*, *95*(11), 3053–3063. doi:10.1111/j.1572-0241.2000.03434.x PMID:11095318

Bozek, J., & Dumic, E. (2009). Bilateral asymmetry detection in digital mammography using B-spline interpolation. In Systems, Signals and Image (pp. 1-4). IEEE.

Bryan, R. N. (2010). *Introduction to the Science of Medical Imaging*. Cambridge, UK: Cambridge University Press.

Buades, A., Coll, B., & Morel, J.-M. J.-M. (2005). A non-local algorithm for image denoising. *Computer Vision and Pattern Recognition, 2005. CVPR 2005. IEEE Computer Society Conference on, 2*, 60–65. 10.1109/CVPR.2005.38

Buck, F. M., Jost, B., & Hodler, J. (2008). Shoulder arthroplasty. *European Radiology*, *18*(12), 2937–2948. doi:10.100700330-008-1093-8 PMID:18618117

Burak, Rubin, Napel, Beaulieu, Greenspan, & Acer. (2011). Content-based image retrieval in radiology: current status and future directions. *Journal of Digital Imaging, 24*(2), 208-222.

Calligaris, D., Caragacianu, D., Liu, X., Norton, I., Thompson, C. J., Richardson, A. L., ... Agar, N. Y. R. (2014). Application of desorption electrospray ionization mass spectrometry imaging in breast cancer margin analysis. *Proceedings of the National Academy of Sciences of the United States of America*, *111*(42), 15184–15189. doi:10.1073/pnas.1408129111 PMID:25246570

Cancer Imaging Archives. (2017). *TCIA Collections*. Retrieved from http://cancerimagingarchive.net

Carter, J. M., Caron, B. L., Dogan, A., & Folpe, A. L. (2015). A novel chromogenic in situ hybridization assay for FGF23 mRNA in phosphaturic mesenchymal tumors. *The American Journal of Surgical Pathology*, *39*(1), 75–83. doi:10.1097/PAS.0000000000000290 PMID:25025444

Casadonte, R., & Caprioli, R. M. (2011). Proteomic analysis of formalin- fixed paraffin-embedded tissue by MALDI imaging mass spectrometry. *Nature Protocols*, *6*(11), 1695–1709. doi:10.1038/nprot.2011.388 PMID:22011652

Casadonte, R., Longuespée, R., Kriegsmann, J., & Kriegsmann, M. (2017). MALDI IMS and Cancer Tissue Microarrays. *Advances in Cancer Research*, *134*, 173–200. doi:10.1016/bs.acr.2016.11.007 PMID:28110650

Cauvin, J. M., Le Guillou, C., Solaiman, B., Robaszkiewicz, M., Le Beux, P., & Roux, C. (2003). Computer-assisted diagnosis system in digestive endoscopy. *IEEE Transactions on Information Technology in Biomedicine*, *7*(4), 256–262. doi:10.1109/TITB.2003.823293 PMID:15000352

Cazares, L. H., Troyer, D., Mendrinos, S., Lance, R. A., & Nyalwidhe, J. O. (2009). Imaging mass spectrometry of a specific fragment of mitogen-activated protein kinase/extracellular signal-regulated kinase 2 discriminates cancer from uninvolved prostate tissue. *Clinical Cancer Research*, *15*, 5541–5551. doi:10.1158/1078-0432.CCR-08-2892 PMID:19690195

Centers for Disease Control and Prevention (CDC). (2011). Vital signs: Colorectal cancer screening, incidence, and mortality--United States, 2002-2010. *MMWR. Morbidity and Mortality Weekly Report*, *60*(26), 884. PMID:21734636

Chan, H. P., Wei, J., Zhang, Y., Helvie, M. A., Moore, R. H., Sahiner, B., & Kopans, D. B. (2008). Computer-aided detection of masses in digital tomosynthesis mammography: Comparison of three approaches. *Medical Physics*, *35*(9), 4087–4095. doi:10.1118/1.2968098 PMID:18841861

Chan, W. Y., Law, N. F., & Siu, W. C. (2003). Multiscale Feature Analysis Using Directional Filter Bank. *International Conference on Information, Communications and Signal Processing*, 2, 822-826. 10.1109/ICICS.2003.1292571

Chaurand, P., Fouchécourt, S., DaGue, B. B., Xu, B. J., Reyzer, M. L., Orgebin-Crist, M. C., & Caprioli, R. M. (2003). Profiling and imaging proteins in the mouse epididymis by imaging mass spectrometry. *Proteomics*, *3*(11), 2221–2239. doi:10.1002/pmic.200300474 PMID:14595821

Chen, D., Abdelmunim, H., Farag, A. A., Falk, R., & Dryden, G. (2008, September). Segmentation of colon tissue in ct colonography using adaptive level sets method. In MICCAI 2008 workshop: computational and visualization challenges in the new era of virtual colonoscopy (pp. 108-115). Academic Press.

Chen, X. W., & Tian, J. W. (2010). Wavelet-contourlet texture image retrieval system. *Computer Engineering and Applications*, *46*, 11–13.

Choi, J. H., Shin, N. R., Moon, H. J., Kwon, C. H., & Kim, G. H. (2012). Identification of S100A8 and S100A9 as negative regulators for lymph node metastasis of gastric adenocarcinoma. *Histology and Histopathology*, *27*, 1439–1448. PMID:23018243

Choras, R. S. (2007). Image feature Extraction techniques and their applications for CBIR and Biometrics system. *International Journal of Biology and Biomedical Engineering, 1*(1), 231-238.

Chowdhury, T. A., Whelan, P. F., & Ghita, O. (2008). A fully automatic CAD-CTC system based on curvature analysis for standard and low-dose CT data. *IEEE Transactions on Biomedical Engineering*, *55*(3), 888–901. doi:10.1109/TBME.2007.909506 PMID:18334380

Chughtai, K., Jiang, L., Greenwood, T. R., Glunde, K., & Heeren, R. M. (2013). Mass spectrometry images acylcarnitines, phosphatidylcholines, and sphingomyelin in MDA-MB-231 breast tumor models. *Journal of Lipid Research*, *54*(2), 333–344. doi:10.1194/jlr.M027961 PMID:22930811

Comaniciu, D., Meer, P., & Foran, D. J. (1999). Image-guided decision support system for pathology. *Machine Vision and Applications*, *11*(4), 213–224. doi:10.1007001380050104

Cornett, D. S., Mobley, J. A., Dias, E. C., Andersson, M., Arteaga, C. L., Sanders, M. E., & Caprioli, R. M. (2006). A novel histology- directed strategy for MALDI-MS tissue profiling that improves throughput and cellular specificity in human breast cancer. *Molecular & Cellular Proteomics*, *5*(10), 1975–1983. doi:10.1074/mcp.M600119-MCP200 PMID:16849436

Cryan, J. B., Haidar, S., Ramkissoon, L. A., Bi, W. L., Knoff, D. S., Schultz, N., ... Ramkissoon, S. H. (2014). Clinical multiplexed exome sequencing distinguishes adult oligodendroglial neoplasms from astrocytic and mixed lineage gliomas. *Oncotarget*, *5*(18), 8083–8092. doi:10.18632/oncotarget.2342 PMID:25257301

Cucoranu, I. C., Parwani, A. V., Vepa, S., Weinstein, R. S., & Pantanowitz, L. (2014). Digital pathology: A systematic evaluation of the patent landscape. *Journal of Pathology Informatics*, *5*(1), 16. doi:10.4103/2153-3539.133112 PMID:25057430

da Cunha, A. L., Zhou, J., & Do, M. N. (2006, October). The Nonsubsampled Contourlet Transform: Theory, Design, and Applications. *IEEE Transactions on Image Processing*, *15*(10), 3089–3101. doi:10.1109/TIP.2006.877507 PMID:17022272

Dash, R., Sa, P. K., & Majhi, B. (2011). *Spatial Variant Deblurring of Images*, International Journal of Computational Vision and Robotics. *Inderscience Publishers*, *2*(1), 80–88.

Dekker, T. J., Balluff, B. D., Jones, E. A., Schöne, C. D., Schmitt, M., Aubele, M., ... McDonnell, L. A. (2014). Multicenter matrix-assisted laser desorption/ionization mass spectrometry imaging (MALDI MSI) identifies proteomic differences in breast-cancer-associated stroma. *Journal of Proteome Research*, *13*(11), 4730–4738. doi:10.1021/pr500253j PMID:24762205

Depeursinge, A., Fischer, B., Müller, H., & Deserno, T. M. (2011). Prototypes for content-based image retrieval in clinical practice. *Journal of Open Medical Informatics*, *5*(1), 58–72. doi:10.2174/1874431101105010058 PMID:21892374

Deselaers, T. (2003). *Features for image retrieval* (Master thesis). University of Rhine-Westphalia Alsiche Technical University of Aachen.

Deutsch, A., Abboud, J. A., Kelly, J., Mody, M., Norris, T., Ramsey, M. L., ... Williams, G. R. (2007). Clinical results of revision shoulder arthroplasty for glenoid component loosening. *Journal of Shoulder and Elbow Surgery*, *16*(6), 706–716. doi:10.1016/j.jse.2007.01.007 PMID:17931898

Diagnostic and Interventional Radiology. (n.d.). Retrieved from www.dirjournal.org

DICOM. (2018). Retrieved from Dicom.nema.org

Dıez, Y., Martı, R., Oliver, A., & Llado, X. (2010). Comparison of registration methods using mamographic images. *Proceedings of the IEEE international conference image process*, 4421–4424. 10.1109/ICIP.2010.5653325

Dimitrovski, I., Kocev, D., Kitanovski, I., Loskovska, S., & Džeroski, S. (2015). Improved medical image modality classification using a combination of visual and textual features. *Computerized Medical Imaging and Graphics*, *39*, 14–26. doi:10.1016/j.compmedimag.2014.06.005 PMID:24997992

Djaafar, Z., & Fouad, B. A. (2018). A cooperative swarm intelligence algorithm based on quantum-inspired and rough sets for feature selection. *Computers & Industrial Engineering*, *115*, 26–36. doi:10.1016/j.cie.2017.10.025

Djidja, M. C., Claude, E., Snel, M. F., Francese, S., Scriven, P., Carolan, V., & Clench, M. R. (2010). Novel molecular tumour classification using MALDI-mass spectrometry imaging of tissue micro-array. *Analytical and Bioanalytical Chemistry*, *397*(2), 587–601. doi:10.100700216-010-3554-6 PMID:20204332

Djidja, M. C., Claude, E., Snel, M. F., Scriven, P., Francese, S., Carolan, V., & Clench, M. R. (2009). MALDI-ion mobility separation-mass spectrometry imaging of glucose-regulated protein 78 kDa (Grp78) in human formalin-fixed, paraffin-embedded pancreatic adenocarcinoma tissue sections. *Journal of Proteome Research*, *8*(10), 4876–4884. doi:10.1021/pr900522m PMID:19673544

Doi, K. (2009). *Computer-aided diagnosis in medical imaging: achievements and challenges*. Paper presented at the World Congress on Medical Physics and Biomedical Engineering, Munich, Germany. 10.1007/978-3-642-03904-1_26

Doi, K. (2014). Current status and future potential of computer-aided diagnosis in medical imaging. *The British Journal of Radiology*, *78*(suppl_1), S3–S19. doi:10.1259/bjr/82933343 PMID:15917443

Do, M. N., & Vetterli, M. (2002). Contourlets: A Directional Multiresolution Image Representation. In *International Conference on Image Processing* (Vol. 1). IEEE. 10.1109/ICIP.2002.1038034

Do, M. N., & Vetterli, M. (2003). The contourlet transform: An efficient directional multiresolution image representation. *IEEE Transactions on Image Processing*, *14*(12), 2091–2106. doi:10.1109/TIP.2005.859376 PMID:16370462

Dorsey, J., & Durand, F. (2002). Fast Bilateral Filtering for the Display of High-Dynamic-Range Images Introduction. *Vine*, 257–266.

Dos Santos Teixeira, R. F. (2012). *Computer analysis of mammography images to aid diagnosis*. MSc in Biomedical Engineering, Faculdade de Engenharia da Universidade do Porto, 35.

Dougherty, D. (2009). *Digital Image Processing for Medical Applications*. Cambridge, UK: Cambridge University Press.

Drak Alsibai, K., Azoulay, S., Languille-Mimoune, O., Poulet, B., Barres, A., & Adem, C. (2013a). Digital Imaging in Breast Cancer: An Ode to Microscopy. USCAP Poster Session V (Abstract 2048). *Modern Patho*logy, *26*(S2), 489-504. doi:10.1038/modpathol.2013.26

Drak Alsibai, K., Denis, B., Bottlaender, J., Kleinclaus, I., Straub, P., & Fabre, M. (2006). Impact of cytopathologist expert on diagnosis and treatment of pancreatic lesions in current clinical practice. A series of 106 endoscopic ultrasound-guided fine needle aspirations. *Cytopathology*, *17*(1), 18–26. doi:10.1111/j.1365-2303.2006.00312.x PMID:16417561

Drak Alsibai, K., & Meseure, D. (2018). Tumor microenvironment and noncoding RNAs as co-drivers of epithelial-mesenchymal transition and cancer metastasis. *Developmental Dynamics*, *247*(3), 405–431. doi:10.1002/dvdy.24548 PMID:28691356

Duraiyan, J., Govindarajan, R., Kaliyappan, K., & Palanisamy, M. (2012). Applications of immunohistochemistry. *Journal of Pharmacy & Bioallied Sciences*, *4*(6Suppl 2), S307–S309. doi:10.4103/0975-7406.100281 PMID:23066277

Eberlin, L. S., Norton, I., Orringer, D., Dunn, I. F., Liu, X., Ide, J. L., ... Cooks, R. G. (2013). Ambient mass spectrometry for the intraoperative molecular diagnosis of human brain tumors. *Proceedings of the National Academy of Sciences of the United States of America*, *110*(5), 1611–1616. doi:10.1073/pnas.1215687110 PMID:23300285

Egmentation, S., Pham, D. L., Xu, C., & Prince, J. L. (2000). Current methods in medical image segmentation. *Annual Review of Biomedical Engineering*, *2*(1), 315–337. doi:10.1146/annurev.bioeng.2.1.315 PMID:11701515

Eikrem, O., Beisland, C., Hjelle, K., Flatberg, A., Scherer, A., Landolt, L., ... Marti, H.-P. (2016). Transcriptome Sequencing (RNAseq) Enables Utilization of Formalin-Fixed, Paraffin-Embedded Biopsies with Clear Cell Renal Cell Carcinoma for Exploration of Disease Biology and Biomarker Development. *PLoS One*, *11*(2), e0149743. doi:10.1371/journal.pone.0149743 PMID:26901863

Elsner, M., Rauser, S., Maier, S., Schone, C., Balluff, B., Meding, S., ... Walch, A. (2012). MALDI imaging mass spectrometry reveals COX7A2, TAGLN2 and S100-A10 as novel prognostic markers in Barrett's adenocarcinoma. *Journal of Proteomics*, *75*(15), 4693–4704. doi:10.1016/j.jprot.2012.02.012 PMID:22365974

Eriksson, C., Masaki, N., Yao, I., Hayasaka, T., & Setou, M. (2013). MALDI Imaging Mass Spectrometry—A Mini Review of Methods and Recent Developments. *Mass Spectrometry (Tokyo, Japan)*, *2*(Spec Iss), S0022. doi:10.5702/massspectrometry.S0022 PMID:24349941

Esbona, K., Inman, D., Saha, S., Jeffery, J., Schedin, P., Wilke, L., & Keely, P. (2016). COX-2 modulates mammary tumor progression in response to collagen density. *Breast Cancer Research : BCR*, *18*(1), 35. doi:10.118613058-016-0695-3 PMID:27000374

Extrahop. (2016). *An Introduction to DICOM (Digital Imaging and Communications in Medicine)*. Retrieved from https://www.extrahop.com/company/blog/2016/introduction-to-dicom-protocol/

Fan, J., & Yau, D. K. Y. (2001). Automatic image segmentation by integrating color-edge extractionand seeded region growing. *IEEE Transactions on Image Processing*, *10*(10), 1454–1466. doi:10.1109/83.951532 PMID:18255490

Fan, Y. W., & Nagy, J. G. (2010). Synthetic boundary conditions for image blurring. *Linear Algebra and Its Applications*, *434*(11), 2244–2268. doi:10.1016/j.laa.2009.12.021

Farahani, N., Braun, A., Jutt, D., Huffman, T., Reder, N., Liu, Z., ... Pantanowitz, L. (2017). Three-dimensional Imaging and Scanning: Current and Future Applications for Pathology. *Journal of Pathology Informatics*, *8*(1), 36. doi:10.4103/jpi.jpi_32_17 PMID:28966836

Farahani, N., Parwani, A. V., & Pantanowitz, L. (2015). Whole slide imaging in pathology: Advantages, limitations, and emerging perspectives. *Pathology and Laboratory Medicine International: PLMI*, *7*, 23–33.

Farshad, M., & Gerber, C. (2010). Reverse total shoulder arthroplasty-from the most to the least common complication. *International Orthopaedics*, *34*(8), 1075–1082. doi:10.100700264-010-1125-2 PMID:20865260

Farsiu, S., Robinson, D., Elad, M., & Milanfar, P. (2004). Advances and Challenges in Super resolution. *International Journal of Imaging Systems and Technology*, *14*(2), 47–57. doi:10.1002/ima.20007

Fiori, M., Musé, P., & Sapiro, G. (2011). *A complete system for polyps flagging in virtual colonoscopy*. Academic Press.

Gautherie, M. (1983). Thermobiological Assessment of Benign and Malignant Breast Diseases. *American Journal of Obstetrics and Gynecology*, *8*(8), 861–869. doi:10.1016/0002-9378(83)90236-3 PMID:6650622

Gayathri Devi, K., & Radhakrishnan, R. (2015). Automatic segmentation of colon in 3D CT images and removal of opacified fluid using cascade feed forward neural network. *Computational and mathematical methods in medicine*.

Gayathri Devi, K., & Radhakrishnan, R. (2014). A Comparative Study on the Automatic Segmentation of Colon in CT Colonography Using K- Means And Fuzzy C-Means Clustering. *Australian Journal of Basic and Applied Sciences*, *8*(9), 422–432.

Geert, L., Thijs, K., Babak, E. B., Arnaud, A. A., Francesco, C., Mohsen, G., ... Clara, I. S. (2017). A survey on deep learning in medical image analysis. *Medical Image Analysis*, *42*, 60–88. doi:10.1016/j.media.2017.07.005 PMID:28778026

Geethu, M. M., & Monica, S. (2018). MRI based medical image analysis: Survey on brain tumor grade classification. *Biomedical Signal Processing and Control*, *39*, 139–161. doi:10.1016/j.bspc.2017.07.007

Gerdes, M. J., Sevinsky, C. J., Sood, A., Adak, S., Bello, M. O., Bordwell, A., ... Ginty, F. (2013). Highly multiplexed single-cell analysis of formalin-fixed, paraffin-embedded cancer tissue. *Proceedings of the National Academy of Sciences of the United States of America*, *110*(29), 11982–11987. doi:10.1073/pnas.1300136110 PMID:23818604

Ghafurian, S., Galdi, B., Bastian, S., Tan, V., & Li, K. (2016). Computerized 3D morphological analysis of glenoid orientation. *Journal of Orthopaedic Research*, *34*(4), 692–698. doi:10.1002/jor.23053 PMID:26400654

Gharipour, A., & Liew, A. W. C. (2013, July). Colon cell image segmentation based on level set and kernel-based fuzzy clustering. In *International Conference on Intelligent Computing* (pp. 120-129). Springer. 10.1007/978-3-642-39482-9_14

Giancardo, Meriaudeau, Karnowski, Li, Garg, Tobin Jr., & Chaum. (2012). Exudate-based diabetic macular edema detection in fundus images using publicly available datasets. *Medical Image Analysis*, *16*(1), 216–226. PMID:21865074

Gletsos, M., Mougiakakou, S. G., Matsopoulos, G. K., Nikita, K. S., Nikita, A. S., & Kelekis, D. (2003). A computer-aided diagnostic system to characterize CT focal liver lesions: Design and optimization of a neural network classifier. *IEEE Transactions on Information Technology in Biomedicine*, *7*(3), 153–162. doi:10.1109/TITB.2003.813793 PMID:14518728

Goatman, K. A., Fleming, A. D., Philip, S., Williams, G. J., Olson, J. A., & Sharp, P. F. (2011). Detection of new vessels on the optic disc using retinal photographs. *IEEE Transactions on Medical Imaging*, *30*(4), 972–979. doi:10.1109/TMI.2010.2099236 PMID:21156389

Godinho. (2016, January). A Routing Mechanism for Cloud Outsourcing of Medical Imaging Repositories. *IEEE Journal of Biomedical and Health Informatics*, *20*(1).

Gonçalves, V. M., Delamaro, M. E., & Nuns, F. L. S. (2014). A systematic review on the evaluation and characteristics of computer-aided diagnosis systems. *Revista Brasileira de Engenharia Biomédica*, *30*(4), 355–383. doi:10.1590/1517-3151.0517

Gondhalekar, C., Rajwa, B., Patsekin, V., Ragheb, K., Sturgis, J., & Robinson, J.P. (2018). Alternatives to current flow cytometry data analysis for clinical and research studies. *Methods*, *1*(134-135), 113-129. doi: 10.1016/j.ymeth.2017.12.009

Gonzalez, R. C., & Woods, R. E. (2002). *Digital Image processing* (2nd ed.). Prentice Hall of India.

Gonzalez, R., & Woods, R. (2008). *Digital image processing* (3rd ed.). Prentice Hall of India.

Gravel, P., Beaudoin, G., & De Guise, J. A. (2004). A method for modeling noise in medical images. *IEEE Transactions on Medical Imaging*, *23*(10), 1221–1232. doi:10.1109/TMI.2004.832656 PMID:15493690

Grigorescu, S. E., Nevo, S. T., Liedenbaum, M. H., Truyen, R., Stoker, J., Van Vliet, L. J., & Vos, F. M. (2010). Automated detection and segmentation of large lesions in CT Colonography. *IEEE Transactions on Biomedical Engineering*, *57*(3), 675–684. doi:10.1109/TBME.2009.2035632 PMID:19884071

Groseclose, M. R., Massion, P. P., Chaurand, P., & Caprioli, R. M. (2008). High-throughput proteomic analysis of formalin-fixed paraffin- embedded tissue microarrays using MALDI imaging mass spectrometry. *Proteomics*, *8*(18), 3715–3724. doi:10.1002/pmic.200800495 PMID:18712763

Grüner, B. M., Winkelmann, I., Feuchtinger, A., Sun, N., Balluff, B., Teichmann, N., ... Siveke, J. T. (2016, May). Modeling Therapy Response and Spatial Tissue Distribution of Erlotinib in Pancreatic Cancer. *Molecular Cancer Therapeutics*, *15*(5), 1145–1152. doi:10.1158/1535-7163.MCT-15-0165 PMID:26823494

Guy, C. (2005). *Introduction to the Principles of Medical Imaging*. London: Imperial College Press. doi:10.1142/p363

Hajiaghayi, M., Groves, E. M., Jafarkhani, H., & Kheradvar, A. (2017, January). A 3-D Active Contour Method for Automated Segmentation of the Left Ventricle From Magnetic Resonance Images. *IEEE Transactions on Biomedical Engineering*, *64*(1), 134–144. doi:10.1109/TBME.2016.2542243 PMID:27046887

Hamdi. (2012). A Comparative Study in Wavelets, Curvelets and Contourlets as Denoising Biomedical Images. *I.J. Image. Graphics and Signal Processing*, *1*, 44–50.

Hammond, J. W., Queale, W. S., Kim, T. K., & McFarland, E. G. (2003). Surgeon experience and clinical and economic outcomes for shoulder arthroplasty. *The Journal of Bone and Joint Surgery. American Volume*, *85–A*(12), 2318–2324. doi:10.2106/00004623-200312000-00008 PMID:14668500

Hampshire, T., Roth, H. R., Helbren, E., Plumb, A., Boone, D., Slabaugh, G., & Hawkes, D. J. (2013). Endoluminal surface registration for CT colonography using haustral fold matching. *Medical Image Analysis*, *17*(8), 946–958. doi:10.1016/j.media.2013.04.006 PMID:23845949

Han, J., & Kamber, M. (2011). *Data mining: Concepts and techniques* (3rd ed.). Burlington, MA: Elsevier.

Hanna, M.G., Pantanowitz, L., & Evans, A.J. (2015). Overview of contemporary guidelines in digital pathology: what is available in 2015 and what still needs to be addressed? *Journal of Clinical Pathology, 68*(7), 499-505. doi: 10.1136/jclinpath-2015-202914

Hardesty, W. M., Kelley, M. C., Mi, D., Low, R. L., & Caprioli, R. M. (2011). Protein signatures for survival and recurrence in metastatic melanoma. *Journal of Proteomics*, *74*(7), 1002–1014. doi:10.1016/j.jprot.2011.04.013 PMID:21549228

Harry's Chest Atlas. (n.d.). *Medical image database*. Retrieved on April 15, 2013 from http://www.Chestatlas.com

Hasan, S. S., Leith, J. M., Smith, K. L., & Matsen, F. A. III. (2003). The distribution of shoulder replacement among surgeons and hospitals is significantly different than that of hip or knee replacement. *Journal of Shoulder and Elbow Surgery*, *12*(2), 164–169. doi:10.1067/mse.2003.23 PMID:12700570

Hegadi, R., Kop, A., & Hangarge, M. (2010). A Survey on Deformable Model and its Applications to Medical Imaging. *International Journal of Computer Applications, RTIPPR*(2), 64–75. Retrieved from http://www.ijcaonline.org/rtippr/number2/SPE101T.pdf%5Cnhttp://files/394/A Survey on Deformable Model and its Applications .pdf%5Cnhttp://files/396/SPE101T.html

Heywang, S. H., Wolf, A., Pruss, E., Hilbertz, T., Eiermann, W., & Permanetter, W. (1989). MR imaging of the breast with Gd-DTPA: Use and limitations. *Radiology*, *171*(1), 95–103. doi:10.1148/radiology.171.1.2648479 PMID:2648479

Higgins, C. (2015, July). Applications and challenges of digital pathology and whole slide imaging. *Biotechnic & Histochemistry*, *90*(5), 341–347. doi:10.3109/10520295.2015.1044566 PMID:25978139

Hill, Batchelor, Holden, & Hawkes. (2001). Medical image registration. *Physics and Medical Biology, 46*, R1-R45.

Hiremath, P. S., & Prema, T. (2010). Speckle Reducing Contourlet Transform for Medical Ultrasound Image. *International Journal of Computer and Information Engineering*, *4*, 4.

Hong, S., Cui, W.-C., & Li, T. (2005). Medical image description in content-based image retrieval. *Proceedings of the IEEE Engineering in Medicine and Biology 27th Annual Conference*, 6336-6339.

Hong, W., Gu, X., Qiu, F., Jin, M., & Kaufman, A. (2006, June). Conformal virtual colon flattening. In *Proceedings of the 2006 ACM symposium on Solid and physical modeling* (pp. 85-93). ACM. 10.1145/1128888.1128901

Horn, C. L., DeKoning, L., Klonowski, P., & Naugler, C. (2014). Current usage and future trends in gross digital photography in Canada. *BMC Medical Education*, *14*(1), 11. doi:10.1186/1472-6920-14-11 PMID:24422898

Huang, A., Li, J., Summers, R. M., Petrick, N., & Hara, A. K. (2010). Improving polyp detection algorithms for CT colonography: Pareto front approach. *Pattern Recognition Letters*, *31*(11), 1461–1469. doi:10.1016/j.patrec.2010.03.013 PMID:20548966

Hunter, D. J., Guermazi, A., Lo, G. H., Grainger, A. J., Conaghan, P. G., Boudreau, R. M., & Roemer, F. W. (2011). Evolution of semi-quantitative whole joint assessment of knee OA: MOAKS (MRI Osteoarthritis Knee Score). *Osteoarthritis and Cartilage*, *19*(8), 990–1002. doi:10.1016/j.joca.2011.05.004 PMID:21645627

Iannotti, J. P., Greeson, C., Downing, D., Sabesan, V., & Bryan, J. A. (2012). Effect of glenoid deformity on glenoid component placement in primary shoulder arthroplasty. *Journal of Shoulder and Elbow Surgery*, *21*(1), 48–55. doi:10.1016/j.jse.2011.02.011 PMID:21600787

Ivan, S., Ilya, I., & Andrey, F. (2016). New Approaches to Parallelization in Filters Aggregation Based Feature Selection Algorithms. *Procedia Computer Science*, *101*, 45–52. doi:10.1016/j.procs.2016.11.007

Iyer, S., & Gogawale, S. V. (2006). *Image enhancemement and restoration techniques in digital image processing*. Computer Society of India Communications.

Jain, A.K. (2005). *Fundamentals of Digital Image Processing* (4th ed.). Pearson Education.

Jain, A.K. (2005). *Fundamentals of Digital Image Processing* (4th ed.). Pearson Education.

James, D., Clymer, B. D., & Schmalbrock, P. (2001). Texture detection of simulated microcalcification susceptibility effects in magnetic resonance imaging of breasts. *Journal of Magnetic Resonance Imaging*, *13*(6), 876–881. doi:10.1002/jmri.1125 PMID:11382947

Jan, J. (2005). *Medical Image Processing, Reconstruction and Restoration: Concepts and Methods*. CRC Press. doi:10.1201/9781420030679

Jatoi, I., & Kaufmann, M. (2010). Management of breast diseases. Springer. doi:10.1007/978-3-540-69743-5

Jayaraman, S., Esakkirajan, S., & Veerakima, T. (2010). Digital Image Processing (3rd ed.). Tata McGraw Hill Education Private Limited.

Jayaraman, S., Esakkirajan, S., & Veerakima, T. (n.d.). *Digital Image Processing* (3rd ed.). Tata McGraw Hill Education Private Limited.

Jefferson, T. O., Huei, D. L., Newton, S., Claudio, S. R. C., & Feng, C. W. (in press). Prototype System for Feature Extraction, Classification and Study of Medical Images. *Expert Systems with Applications.*

Jeong, J. W., Chae, S. H., Chae, E. Y., Kim, H. H., Choi, Y. W., & Lee, S. (2016). Three-Dimensional Computer-Aided Detection of Microcalcification Clusters in Digital Breast Tomosynthesis. *BioMed Research International*, *2016*, 1–8. doi:10.1155/2016/8651573 PMID:27274993

Jiang, Fang, & Tang. (2010). Texture Image Retrieval by Multi-directional Information Fusion of Wavelet Domain. *Computer Engineering*, 215-217.

Jinsamol, K., Shiji, T., & Thomas, V. (2015). CAD system for breast ultrasound images using multi-scale blob detection and active contour segmentation algorithm. *International Conference on Information Science (ICIS' 14).*

Kainz, P., Pfeiffer, M., & Urschler, M. (2017). Segmentation and classification of colon glands with deep convolutional neural networks and total variation regularization. *PeerJ*, *5*, e3874. doi:10.7717/peerj.3874 PMID:29018612

Kamavisdar, P., Saluja, S., & Agrawal, S. (2013). A survey on image classification approaches and techniques. *International Journal of Advertising*, *2*(1), 1005–1009. Retrieved from http://ijarcce.com/upload/january/22-A Survey on Image Classification.pdf

Kampf, C., Olsson, I., Ryberg, U., Sjöstedt, E., & Pontén, F. (2012). Production of Tissue Microarrays, Immunohistochemistry Staining and Digitalization Within the Human Protein Atlas. *Journal of Visualized Experiments*, *3620*(63). doi:10.3791/3620 PMID:22688270

Kamran, Nasri, Nezamabadi-Pour, & Saryazdi. (2012). Image denoising in the wavelet domain using Improved Neigh-shrink. *National Conference New Idea In Electrical Engineering (NCNIEE).*

Kang, S., Shim, H. S., Lee, J. S., Kim, D. S., Kim, H. Y., Hong, S. H., ... Cho, N. H. (2010). Molecular proteomics imaging of tumor interfaces by mass spectrometry. *Journal of Proteome Research*, *9*(2), 1157–1164. doi:10.1021/pr900666q PMID:19821573

Karelse, A., Leuridan, S., Van Tongel, A., Piepers, I. M., Debeer, P., & De Wilde, L. F. (2014). A glenoid reaming study: How accurate are current reaming techniques? *Journal of Shoulder and Elbow Surgery*, *23*(8), 1120–1127. doi:10.1016/j.jse.2013.11.023 PMID:24582954

Kårsnäs, A., Dahl, A. L., & Larsen, R. (2011). Learning histopathological patterns. *Journal of Pathology Informatics*, *2*(2), S12. doi:10.4103/2153-3539.92033 PMID:22811956

Kim, D. H., Kim, S. T., & Ro, Y. M. (2015). Improving mass detection using combined feature representations from projection views and reconstructed volume of DBT and boosting based classification with feature selection. *Physics in Medicine and Biology*, *60*(22), 8809–8832. doi:10.1088/0031-9155/60/22/8809 PMID:26529080

Kim, H. K., Reyzer, M. L., Choi, I. J., Kim, C. G., Kim, H. S., Oshima, A., ... Green, J. E. (2010). Gastric cancer-specific protein profile identified using endoscopic biopsy samples via MALDI mass spectrometry. *Journal of Proteome Research*, *9*(8), 4123–4130. doi:10.1021/pr100302b PMID:20557134

Kim, M. S., Kwon, S., & Park, J. K. (2013). Breast cancer diagnostics using microfluidic multiplexed immunohistochemistry. *Methods in Molecular Biology (Clifton, N.J.)*, *949*, 349–364. doi:10.1007/978-1-62703-134-9_22 PMID:23329453

Kim, S. H., Wise, B. L., Zhang, Y., & Szabo, R. M. (2011). Increasing incidence of shoulder arthroplasty in the United States. *The Journal of Bone and Joint Surgery. American Volume*, *93*(24), 2249–2254. doi:10.2106/JBJS.J.01994 PMID:22258770

Kim, S. T., Kim, D. H., & Ro, Y. M. (2014). Breast mass detection using slice conspicuity in 3D reconstructed digital breast volumes. *Physics in Medicine and Biology*, *59*(17), 5003–5023. doi:10.1088/0031-9155/59/17/5003 PMID:25119017

Kim, Y., & Horii, S. C. (2000). Handbook of Medical Imaging: Vol. 3. *Display and PACS*. Bellingham: SPIE Press.

Klein, S., Staring, M., & Pluim, J. P. W. (2007). Evaluation of optimization methods for non-rigid medical image registration using mutual information and B-Splines. *IEEE Transactions on Image Processing*, *16*(12), 2879–2890. doi:10.1109/TIP.2007.909412 PMID:18092588

Kosus, N., Kosus, A., & Turhan, N. (2010). Comparison of standard mammography with digital mammography and digital infrared thermal imaging for breast cancer screening. *Journal of Turk Ger Gynecol Assoc.*, 152–157.

Kriegsmann, J., Kriegsmann, M., & Casadonte, R. (2015, March). MALDI TOF imaging mass spectrometry in clinical pathology: A valuable tool for cancer diagnostics. *International Journal of Oncology*, *46*(3), 893–906. doi:10.3892/ijo.2014.2788 PMID:25482502

Kriegsmann, M., Arens, N., Endris, V., Weichert, W., & Kriegsmann, J. (2015). Detection of KRAS, NRAS and BRAF by mass spectrometry - a sensitive, reliable, fast and cost-effective technique. *Diagnostic Pathology*, *10*(1), 132. doi:10.118613000-015-0364-3 PMID:26220423

Kuboki, Y., Schatz, C. A., Koechert, K., Schubert, S., Feng, J., Wittemer-Rump, S., ... Ochiai, A. (2017, August 29). In situ analysis of FGFR2 mRNA and comparison with FGFR2 gene copy number by dual-color in situ hybridization in a large cohort of gastric cancer patients. *Gastric Cancer*. doi:10.100710120-017-0758-x PMID:28852882

Kuhl, C. K. (2007). Current status of breast MR imaging, Pt. 2:Clinical applications. *Radiology*, *244*, 672–691. doi:10.1148/radiol.2443051661 PMID:17709824

Kwak, D. M. (2003). „Content-based ultrasound image retrieval using a coarse to fine approach. *Annals of the New York Academy of Sciences*, 212–224. PMID:12594091

Lai, Y-H., & Wang, Y-S. (2017). Matrix-Assisted Laser Desorption/Ionization Mass Spectrometry: Mechanistic Studies and Methods for Improving the Structural Identification of Carbohydrates. *Mass Spectrometry*, *6*(2), S0072. doi:.10.5702/massspectrometry.S0072

Lal, S., Chandra, M., & Upadhyay, G. K. (2011). *Removal of Additive Gaussian Noise by Complex Double Density Dual Tree Discrete Wavelet Transform*. Academic Press.

Laouirem, S., Le Faouder, J., Alexandrov, T., Mestivier, D., Léger, T., Baudin, X., ... Bedossa, P. (2014). Progression from cirrhosis to cancer is associated with early ubiquitin post-translational modifications: Identification of new biomarkers of cirrhosis at risk of malignancy. *The Journal of Pathology*, *234*(4), 452–463. doi:10.1002/path.4398 PMID:24979321

Larsson, C., Koch, J., Nygren, A., Janssen, G., Raap, A. K., Landegren, U., & Nilsson, M. (2004). In situ genotyping individual DNA molecules by target-primed rolling-circle amplification of padlock probes. *Nature Methods*, *1*(3), 227–232. doi:10.1038/nmeth723 PMID:15782198

Law, G. (2013). Quantitative Comparison of Flood Fill and Modified Flood Fill Algorithms. *International Journal of Computer Theory and Engineering*, *5*(3), 503–508. doi:10.7763/IJCTE.2013.V5.738

Lazar, I., & Hajdu, A. (2013). Retinal microaneurysm detection through local rotating cross-section profile analysis. *IEEE Transactions on Medical Imaging*, *32*(2), 400–407. doi:10.1109/TMI.2012.2228665 PMID:23192523

Lazova, R., Seeley, E. H., Keenan, M., Gueorguieva, R., & Caprioli, R. M. (2012). Imaging mass spectrometry - a new and promising method to differentiate Spitz nevi from Spitzoid malignant melanomas. *The American Journal of Dermatopathology*, *34*(1), 82–90. doi:10.1097/DAD.0b013e31823df1e2 PMID:22197864

Le Faouder, J., Laouirem, S., Chapelle, M., Albuquerque, M., Belghiti, J., Degos, F., ... Bedossa, P. (2011). Imaging mass spectrometry provides fingerprints for distinguishing hepatocellular carcinoma from cirrhosis. *Journal of Proteome Research*, *10*(8), 3755–3765. doi:10.1021/pr200372p PMID:21675781

Lee, G. K., Lee, H. S., Park, Y. S., Lee, J. H., Lee, S. C., Lee, J. H., ... Kim, H. K. (2012). Lipid MALDI profile classifies non-small cell lung cancers according to the histologic type. *Lung Cancer (Amsterdam, Netherlands)*, *76*(2), 197–203. doi:10.1016/j.lungcan.2011.10.016 PMID:22099218

Lee, J. G., Kim, J. H., Kim, S. H., Park, H. S., & Choi, B. I. (2011). A straightforward approach to computer-aided polyp detection using a polyp-specific volumetric feature in CT colonography. *Computers in Biology and Medicine*, *41*(9), 790–801. doi:10.1016/j.compbiomed.2011.06.015 PMID:21762887

Lee, J. H. (2017). Quantitative approaches for investigating the spatial context of gene expression. *Wiley Interdisciplinary Reviews. Systems Biology and Medicine*, *9*(2), e1369. doi:10.1002/wsbm.1369 PMID:28001340

Lee, J. H., Daugharthy, E. R., Scheiman, J., Kalhor, R., Ferrante, T. C., Terry, R., ... Church, G. M. (2015). Fluorescent in situ sequencing (FISSEQ) of RNA for gene expression profiling in intact cells and tissues. *Nature Protocols*, *10*(3), 442–458. doi:10.1038/nprot.2014.191 PMID:25675209

Lee, J. H., Daugharthy, E. R., Scheiman, J., Kalhor, R., Yang, J. L., Ferrante, T. C., ... Church, G. M. (2014). Highly multiplexed subcellular RNA sequencing *in situ*. *Science*, *343*(6177), 1360–1363. doi:10.1126cience.1250212 PMID:24578530

Lehmann, T. M., Wein, B., Dhaman, J., Bredno, J., Vogelsang, F., & Kohnen, M. (2000). Content Based image retrival in medical applications: A novel multistep approach. *Proceedings of the Society for Photo-Instrumentation Engineers*, *3972*, 312–320. doi:10.1117/12.373563

Lemaire, R., Menguellet, S. A., Stauber, J., Marchauadon, V., & Lucot, J. P. (2007). Specific MALDI imaging and profiling for biomarker hunting and validation: Fragment of the 11S proteasome activator complex, Reg alpha fragment, is a new potential ovary cancer biomarker. *Journal of Proteome Research*, *6*(11), 4127–4134. doi:10.1021/pr0702722 PMID:17939699

Lewis, G. S., & Armstrong, A. D. (2011). Glenoid spherical orientation and version. *Journal of Shoulder and Elbow Surgery*, *20*(1), 3–11. doi:10.1016/j.jse.2010.05.012 PMID:20932782

Lichman, M. (2013). *UCI Machine Learning Repository*. Irvine, CA: University of California, School of Information and Computer Science.

Li, F., Zou, Y. G., Zhou, Q. Z., Li, T. Q., Guo, W. B., Jing, X. W., ... Zheng, S. B. (2009). Identification of human testicular embryonal carcinoma proteins by two-dimensional gel electrophoresis and mass spectrometry. *Nan Fang Yi Ke da Xue Xue Bao*, *29*(8), 1585–1587. PMID:19726299

Liu, X., Ide, J.L., Norton, I., Marchionni, M.A., Ebling, M.C., ... Agar, N.Y.R. (2013) Molecular imaging of drug transit through the blood-brain barrier with MALDI mass spectrometry imaging. *Sci Rep.*, *4*(3), 2859. doi: 10.1038rep02859

Liu, Y., Chen, Y., Momin, A., Shaner, R., Wang, E., Bowen, N. J., ... Merrill, A. H. (2010). Elevation of sulfatides in ovarian cancer: An integrated transcriptomic and lipidomic analysis including tissue-imaging mass spectrometry. *Molecular Cancer*, *9*(1), 186. doi:10.1186/1476-4598-9-186 PMID:20624317

Liu, Y., Tan, Y. R., Sun, W. W., Ju, W. T., Fu, Y., Wang, L. Z., ... Zhong, L. P. (2018, February 20). Identification of SCARA5 as a potential biomarker for oral squamous cell carcinoma using MALDI TOF MS analysis. *Proteomics. Clinical Applications*. doi:10.1002/prca.201700180 PMID:29461673

Liu, Y., Zhang, D., Lu, G., & Ma, W. Y. (2007). A survey of content-based image retrieval with high-level semantics. *Pattern Recognition*, *40*(1), 262–282. doi:10.1016/j.patcog.2006.04.045

Loeser, H., Schallenberg, S., von Winterfeld, M., Tharun, L., Alakus, H., Hölscher, A., ... Quaas, A. (2017). High protein and mRNA expression levels of TUBB3 (class III ß-tubulin) are associated with aggressive tumor features in esophageal adenocarcinomas. *Oncotarget*, *8*(70), 115179–115189. doi:10.18632/oncotarget.23112 PMID:29383151

Lokhande, R., Arya, K. V., & Gupta, P. (2006). Identification of parameters and restoration of motion blurred images. *Proceedings of the 2006 ACM Symposium on Applied Computing, 9*, 301-305.

Longuespée, R., Casadonte, R., Kriegsmann, M., Pottier, C., Picard de Muller, G., Delvenne, P., ... De Pauw, E. (2016). MALDI mass spectrometry imaging: A cutting-edge tool for fundamental and clinical histopathology. *Proteomics. Clinical Applications*, *10*(7), 701–719. doi:10.1002/prca.201500140 PMID:27188927

Longuespée, R., Casadonte, R., Schwamborn, K., Reuss, D., Kazdal, D., Kriegsmann, K., ... Kriegsmann, M. (2018). Proteomics in Pathology. *Proteomics*, *18*(2), 1700361. doi:10.1002/pmic.201700361 PMID:29236356

Lou, S., Balluff, B., Cleven, A. H. G., Bovée, J. V. M. G., & McDonnell, L. A. (2017). Prognostic Metabolite Biomarkers for Soft Tissue Sarcomas Discovered by Mass Spectrometry Imaging. *Journal of the American Society for Mass Spectrometry*, *28*(2), 376–383. doi:10.100713361-016-1544-4 PMID:27873216

Maes, F., Collignon, A., Vandermeulen, D., Marchal, G., & Suetens, P. (1997). Multimodality image registration by maximization of mutual information. *IEEE Transactions on Medical Imaging*, *16*(2), 187–198. doi:10.1109/42.563664 PMID:9101328

Maier, S. K., Hahne, H., Gholami, A. M., Balluff, B., Meding, S., Schoene, C., ... Kuster, B. (2013). Comprehensive identification of proteins from MALDI imaging. *Molecular & Cellular Proteomics*, *12*(10), 2901–2910. doi:10.1074/mcp.M113.027599 PMID:23782541

Majdi, M., & Seyedali, M. (2018). Whale optimization approaches for wrapper feature selection. *Applied Soft Computing*, *62*, 441–453. doi:10.1016/j.asoc.2017.11.006

Malvia, S., Bagadi, S. A., Dubey, U. S., & Saxena, S. (2017). Epidemiology of breast cancer in Indian women. *Asia Pacific Journal of Clinical Oncology*, *13*(4), 289–295. doi:10.1111/ajco.12661 PMID:28181405

Manivannan, S., Cobb, C., Burgess, S., & Trucco, E. (2017). Sub-category classifiers for multiple-instance learning and its application to retinal nerve fiber layer visibility classification. *IEEE Transactions on Medical Imaging*, *36*(5), 1140–1150. doi:10.1109/TMI.2017.2653623 PMID:28092529

Manizheh, G., & Mohammad-Reza, F. (2016). Feature selection using Forest optimization Algorithm. *Pattern Recognition*, *60*, 121–129. doi:10.1016/j.patcog.2016.05.012

Manjunath, B. S., & Ma, W. Y. (1996). Texture features for browsing and retrieval of image data. *IEEE Transactions on Pattern Analysis and Machine Intelligence*, *8*(8), 837–842. doi:10.1109/34.531803

Marin, D., Aquino, A., Gegundez-Arias, M. E., & Bravo, J. M. (2011). A new supervised method for blood vessel segmentation in retinal images by using gray-level and moment invariants-based features. *IEEE Transactions on Medical Imaging*, *30*(1), 146–158. doi:10.1109/TMI.2010.2064333 PMID:20699207

Mark, S. N., & Alberto, S. A. (2008). *Feature Extraction and Image Processing* (2nd ed.). Elsevier.

Mathworks. (2017). *Image Processing Toolbox User's Guide*. Retrieved September 26, 2017, from https://www.mathworks.com/help/images/ref/dicomread.html

Matsen, F. A. III, Clinton, J., Lynch, J., Bertelsen, A., Richardson, M. L., & Matsen Iii, F. A. (2008). Glenoid Component Failure in Total Shoulder Arthroplasty. *The Journal of Bone and Joint Surgery. American Volume*, *90*(4), 885–896. doi:10.2106/JBJS.G.01263 PMID:18381328

Mauricio Botto de Barros Garcia, J., Leonardo Cruvinel Isaac, D., & Avila, M. (2017). Diabetic retinopathy and OCT angiography: Clinical findings and future perspectives. *International Journal of Retina and Vitreous*, *3*(14), 1–10. PMID:28078103

Max, A. (2016). A survey of medical image registration-under review, Medical Image Analysis. *Medical Image Analysis*, *33*, 140–144. PMID:27427472

Ma, Y., Xie, J., & Luo, J. (2009). Image Enhancement Based on Nonsubsampled Contourlet Transform. *Fifth International Conference on Information Assurance and Security*. 10.1109/IAS.2009.44

McDonnell, L. A., Walch, A., Stoeckli, M., & Corthals, G. L. (2014). MSiMass list: A public database of identifications for protein MALDI MS imaging. *Journal of Proteome Research*, *13*(2), 1138–1142. doi:10.1021/pr400620y PMID:24313301

McKenna, M. T., Wang, S., Nguyen, T. B., Burns, J. E., Petrick, N., & Summers, R. M. (2012). Strategies for improved interpretation of computer-aided detections for CT colonography utilizing distributed human intelligence. *Medical Image Analysis*, *16*(6), 1280–1292. doi:10.1016/j.media.2012.04.007 PMID:22705287

Meding, S., Martin, K., Gustafsson, O. J., Eddes, J. S., Hack, S., Oehler, M. K., & Hoffmann, P. (2013). Tryptic peptide reference data sets for MALDI imaging mass spectrometry on formalin-fixed ovarian cancer tissues. *Journal of Proteome Research*, *12*(1), 308–315. doi:10.1021/pr300996x PMID:23214983

Meeuwis, C., van de Ven, S. M., Stapper, G., Fernandez Gallardo, A. M., van den Bosch, M. A. A. J., Mali, W. P. T. M., & Veldhuis, W. B. (2010). Computer-aided detection (CAD) for breast MRI:evaluation of efficacy at 3.0 T. *European Radiology*, *20*(3), 522–528. doi:10.100700330-009-1573-5 PMID:19727750

Mendonc, Sousaa, Mendonc¸ & Campilhoa. (2013). Automatic localization of the optic disc by combining vascular and intensity information. *Computerized Medical Imaging and Graphics*, *37*(5–6), 409–417. PMID:23726437

Meseure, D., Drak Alsibai, K., & Nicolas, A. (2014). Pivotal Role of Pervasive Neoplastic and Stromal Cells Reprogramming in Circulating Tumor Cells Dissemination and Metastatic Colonization. *Cancer Microenvironment*, *7*(3), 95–115. doi:10.100712307-014-0158-2 PMID:25523234

Meseure, D., Vacher, S., Lallemand, F., Drak Alsibai, K., Hatem, R., Chemlali, W., ... Bieche, I. (2016). Prognostic value of a newly identified MALAT1 alternatively spliced transcript in breast cancer. *British Journal of Cancer, 114*(12), 1395–1404. doi:10.1038/bjc.2016.123 PMID:27172249

Meyerbaese, A. (2003). *Pattern Recognition in Medical Imaging*. San Diego, CA: Academic Press.

Michael, F. (2015). Assessing the scale of tumor heterogeneity by complete hierarchical segmentation of MRI. *Physics in Medicine and Biology, 60*(3), 977–993. doi:10.1088/0031-9155/60/3/977 PMID:25575341

Mignardi, M., Mezger, A., Qian, X., La Fleur, L., Botling, J., Larsson, C., & Nilsson, M. (2015). Oligonucleotide gap-fill ligation for mutation detection and sequencing *in situ*. *Nucleic Acids Research, 43*(22), e151. doi:10.1093/nar/gkv772 PMID:26240388

Mildenberger, P., Eichelberg, M., & Martin, E. (2002). Introduction to the DICOM standard. *European Radiology, 12*(4), 920–927. doi:10.1007003300101100 PMID:11960249

Mlecnik, B., Bindea, G., Kirilovsky, A., Angell, H. K., Obenauf, A. C., Tosolini, M., ... Galon, J. (2016). The tumor microenvironment and Immunoscore are critical determinants of dissemination to distant metastasis. *Science Translational Medicine, 8*(327), 327ra26. doi:10.1126citranslmed.aad6352 PMID:26912905

Moineau, G., Levigne, C., Boileau, P., Young, A., & Walch, G. (2012). Three-dimensional measurement method of arthritic glenoid cavity morphology: Feasibility and reproducibility. *Orthopaedics & Traumatology: Surgery & Research, 98*(S6), S139–S145. doi:10.1016/j.otsr.2012.06.007 PMID:22964089

Mookiah, M. R. K., Acharya, U. R., Chua, C. K., Min, L. C., Ng, E. Y. K., Mushrif, M. M., & Laude, A. (2013b). Automated detection of optic disk in retinal fundus images using intuitionistic fuzzy histon segmentation. *Proceedings of the Institution of Mechanical Engineers, Part H., 227*(1), 37–49. doi:10.1177/0954411912458740 PMID:23516954

Mookiah, M. R. K., Acharya, U. R., Martis, R. J., Chua, C. K., Min, L. C., Ng, E. Y. K., & Laude, A. (2013a). Evolutionary algorithm based classifier parameter tuning for automatic diabetic retinopathy grading: A hybrid feature extraction approach. *Knowledge-Based Systems, 39*(0), 9–22. doi:10.1016/j.knosys.2012.09.008

Morita, Y., Ikegami, K., Goto-Inoue, N., Hayasaka, T., Zaima, N., Tanaka, H., ... Konno, H. (2010). Imaging mass spectrometry of gastric carcinoma in formalin-fixed paraffin-embedded tissue microarray. *Cancer Science, 101*(1), 267–273. doi:10.1111/j.1349-7006.2009.01384.x PMID:19961487

Muller, H., Muller, W., Squire, D. M., Marchand, S., Maillet, & Pun, T. (2000). Strategies for positive and negative relevance feedback in image retrieval. In *Proceedings of the 15th International Conference on Pattern Recognition (ICPR2000)*. IEEE. 10.1109/ICPR.2000.905650

Muller, H., Michoux, N., Bandon, D., & Geissbuhler, A. (2004). A review of content-based image retrieval applications-clinical benefits and future directions. *International Journal of Medical Informatics*, *73*(1), 1–23. doi:10.1016/j.ijmedinf.2003.11.024 PMID:15036075

Murakami, Y., Kakeda, S., Kamada, K., Ohnari, N., Nishimura, J., Ogawa, M., ... Korogi, Y. (2010). Effect of tube voltage on image quality in 64-section multidetector 3D CT angiography: Evaluation with a vascular phantom with superimposed bone skull structures. *AJNR. American Journal of Neuroradiology*, *31*(4), 620–625. doi:10.3174/ajnr.A1871 PMID:19942711

Mustra, M., Delac, K., & Grgic, M. (2008). Overview of the DICOM standard. *2008 50th International Symposium ELMAR, 1*, 39–44.

Naishadham, D., Lansdorp-Vogelaar, I., Siegel, R., Cokkinides, V., & Jemal, A. (2011). State disparities in colorectal cancer mortality patterns in the United States. *Cancer Epidemiology, Biomarkers & Prevention*, *20*(7), 1296–1302. doi:10.1158/1055-9965.EPI-11-0250 PMID:21737410

Nayebifar, B., & Moghaddam, H. A. (2013). A novel method for retinal vessel tracking using particle filters. *Computers in Biology and Medicine*, *43*(5), 541–548. doi:10.1016/j.compbiomed.2013.01.016 PMID:23434235

Newman, T. S., & Yi, H. (2006). A survey of the marching cubes algorithm. *Computers and Graphics (Pergamon)*, *30*(5), 854–879. doi:10.1016/j.cag.2006.07.021

Nguyen, D., Ferreira, L. M., Brownhill, J. R., King, G. J. W., Drosdowech, D. S., Faber, K. J., & Johnson, J. A. (2009). Improved accuracy of computer assisted glenoid implantation in total shoulder arthroplasty: An in-vitro randomized controlled trial. *Journal of Shoulder and Elbow Surgery*, *18*(6), 907–914. doi:10.1016/j.jse.2009.02.022 PMID:19482490

Nie, K. (2009). *Development of breast MRI computer-aided diagnosis system* (Thesis). Irvine, CA: University of California.

Nipp, M., Elsner, M., Balluff, B., Meding, S., Sarioglu, H., Ueffing, M., ... Zitzelsberger, H. (2012). S100-A10, thioredoxin, and S100-A6 as biomarkers of papillary thyroid carcinoma with lymph node metastasis identified by MALDI imaging. *Journal of Molecular Medicine*, *90*(2), 163–174. doi:10.100700109-011-0815-6 PMID:21938494

Nirmalan, N.J., Harnden, P., Selby, P.J., & Banks, R.E. (2009). Development and validation of a novel protein extraction methodology for quantitation of protein expression in formalin-fixed paraffin-embedded tissues using western blotting. *J Pathol*, *217*, 497-506.

Nowak, R. D. (1999). Wavelet-based Rician noise removal for magnetic resonance imaging. *IEEE Transactions on Image Processing*, *8*(10), 1408–1419. doi:10.1109/83.791966 PMID:18267412

Nyirjesy, M. D. (1986). Clinical Evaluation, Mammography and Thermography in the Diagnosis of Breast Carcinoma. *Thermology*, *1*, 170–173.

Olga, D., Herbert, E., Anton, L., Michael, M., Daria, M., Roman, K., & Sergey, K. (in press). The classification of endoscopy images with persistent homology. *Pattern Recognition Letters*.

Oppenheimer, S. R., Mi, D., Sanders, M. E., & Caprioli, R. M. (2010). Molecular analysis of tumor margins by MALDI mass spectrometry in renal carcinoma. *Journal of Proteome Research*, *9*(5), 2182–2190. doi:10.1021/pr900936z PMID:20141219

Pagni, F., Mainini, V., Garancini, M., Bono, F., Vanzati, A., Giardini, V., ... Magni, F. (2015). Proteomics for the diagnosis of thyroid lesions: Preliminary report. *Cytopathology*, *26*(5), 318–324. doi:10.1111/cyt.12166 PMID:25040579

Palma, G., Bloch, I., & Muller, S. (2014). Detection of masses and architectural distortions in digital breast tomosynthesis images using fuzzy and a contrario approaches. *Pattern Recognition*, *47*(7), 2467–2480. doi:10.1016/j.patcog.2014.01.009

Pantanowitz, L., Valenstein, P. N., Evans, A. J., Kaplan, K. J., & Pfeifer, J. D. (2011). Review of the current state of whole slide imaging in pathology. *Journal of Pathology Informatics*, *2*(1), 36. doi:10.4103/2153-3539.83746 PMID:21886892

Pickhardt, P. J., Kim, D. H., Pooler, B. D., Hinshaw, J. L., Barlow, D., Jensen, D., ... Cash, B. D. (2013). Assessment of volumetric growth rates of small colorectal polyps with CT colonography: A longitudinal study of natural history. *The Lancet Oncology*, *14*(8), 711–720. doi:10.1016/S1470-2045(13)70216-X PMID:23746988

Pluim, J. P. W., Maintz, J. B. A., & Viergever, M. A. (2000). Interpolation artefacts in mutual information-based image registration. *Computer Vision and Image Understanding*, *77*(2), 211–232. doi:10.1006/cviu.1999.0816

Po, D. D.-Y., & Do, M. N. (2006). Directional multiscale modeling of images using the contourlet transform. *IEEE Transactions on Image Processing*, *15*(6), 1610–1620. doi:10.1109/TIP.2006.873450 PMID:16764285

Pokrajac, D., Megalooikonomou, V., Lazarevic, A., Kontos, D., & Obradovic, Z. (2005). Applying spatial distribution analysis techniques to classification of 3D medical images. *Artificial Intelligence in Medicine*, *33*(3), 261–280. doi:10.1016/j.artmed.2004.07.001 PMID:15811790

Pratt, W. K. (2002). *Digital Iamge Processing*. John Wiley & Sons.

Preim, B., & Bartz, D. (2007). *Visualization in Medicine: Theory, Algorithms, and Applications*. Amsterdam: Morgan Kaufmann.

Qian, X. N., & Tagare, H. D. (2005). *Optimal embedding for shape indexing in medical image databases*. Medical Image Computing and Computer Assisted. doi:10.1007/11566489_47

Querido, E., Dekakra-Bellili, L., & Chartrand, P. (2017). RNA fluorescence in situ hybridization for high-content screening. *Methods (San Diego, Calif.)*, *15*(126), 149–155. doi:10.1016/j.ymeth.2017.07.005 PMID:28694064

Qureshi, Kovacs, Harangi, Nagy, Peto, & Hajdu. (2012). Combining algorithms for automatic detection of optic disc and macula in fundus images. *Computer Vision and Image Understanding*, *116*(1), 138-145.

RadiologyInfo.org. (2013). *Medical image database.* Retrieved on April 5, 2013 from www.radiologyinfo.org

Rahman, M., Bhattacharya, P., & Desai, B. C. (2007). A framework for medical image retrieval using machine learning and statistical content-based image retrieval in radiology similarity matching techniques with relevance feedback. *IEEE Transactions on Information Technology in Biomedicine, 11*(1), 58–69. doi:10.1109/TITB.2006.884364 PMID:17249404

Ram, K., Joshi, G. D., & Sivaswamy, J. (2011). A Successive Clutter-Rejection-Based Approach for Early Detection of Diabetic Retinopathy. *IEEE Transactions on Biomedical Engineering, 58*(3), 664–673. doi:10.1109/TBME.2010.2096223 PMID:21134810

Rattanawadee, P., & Anongnart, S. (2015). Wrapper Feature Subset Selection for Dimension Reduction Based on Ensemble Learning Algorithm. *Procedia Computer Science, 72*, 162–169. doi:10.1016/j.procs.2015.12.117

Remark, R., Merghoub, T., Grabe, N., Litjens, G., Damotte, D., Wolchok, J.D., … Gnjatic, S. (2016). In-depth tissue profiling using multiplexed immunohistochemical consecutive staining on single slide. *Science Immunology, 14*(1). doi: 10.1126ciimmunol.aaf6925

Reported Shoulder Procedures. (2017). Retrieved September 26, 2017, from https://aoanjrr.sahmri.com/shoulders

Reyzer, M. L., Hsieh, Y., Ng, K., Korfmacher, W. A., & Caprioli, R. M. (2003). Direct analysis of drug candidates in tissue by matrix-assisted laser desorption/ionization mass spectrometry. *Journal of Mass Spectrometry, 38*(10), 1081–1092. doi:10.1002/jms.525 PMID:14595858

Riazifar, N., & Yazdi, M. (2009). Effectiveness of Contourlet vs. Wavelet Transform on Medical Image Compression: A Comparative Study. *World Academy of Science, Engineering and Technology.*

Rocha, A., Carvalho, T., Jelinek, H. F., Goldenstein, S., & Wainer, J. (2012). Points of Interest and Visual Dictionaries for Automatic Retinal Lesion Detection. *IEEE Transactions on Biomedical Engineering, 59*(8), 2244–2253. doi:10.1109/TBME.2012.2201717 PMID:22665502

Rossant, F., Badellino, M., Chavillon, A., Bloch, I., & Paques, M. (2011). A morphological approach for vessel segmentation in eye fundus images, with quantitative evaluation. *Journal of Medical Imaging and Health Informatics., 1*(1), 42–49. doi:10.1166/jmihi.2011.1006

Roy & Bandyopadhyay. (2012). Detection and Quantification of Brain Tumor from MRI of Brain and it's Symmetric Analysis. *International Journal of Information and Communication Technology Research, 2*(6).

Ruijie, Z., Jian, S., Fushan, W., Xiong, L., & Arun, K. S. (in press). Medical image classification based on multi-scale non-negative sparse coding. *Artificial Intelligence in Medicine.*

Rui, Y., Huang, T. S., & Chang, S. F. (1999). Image retrieval: Current techniques, promising directions, and open issues. *Journal of Visual Communication and Image Representation, 10*(1), 39–62. doi:10.1006/jvci.1999.0413

Sahiner, B., Chan, H. P., Hadjiiski, L. M., Helvie, M. A., Wei, J., Zhou, C., & Lu, Y. (2012). Computer-aided detection of clustered microcalcifications in digital breast tomosynthesis: A 3D approach. *Medical Physics*, *39*(1), 28–39. doi:10.1118/1.3662072 PMID:22225272

Saki, F., & Tahmasbi, A. (2010). *A novel opposition-based classifier for mass diagnosis in mammography images.* ICBME.

Salphati, L., Shahidi-Latham, S., Quiason, C., Barck, K., Nishimura, M., Alicke, B., ... Phillips, H. S. (2014). ... Distribution of the phosphatidylinositol 3-kinase inhibitors Pictilisib (GDC-0941) and GNE-317 in U87 and GS2 intracranial glioblastoma models-assessment by matrix-assisted laser desorption ionization imaging. *Drug Metabolism and Disposition: the Biological Fate of Chemicals*, *42*(7), 1110–1116. doi:10.1124/dmd.114.057513 PMID:24754926

Salto-Tellez, M., James, J. A., & Hamilton, P. W. (2014). Molecular pathology – The value of an integrative approach. *Molecular Oncology*, *8*(7), 1163–1168. doi:10.1016/j.molonc.2014.07.021 PMID:25160635

Salto-Tellez, M., & Kennedy, R. D. (2015, December). Integrated molecular pathology: The Belfast model. *Drug Discovery Today*, *20*(12), 1451–1454. doi:10.1016/j.drudis.2015.10.011 PMID:26499202

Samala, R. K., Chan, H. P., Hadjiiski, L., Helvie, M. A., Wei, J., & Cha, K. (2016). Mass detection in digital breast tomosynthesis: Deep convolutional neural network with transfer learning from mammography. *Medical Physics*, *43*(12), 6654–6666. doi:10.1118/1.4967345 PMID:27908154

Schwamborn, K., Krieg, R. C., Jirak, P., Ott, G., Knuchel, R., Rosenwald, A., & Wellmann, A. (2010). Application of MALDI imaging for the diagnosis of classical Hodgkin lymphoma. *Journal of Cancer Research and Clinical Oncology*, *136*(11), 1651–1655. doi:10.100700432-010-0823-x PMID:20865362

Schwamborn, K., Krieg, R. C., Reska, M., Jakse, G., Knuechel, R., & Wellmann, A. (2007). Identifying prostate carcinoma by MALDI-Imaging. *International Journal of Molecular Medicine*, *20*, 155–159. PMID:17611632

Schwamborn, K., Krieg, R. C., Uhlig, S., Ikenberg, H., & Wellmann, A. (2011). MALDI imaging as a specific diagnostic tool for routine cervical cytology specimens. *International Journal of Molecular Medicine*, *27*(3), 417–421. doi:10.3892/ijmm.2010.587 PMID:21174066

Schwartz, S. A., Reyzer, M. L., & Caprioli, R. M. (2003). Direct tissue analysis using matrix-assisted laser desorption/ionization mass spectrometry: Practical aspects of sample preparation. *Journal of Mass Spectrometry*, *38*(7), 699–708. doi:10.1002/jms.505 PMID:12898649

Seeley, E. H., & Caprioli, R. M. (2011). MALDI imaging mass spectrometry of human tissue: Method challenges and clinical perspectives. *Trends in Biotechnology*, *29*(3), 136–143. doi:10.1016/j.tibtech.2010.12.002 PMID:21292337

Selvanayaki & Kalugasalam. (2013). Intelligent Brain Tumor Tissue Segmentation From Magnetic Resonance Image (MRI) Using Meta Heuristic Algorithms. *Journal of Global Research in Computer Science, 4*(2).

Sergei, K. (2007). Using hard and soft models for classification of medical images. *Chemometrics and Intelligent Laboratory Systems, 88*(1), 100–106. doi:10.1016/j.chemolab.2006.08.012

Serief, C., Barkat, M., & Bentoutou, Y. (2007). An automatic image registration scheme based on the nonsubsampled contourlet transform. *Proceedings of the 9th International Symposium on Signal Processing and Its Applications*, 1–4. 10.1109/ISSPA.2007.4555446

Sezgin, M., & Sankur, B. (2004). Survey over image thresholding techniques and quantitative performance evaluation. *Journal of Electronic Imaging, 13*(1), 146–165. doi:10.1117/1.1631315

Shahbazi, M., Sattari, M., & Ghazic, M. (2008). Automatic polyp detection from CT colonography using mathematical morphology. In *Proceedings of the 21st ISPRS Congress* (pp. 823-828). Academic Press.

Shanthi, S., & Muralibhaskaran, V. (2014). Automatic Detection and Classification of Microcalcification, Mass, Architectural Distortion and Bilateral Asymmetry in Digital Mammogram. *World Academy of Science, Engineering and Technology, International Journal of Medical, Health, Biomedical, Bioengineering and Pharmaceutical Engineering, 8*(11), 822–827.

Sharif, M. S., Qahwaji, R., Ipsona, S., & Brahma, A. (2015). Medical image classification based on artificial intelligence approaches: A practical study on normal and abnormal confocal corneal images. *Applied Soft Computing, 36*, 269–282. doi:10.1016/j.asoc.2015.07.019

Sheffield, B. S. (2016). Immunohistochemistry as a Practical Tool in Molecular Pathology. *Archives of Pathology & Laboratory Medicine, 140*(8), 766–769. doi:10.5858/arpa.2015-0453-RA PMID:27472235

Shirinifard, A., Thiagarajan, S., Vogel, P., & Sablauer, A. (2016). Detection of Phenotypic Alterations Using High-Content Analysis of Whole-Slide Images. *The Journal of Histochemistry and Cytochemistry, 64*(5), 301–310. doi:10.1369/0022155416639884 PMID:27026297

Shyu, C. R., Brodley, C. E., Kak, A. C., Kosaka, A., Aisen, A. M., & Broderick, L. S. (1999). ASSERT: A physician-in-the-loop content-based image retrieval system for HRCT image databases. *Computer Vision and Image Understanding, 75*(2), 111–132. doi:10.1006/cviu.1999.0768

Shyu, C. R., Kak, A., Brodley, C., & Broderick, L. S. (1999). Testing for human perceptual categories in a physician-in-the-loop CBIR system for medical imagery. *Proceedings of the IEEE Workshop on Content-based Access of Image and Video Libraries (CBAIVL)*, 102-108. 10.1109/IVL.1999.781132

Siegel, R. L., Miller, K. D., & Jemal, A. (2015). Cancer statistics, 2015. *CA: A Cancer Journal for Clinicians, 65*(1), 5–29. doi:10.3322/caac.21254 PMID:25559415

Skripcak, T., Just, U., Simon, M., Buttner, D., Luhr, A., Baumann, M., & Krause, M. (2016, September). Toward Distributed Conduction of Large-Scale Studies in Radiation Therapy and Oncology: Open-Source System Integration Approach. *IEEE Journal of Biomedical and Health Informatics*, *20*(5), 1397–1403. doi:10.1109/JBHI.2015.2450833

Smeulders, A. W. M., Worring, M., Santini, S., Gupta, A., & Jain, R. (2000). Content-based image retrieval at the end of the early years. *IEEE Transactions on Pattern Analysis and Machine Intelligence*, *22*(12), 1349–1380. doi:10.1109/34.895972

Sopharak, Uyyanonvara, & Barmanb, & Williamson. (2008). Automatic detection of diabetic retinopathy exudates from non-dilated retinal images using mathematical morphology methods. *Computerized Medical Imaging and Graphics*, *32*(8), 720–727. PMID:18930631

Sotiras, Davatzikos, & Paragios. (2013). Deformable Medical Image Registration: A Survey. IEEE Transactions on Medical Imaging, 32(7), 1153-1190.

Stack, E. C., Wang, C., Roman, K. A., & Hoyt, C. C. (2014). Multiplexed immunohistochemistry, imaging, and quantitation: A review, with an assessment of Tyramide signal amplification, multispectral imaging and multiplex analysis. *Methods (San Diego, Calif.)*, *70*(1), 46–58. doi:10.1016/j.ymeth.2014.08.016 PMID:25242720

Steurer, S., Borkowski, C., Odinga, S., Buchholz, M., Koop, C., Huland, H., ... Schlüter, H. (2013). MALDI mass spectrometric imaging based identification of clinically relevant signals in prostate cancer using large-scale tissue microarrays. *International Journal of Cancer*, *133*(4), 920–928. doi:10.1002/ijc.28080 PMID:23381989

Steurer, S., Seddiqi, A. S., Singer, J. M., Bahar, A. S., & Eichelberg, C. (2014). MALDI imaging on tissue microarrays identifies molecular features associated with renal cell cancer phenotype. *Anticancer Research*, *34*, 2255–2261. PMID:24778028

Steurer, S., Singer, J. M., Rink, M., Chun, F., & Dahlem, R. (2014). MALDI imaging-based identification of prognostically relevant signals in bladder cancer using large-scale tissue microarrays. *Urologic Oncology*, *32*(8), 1225–1233. doi:10.1016/j.urolonc.2014.06.007 PMID:25131659

Stomp, W., Reijnierse, M., Kloppenburg, M., de Mutsert, R., Bovée, J. V. M. G., den Heijer, M., & Bloem, J. L. (2015). Prevalence of cartilaginous tumours as an incidental finding on MRI of the knee. *European Radiology*, *25*(12), 3480–3487. doi:10.100700330-015-3764-6 PMID:25994192

Sufyan, Y. (2011). Automatic graph-cut based segmentation of bones from knee magnetic resonance images for osteoarthritis research. *Medical Image Analysis*, *15*(4), 438–448. doi:10.1016/j.media.2011.01.007 PMID:21474362

Sugihara, Y. (2014). A new look at drugs targeting malignant melanoma - an application for mass spectrometry imaging. *Proteomics*, *14*, 1963–1970. doi:10.1002/pmic.201300476 PMID:25044963

Sundaram, P., Zomorodian, A., Beaulieu, C., & Napel, S. (2008). Colon polyp detection using smoothed shape operators: Preliminary results. *Medical Image Analysis, 12*(2), 99–119. doi:10.1016/j.media.2007.08.001 PMID:17910934

Svensson, W. (1997). A review of the current status of breast ultrasound. *European Journal of Ultrasound, 6*(2), 77–101. doi:10.1016/S0929-8266(97)10009-X

Swamidoss, I. N., Kårsnäs, A., Uhlmann, V., Ponnusamy, P., & Kampf, C. (2013). Automated classification of immunostaining patterns in breast tissue from the human protein atlas. *Journal of Pathology Informatics, 4*(2Suppl), S14. doi:10.4103/2153-3539.109881 PMID:23766936

Tabata, K., Mori, I., Sasaki, T., Itoh, T., Shiraishi, T., Yoshimi, N., ... Fukuoka, J. (2017, November). Whole-slide imaging at primary pathological diagnosis: Validation of whole-slide imaging-based primary pathological diagnosis at twelve Japanese academic institutes. *Pathology International, 67*(11), 547–554. doi:10.1111/pin.12590 PMID:28980740

Takats, Z., Strittmatter, N., & McKenzie, J. S. (2017). Ambient Mass Spectrometry in Cancer Research. *Advances in Cancer Research, 134*, 231–256. doi:10.1016/bs.acr.2016.11.011 PMID:28110652

Tang, L., Zhao, F., & Zhao, Z. G. (2007). The nonsubsampled contourlet transform for image fusion. *International Conference on Wavelet Analysis and Pattern Recognition (ICWAPR '07)*, 305–310.

Tanvi, G., Tapan, K. G., Gupta, R. K., & Panigrahi, B. K. (in press). Classification of patients with tumor using MR FLAIR images. *Pattern Recognition Letters.*

Thirion, J. P. (1998). Image matching as a diffusion process: An analogy with Maxwell's demons. *Medical Image Analysis, 2*(3), 243–260. doi:10.1016/S1361-8415(98)80022-4 PMID:9873902

Thomas, A., Patterson, N. H., Marcinkiewicz, M. M., Lazaris, A., Metrakos, P., & Chaurand, P. (2013). Histology-driven data mining of lipid signatures from multiple imaging mass spectrometry analyses: Application to human colorectal cancer liver metastasis biopsies. *Analytical Chemistry, 85*(5), 2860–2866. doi:10.1021/ac3034294 PMID:23347294

Tiffen, J., Wilson, S., Gallagher, S. J., Hersey, P., & Filipp, F. V. (2016). Somatic Copy Number Amplification and Hyperactivating Somatic Mutations of EZH2 Correlate With DNA Methylation and Drive Epigenetic Silencing of Genes Involved in Tumor Suppression and Immune Responses in Melanoma. *Neoplasia (New York, N.Y.), 18*(2), 121–132. doi:10.1016/j.neo.2016.01.003 PMID:26936398

Toews, M., & Arbel, T. (2007). A statistical parts-based model of anatomical variability. *IEEE Transactions on Medical Imaging, 26*(4), 497–508. doi:10.1109/TMI.2007.892510 PMID:17427737

Tomasi, C., & Manduchi, R. (1988). Bilateral filtering for gray and color images. *Sixth International Conference on Computer Vision* (IEEE Cat. No.98CH36271), 839–846. 10.1109/ICCV.1998.710815

Toriyama, A., Mori, T., Sekine, S., Yoshida, A., Hino, O., & Tsuta, K. (2014). Utility of PAX8 mouse monoclonal antibody in the diagnosis of thyroid, thymic, pleural and lung tumours: A comparison with polyclonal PAX8 antibody. *Histopathology*, *65*(4), 465–472. doi:10.1111/his.12405 PMID:24592933

Trofa, D., Rajaee, S. S., & Smith, E. L. (2014). Nationwide trends in total shoulder arthroplasty and hemiarthroplasty for osteoarthritis. *American Journal of Orthopedics (Belle Mead, N.J.)*, *43*(4), 166–172. PMID:24730001

Uligoj, F. (2017). *Automated Marker Localization in the Planning Phase of Robotic Neurosurgery* (Vol. 5). IEEE Access.

Uligoj, F., Vaco, M., Jerbi, B., Ekoranja, B., & Vidakovi, J. (2017). Automated Marker Localization in the Planning Phase of Robotic Neurosurgery. *IEEE Access*, *5*, 12265–12274. doi:10.1109/ACCESS.2017.2718621

van den Elsen, P. A., Maintz, J. B. A., Pol, E.-J. D., & Viergever, M. A. (1995). Automatic registration of CT and MR brain images using correlation of geometrical features. *IEEE Transactions on Medical Imaging*, *14*(2), 384–396. doi:10.1109/42.387719 PMID:18215841

Van Kitanovski, I. D., Madjarov, G., & Loskovska, S. (2017, January). Multimodal medical image retrieval system. *Multimedia Tools and Applications*, *76*(2), 2955–2978. doi:10.100711042-016-3261-1

Van Ravesteijn, V. F., Van Wijk, C., Vos, F. M., Truyen, R., Peters, J. F., Stoker, J., & Van Vliet, L. J. (2010). Computer-aided detection of polyps in CT colonography using logistic regression. *IEEE Transactions on Medical Imaging*, *29*(1), 120–131. doi:10.1109/TMI.2009.2028576 PMID:19666332

Verborgt, O., De Smedt, T., Vanhees, M., Clockaerts, S., Parizel, P. M., & Van Glabbeek, F. (2011). Accuracy of placement of the glenoid component in reversed shoulder arthroplasty with and without navigation. *Journal of Shoulder and Elbow Surgery*, *20*(1), 21–26. doi:10.1016/j.jse.2010.07.014 PMID:21134663

Vyas, N. S., Markow, M., Prieto-Granada, C., Gaudi, S., Turner, L., Rodriguez-Waitkus, P., ... Jukic, D. M. (2016). Comparing whole slide digital images versus traditional glass slides in the detection of common microscopic features seen in dermatitis. *Journal of Pathology Informatics*, *7*(1), 30. doi:10.4103/2153-3539.186909 PMID:27563489

Walch, G., Boileau, P., & Noël, E. (2010). Shoulder arthroplasty: Evolving techniques and indications. *Joint, Bone, Spine*, *77*(6), 501–505. doi:10.1016/j.jbspin.2010.09.004 PMID:20961793

Wang, H., He, C., & Wei, L. (2010). Locally adaptive bivariate shrinkage algorithm for image denoising based on Nonsubsampled Contourlet Transform. *International Conference on Computer, Mechatronics, Control and Electronic Engineering (CMCE)*, 5.

Wang, J. Z. (2000). Pathfinder: Multiresolution region based searching of pathology images using IRM. *Proceedings of the AMIA Symposium*, 883-887.

Wang, L. C., DeMartini, W. B., Partridge, S. C., Peacock, S., & Lehman, C. D. (2009). MRI-detected suspicious breast lesions: Predictive values of kinetic features measured by computer-aided evaluation. *AJR. American Journal of Roentgenology, 193*(3), 826–831. doi:10.2214/AJR.08.1335 PMID:19696298

Warwick. (2013). Retrieved in 2013 from www.warwick.ac.uk

Wikipedia. (2018). *DICOM*. Retrieved from https://en.wikipedia.org/wiki/DICOM

Willems, S. M., van Remoortere, A., van Zeijl, R., Deelder, A. M., McDonnell, L. A., & Hogendoorn, P. C. (2010). Imaging mass spectrometry of myxoid sarcomas identifies proteins and lipids specific to tumour type and grade, and reveals biochemical intratumour heterogeneity. *The Journal of Pathology, 222*(4), 400–409. doi:10.1002/path.2771 PMID:20839361

Winawer, S. J., & Zauber, A. G. (2002). The advanced adenoma as the primary target of screening. *Gastrointestinal Endoscopy Clinics, 12*(1), 1–9. doi:10.1016/S1052-5157(03)00053-9 PMID:11916153

Winnemöller, H., Olsen, S. C., & Gooch, B. (2006). Real-time video abstraction. *ACM SIGGRAPH 2006 Papers on - SIGGRAPH '06*, 1221. 10.1145/1179352.1142018

Witten, I. H., Frank, E., & Hall, M. A. (2011). *Data mining: Practical machine learning tools and techniques*. Burlington, MA: Morgan Kaufmann.

Worring, M., Smeulders, W. M., & Santini, S. (2000). Interaction in content-based image retrieval: an evaluation of the state of the art. In R. Laurini (Ed.), *Proceedings of the Fourth International Conference On Visual Information Systems (VISUAL)*. Springer-Verlag. 10.1007/3-540-40053-2_3

Wu, Y. Q., & Wu, Y. Y. (2011). Image Retrieval Based on NSCT and Krawtchouk Moments. *Wuhan Daxue Xuebao. Xinxi Kexue Ban*, 691–694.

Xie, Z., & Farin, G. E. (2004). Image registration using hierarchical B-Splines. *IEEE Transactions on Visualization and Computer Graphics, 10*(1), 85–94. doi:10.1109/TVCG.2004.1260760 PMID:15382700

Xu, Y., Cai, W., Nappi, J., & Yoshida, H. (2012). Fecal-tagging CT colonography with structure-analysis electronic cleansing for detection of colorectal flat lesions. *European Journal of Radiology, 81*(8), 1712–1716. doi:10.1016/j.ejrad.2011.04.051 PMID:21596500

Yadav, N.K., Shukla, P., Omer, A., Pareek, S., & Singh, R.K. (2014). Next Generation Sequencing: Potential and Application in Drug Discovery. *The Scientific World Journal*. doi:10.1155/2014/802437

Yagel, R., & Cohen, D. (2000). Volume Graphics. In Computer (Vol. 26). London: Springer London. doi:10.1007/978-1-4471-0737-8

Yanagisawa, K., Shyr, Y., Xu, B. J., Massion, P. P., Larsen, P. H., White, B. C., ... Carbone, D. P. (2003). Proteomic patterns of tumour subsets in non-small-cell lung cancer. *Lancet, 362*(9382), 433–439. doi:10.1016/S0140-6736(03)14068-8 PMID:12927430

Yang & Bo. (2013). Image De-Noising Algorithm Using Adaptive Bayes Threshold by subband Based on Nonsubsampled Contourlet Transform. *Third International Conference on Intelligent System Design and Engineering Applications*.

Yang, A., Meng, L., Luo, J., & Lin, C. (2007). A rapid registration framework for medical images. *Proceedings of fourth international conference on images and graphics*, 731–736. 10.1109/ICIG.2007.78

Yang, C. C. (2006). Image enhancement by modified contrast-stretching manipulation. *Optics & Laser Technology*, *38*(3), 196–201. doi:10.1016/j.optlastec.2004.11.009

Yang, S., Weidong, C., Heng, H., Yun, Z., Yue, W., & David, D. (in press). FengLocality-constrained Subcluster Representation Ensemble for Lung Image Classification. *Medical Image Analysis*.

Yang, Z., & Cohen, F. S. (1999). Image registration and object recognition using affine invariants and convex hills. *IEEE Transactions on Image Processing*, *8*(7), 934–946. doi:10.1109/83.772236 PMID:18267506

Yan, Z., Zhan, Y., Peng, Z., & Shu, L. (2016, May). Multi-Instance Deep Learning: Discover Discriminative Local Anatomies for Bodypart Recognition. *IEEE Transactions on Medical Imaging*, *35*(5), 1332–1343. doi:10.1109/TMI.2016.2524985

Yao, J., & Summers, R. M. (2007, April). Detection and segmentation of colonic polyps on haustral folds. In *Biomedical Imaging: From Nano to Macro, 2007. ISBI 2007. 4th IEEE International Symposium on* (pp. 900-903). IEEE. 10.1109/ISBI.2007.356998

Yao, J., Miller, M., Franaszek, M., & Summers, R. M. (2004). Colonic polyp segmentation in CT colonography-based on fuzzy clustering and deformable models. *IEEE Transactions on Medical Imaging*, *23*(11), 1344–1352. doi:10.1109/TMI.2004.826941 PMID:15554123

Yoshida, H., & Nappi, J. (2001). Three-dimensional computer-aided diagnosis scheme for detection of colonic polyps. *IEEE Transactions on Medical Imaging*, *20*(12), 1261–1274. doi:10.1109/42.974921 PMID:11811826

Yuan, J., Zhang, J., Zhu, Y., Li, N., Tian, T., Li, Y., ... Shen, L. (2016). Programmed death-ligand-1 expression in advanced gastric cancer detected with RNA in situ hybridization and its clinical significance. *Oncotarget*, *7*(26), 39671–39679. doi:10.18632/oncotarget.9381 PMID:27191996

Zenteno, Rojas, Chang, & Castaneda. (2016). SonicCare: Performance of a New Low-Cost and Portable Device for Medical Tele-Ultrasonography on Underserved Areas. *IEEE Latin America Transactions, 14*(7).

Zhao, H., Xu, W., Li, L., & Zhang, J. (2011). Classification of Breast Masses Based on Multi-View Information Fusion Using Multi-Agent Method. In *2011 5th International Conference on Bioinformatics and Biomedical Engineering* (pp. 1-4). IEEE.

Zheng, Y., Coltharp, C., Dilworth, R., Liu, L., Unfricht, D., Hoyt, C., ... Miller, P. (2017). Optimization strategy for fluorescent multiplex immunohistochemistry tissue staining. Abstract 3832. *Cancer Research, 77*(13S), 3832.

Zheng, Y., Coltharp, C., Dilworth, R., Liu, L., Unfricht, D., Hoyt, C., ... Peter Miller, P. Optimization strategy for fluorescent multiplex immunohistochemistry tissue staining. In *Proceedings of the American Association for Cancer Research Annual Meeting 2017*. Philadelphia: AACR. doi:10.1158/1538-7445.AM2017-3832

Zhou, Cunha, & Do. (2005). Nonsubsampled contourlet transform: construction and application in enhancement. *IEEE International Conference on Image Processing*, 11-14.

Zhou, D., & Cheng, W. (2008). Image denoising with an optimal threshold and neighbouring window. *Pattern Recognition Letters*, *29*(11), 1694–1697. doi:10.1016/j.patrec.2008.04.014

Zhu, H., Duan, C., Pickhardt, P., Wang, S., & Liang, Z. (2009). Computer-aided detection of colonic polyps with level set-based adaptive convolution in volumetric mucosa to advance CT colonography toward a screening modality. *Cancer Management and Research*, *1*, 1–13. doi:10.2147/CMAR.S4546 PMID:20428331

Zitova, B., & Flusser, J. (2003). Image registration methods: A survey. *Image and Vision Computing, Elsevier*, *21*(11), 977–1000. doi:10.1016/S0262-8856(03)00137-9

Zumstein, M. A., Pinedo, M., Old, J., & Boileau, P. (2011). Problems, complications, reoperations, and revisions in reverse total shoulder arthroplasty: A systematic review. *Journal of Shoulder and Elbow Surgery*, *20*(1), 146–157. doi:10.1016/j.jse.2010.08.001 PMID:21134666

Index

I

K

M

N

O

P

R

S

T

W

X

www.ingramcontent.com/pod-product-compliance
Lightning Source LLC
LaVergne TN
LVHW061548290926
849162LV00004B/943